T0226812

Complications of Cirrhosis

Editors

ANDRES CARDENAS
THOMAS REIBERGER

CLINICS IN LIVER DISEASE

www.liver.theclinics.com

Consulting Editor
NORMAN GITLIN

May 2021 • Volume 25 • Number 2

ELSEVIER

1600 John F. Kennedy Boulevard • Suite 1800 • Philadelphia, Pennsylvania, 19103-2899

http://www.theclinics.com

CLINICS IN LIVER DISEASE Volume 25, Number 2
May 2021 ISSN 1089-3261, ISBN-13: 978-0-323-79387-2

Editor: Kerry Holland
Developmental Editor: Ann Gielou M. Posedio

Clinics in Liver Disease (ISSN 1089-3261) is published quarterly by Elsevier Inc., 360 Park Avenue South, New York, NY 10010-1710. Months of issue are February, May, August, and November. Business and Editorial Offices: 1600 John F. Kennedy Blvd., Ste. 1800, Philadelphia, PA 19103-2899. Customer Service Office: 3251 Riverport Lane, Maryland Heights, MO 63043. Periodicals postage paid at New York, NY and additional mailing offices. Subscription prices are $319.00 per year (U.S. individuals), $100.00 per year (U.S. student/resident), $752.00 per year (U.S. institutions), $409.00 per year (international individuals), $200.00 per year (international student/resident), $790.00 per year (international instituitions), $371.00 per year (Canadian individuals), $100.00 per year (Canadian student/resident), and $790.00 per year (Canadian institutions). Foreign air speed delivery is included in all *Clinics* subscription prices. All prices are subject to change without notice. **POSTMASTER:** Send address changes to *Clinics in Liver Disease*, Elsevier Health Sciences Division, Subscription Customer Service, 3251 Riverport Lane, Maryland Heights, MO 63043. **Customer Service: Telephone: 1-800-654-2452 (U.S. and Canada); 314-447-8871 (outside U.S. and Canada). Fax: 314-447-8029. E-mail: journalscustomer service-usa@elsevier.com (for print support); journalsonlinesupport-usa@elsevier.com (for online support).**

Reprints. For copies of 100 or more of articles in this publication, please contact the Commercial Reprints Department, Elsevier Inc., 360 Park Avenue South, New York, NY 10010-1710. Tel.: 212-633-3874; Fax: 212-633-3820; E-mail: reprints@elsevier.com.

Clinics in Liver Disease is covered in *MEDLINE/PubMed (Index Medicus)*, Science Citation Index Expanded, Journal Citation Reports/Science Edition, and Current Contents/Clinical Medicine.

Contributors

CONSULTING EDITOR

NORMAN GITLIN, MD, FRCP (LONDON), FRCPE (EDINBURGH), FAASLD, FACP, FACG
Head of Hepatology, Southern California Liver Centers, San Clemente, California, USA

EDITORS

ANDRES CARDENAS, MD, MMSc, PhD, AGAF, FAASLD
GI/Liver Unit, Institut Clínic de Malalties Digestives i Metabòliques, Hospital Clínic, Institut d'Investigacions Biomèdiques August Pi-Sunyer (IDIBAPS) and Ciber de Enfermedades Hepáticas y Digestivas (CIBEREHD), Department of Medicine, Associate Professor of Medicine, University of Barcelona, Barcelona, Spain

THOMAS REIBERGER, MD
Associate Professor of Gastroenterology and Hepatology, Medical University of Vienna, Division of Gastroenterology and Hepatology, Department of Medicine III, Head of the Christian Doppler Lab for Portal Hypertension and Liver Fibrosis, Medical University of Vienna, Vienna, Austria

AUTHORS

JUAN G. ABRALDES, MD, MMSc
Professor of Medicine, Division of Gastroenterology, University of Alberta, CEGIIR, Edmonton, Alberta, Canada

PAOLO ANGELI, MD, PhD
Unit of Internal Medicine and Hepatology (UIMH), Department of Medicine – DIMED, University and Hospital of Padova, Padova, Italy

ANNA BAIGES, MD, PhD
Barcelona Hepatic Hemodynamic Laboratory, Liver Unit, Hospital Clínic, Institut de Investigacions Biomèdiques August Pi i Sunyer (IDIBAPS), University of Barcelona, Barcelona, Spain; CIBEREHD (Centro de Investigación Biomédica en Red Enfermedades Hepáticas y Digestivas), HealthCare Provider of the European Reference Network on Rare Liver Disorders (ERN-Liver)

ITAY BENTOV, MD, PhD
Department of Anesthesiology and Pain Medicine, University of Washington, Seattle, Washington, USA

ANNALISA BERZIGOTTI, MD, PhD
Head of Hepatology and Associate Professor of Hepatology, University Clinic for Visceral Surgery and Medicine (UVCM), Inselspital, University Hospital of Bern, Department of Biomedical Research, University of Bern, Switzerland

ANNABEL BLASI, MD, PhD
Anesthesia Department, Hospital Clínic of Barcelona, Institut d'Investigacions
Biomèdiques August Pi-Sunyer (IDIBAPS) and Ciber de Enfermedades Hepáticas y
Digestivas (CIBEREHD), Barcelona, Spain

CHARLOTTE BOUZBIB, MD
Brain Liver Salpêtrière Study Group, Sorbonne Université, INSERM UMR_S 938, Centre
de Recherche Saint-Antoine & Institute of Cardiometabolism and Nutrition (ICAN), AP-HP,
Sorbonne Université, Liver Intensive Care Unit, Hepatogastroenterology Department,
Pitié-Salpêtrière Hospital, Paris, France

ELIZABETH BUGANZA, MD
Division of Gastroenterology, Zeidler Ledcor Centre, University of Alberta, Edmonton,
Alberta, Canada

CHRISTOPHE BUREAU, MD, PhD
Service d'Hépatologie Hôpital Rangueil, CHU Toulouse France and Université Toulouse
III-Paul Sabatier, France

ANDRES CARDENAS, MD, MMSc, PhD, AGAF, FAASLD
GI/Liver Unit, Institut Clínic de Malalties Digestives i Metabòliques, Hospital Clínic, Institut
d'Investigacions Biomèdiques August Pi-Sunyer (IDIBAPS) and Ciber de Enfermedades
Hepáticas y Digestivas (CIBEREHD), Department of Medicine, Associate Professor of
Medicine, University of Barcelona, Barcelona, Spain

LIAT DEUTSCH, MD
Liver Unit, Department of Gastroenterology, Tel Aviv Medical Center, Sackler Faculty of
Medicine, Tel Aviv University, Tel Aviv, Israel

PHILIP FERSTL, MD
Departments for Internal Medicine I, and Gastroenterology and Hepatology, University
Hospital, Goethe University, Frankfurt am Main, Germany

JUAN CARLOS GARCÍA-PAGÁN, MD, PhD
Professor, Barcelona Hepatic Hemodynamic Laboratory, Liver Unit, Hospital Clínic,
Institut de Investigacions Biomèdiques August Pi i Sunyer (IDIBAPS), University of
Barcelona, Barcelona, Spain; CIBEREHD (Centro de Investigación Biomédica en Red
Enfermedades Hepáticas y Digestivas), HealthCare Provider of the European Reference
Network on Rare Liver Disorders (ERN-Liver)

PERE GINÈS, MD, PhD
Professor and Chairman, Liver Unit, Hospital Clínic de Barcelona, Institut d'Investigacions
Biomèdiques August Pi i Sunyer (IDIBAPS), Centro de Investigación Biomédica en Red de
Enfermedades Hepáticas y Digestivas (CIBEREHD), Barcelona, Spain; Faculty of
Medicine and Health Sciences, University of Barcelona, Barcelona, Catalonia, Spain

VIRGINIA HERNÁNDEZ-GEA, MD, PhD
Professor, Barcelona Hepatic Hemodynamic Laboratory, Liver Unit, Hospital Clínic,
Institut de Investigacions Biomèdiques August Pi i Sunyer (IDIBAPS), University of
Barcelona, Barcelona, Spain; CIBEREHD (Centro de Investigación Biomédica en Red
Enfermedades Hepáticas y Digestivas), HealthCare Provider of the European Reference
Network on Rare Liver Disorders (ERN-Liver)

DANA IVANCOVSKY-WAJCMAN, RD
School of Public Health, University of Haifa, Haifa, Israel

MANHAL J. IZZY, MD
Assistant Professor, Department of Medicine, Division of Gastroenterology, Hepatology, and Nutrition, Vanderbilt University School of Medicine, Nashville, Tennessee, USA

MATHIAS JACHS, MD
Division of Gastroenterology and Hepatology, Department of Medicine III, Vienna Hepatic Hemodynamic Lab, Christian Doppler Lab for Portal Hypertension and Liver Fibrosis, Medical University of Vienna, Vienna, Austria

ADRIÀ JUANOLA, MD
Liver Unit, Hospital Clínic de Barcelona, Barcelona, Spain; Institut d'Investigacions Biomèdiques August Pi i Sunyer (IDIBAPS), Barcelona, Spain

HÉLÈNE LARRUE, MD
Service d'Hépatologie Hôpital Rangueil, CHU Toulouse France and Université Toulouse III-Paul Sabatier, France

MARTA MAGAZ, MD
Barcelona Hepatic Hemodynamic Laboratory, Liver Unit, Hospital Clínic, Institut de Investigacions Biomèdiques August Pi i Sunyer (IDIBAPS), University of Barcelona, Barcelona, Spain; CIBEREHD (Centro de Investigación Biomédica en Red Enfermedades Hepáticas y Digestivas), HealthCare Provider of the European Reference Network on Rare Liver Disorders (ERN-Liver)

MATTIAS MANDORFER, MD, PhD
Division of Gastroenterology and Hepatology, Department of Internal Medicine III, Vienna Hepatic Hemodynamic Lab, Medical University of Vienna, Vienna, Austria

SALVATORE PIANO, MD, PhD
Unit of Internal Medicine and Hepatology (UIMH), Department of Medicine – DIMED, University and Hospital of Padova, Padova, Italy

LIANE RABINOWICH, MD
Liver Unit, Department of Gastroenterology, Tel Aviv Medical Center, Sackler Faculty of Medicine, Tel Aviv University, Tel Aviv, Israel

THOMAS REIBERGER, MD
Associate Professor of Gastroenterology and Hepatology, Medical University of Vienna, Division of Gastroenterology and Hepatology, Department of Medicine III, Head of the Christian Doppler Lab for Portal Hypertension and Liver Fibrosis, Medical University of Vienna, Vienna, Austria

SUSANA G. RODRIGUES, MD
Attending Hepatologist, University Clinic for Visceral Surgery and Medicine (UVCM), Inselspital, University Hospital of Bern, Department of Biomedical Research, University of Bern, Switzerland

MARIKA RUDLER, MD, PhD
Brain Liver Salpêtrière Study Group, Sorbonne Université, INSERM UMR_S 938, Centre de Recherche Saint-Antoine & Institute of Cardiometabolism and Nutrition (ICAN), AP-HP, Sorbonne Université, Liver Intensive Care Unit, Hepatogastroenterology Department, Pitié-Salpêtrière Hospital, Paris, France

BENEDIKT SIMBRUNNER, MD
Division of Gastroenterology and Hepatology, Department of Internal Medicine III, Vienna Hepatic Hemodynamic Lab, Medical University of Vienna, Vienna, Austria

ELSA SOLÀ, MD, PhD
Liver Unit, Hospital Clínic de Barcelona, Institut d'Investigacions Biomèdiques August Pi i
Sunyer (IDIBAPS), Centro de Investigación Biomédica en Red de Enfermedades
Hepáticas y Digestivas (CIBEREHD), Barcelona, Spain; Faculty of Medicine and Health
Sciences, University of Barcelona, Barcelona, Catalonia, Spain

CRISTINA SOLÉ, MD, PhD
Liver Unit, Hospital Clínic de Barcelona, Institut d'Investigacions Biomèdiques August Pi i
Sunyer (IDIBAPS), Centro de Investigación Biomédica en Red de Enfermedades
Hepáticas y Digestivas (CIBEREHD), Barcelona, Spain

DOMINIQUE THABUT, MD, PhD
Brain Liver Salpêtrière Study Group, Sorbonne Université, INSERM UMR_S 938, Centre
de Recherche Saint-Antoine & Institute of Cardiometabolism and Nutrition (ICAN), AP-HP,
Sorbonne Université, Liver Intensive Care Unit, Hepatogastroenterology Department,
Pitié-Salpêtrière Hospital, Sorbonne Université, Paris, France

DAVID TOAPANTA, MD
Liver Unit, Hospital Clínic de Barcelona, Barcelona, Spain

JONEL TREBICKA, MD, PhD
Departments for Internal Medicine I, and Gastroenterology and Hepatology, University
Hospital, Goethe University, Frankfurt am Main, Germany; European Foundation for the
Study of Chronic Liver Failure, Barcelona, Spain

FANNY TURON, MD
Barcelona Hepatic Hemodynamic Laboratory, Liver Unit, Hospital Clínic, Institut de
Investigacions Biomèdiques August Pi i Sunyer (IDIBAPS), University of Barcelona,
Barcelona, Spain; CIBEREHD (Centro de Investigación Biomédica en Red Enfermedades
Hepáticas y Digestivas), HealthCare Provider of the European Reference Network on Rare
Liver Disorders (ERN-Liver)

LISA B. VANWAGNER, MD, MSc
Assistant Professor, Department of Medicine, Division of Gastroenterology and
Hepatology, Department of Preventive Medicine, Division of Epidemiology, Northwestern
University Feinberg School of Medicine, Chicago, Illinois, USA

DANIEL VELDHUIJZEN VAN ZANTEN, MD, MBA
Department of Medicine, University of Alberta, Edmonton, Alberta, Canada

JEAN PIERRE VINEL, MD
Service d'Hépatologie Hôpital Rangueil, CHU Toulouse France and Université Toulouse
III-Paul Sabatier, France

ÉLISE VUILLE-LESSARD, MD
Clinical and Research Fellow, Hepatology, University Clinic for Visceral Surgery and
Medicine (UVCM), Inselspital, University Hospital of Bern, Department of Biomedical
Research, University of Bern, Switzerland

NICOLAS WEISS, MD, PhD
Brain Liver Salpêtrière Study Group, Sorbonne Université, INSERM UMR_S 938, Centre
de Recherche Saint-Antoine & Institute of Cardiometabolism and Nutrition (ICAN), AP-HP,
Sorbonne Université, Neurological Intensive Care Unit, Neurology Department, Pitié-
Salpêtrière Hospital, Sorbonne Université, Paris, France

SHIRA ZELBER-SAGI, RD, PhD
School of Public Health, University of Haifa, Haifa, Israel; Liver Unit, Department of
Gastroenterology, Tel Aviv Medical Center, Tel Aviv, Israel

Contents

Patients with compensated advanced chronic liver disease have different prognoses depending on the presence of portal hypertension. Current non-invasive diagnostic methods allow identification of clinically significant portal hypertension. Portosystemic collaterals on imaging or liver stiffness of more than 20 to 25 kPa by using transient elastography identifies patients with clinically significant portal hypertension. Patients with liver stiffness of less than 20 kPa and platelet count of greater than 150 g/L can avoid endoscopy. This rule could be expanded using spleen stiffness. Methods to risk stratify for portal hypertension in compensated advanced chronic liver disease and successfully treated chronic hepatitis C and B are subject of research.

The first occurrence of decompensation constitutes a watershed moment in the natural history of chronic liver disease; it denotes a point of no return in a relevant proportion of patients. Preventive strategies may profoundly decrease cirrhosis-related morbidity and mortality. Removing the primary etiologic factor and cofactors, is key; however, a considerable proportion of patients require additional etiology-independent treatment strategies that target important pathomechanisms promoting decompensation (ie, portal hypertension and systemic inflammation). This article explains the importance of preventing first decompensation and summarizes the evidence for etiologic and etiology-independent (most important, nonselective beta-blockers and statins) therapies.

Nonselective beta-blockers represent the mainstay of medical therapy in the prophylaxis of variceal bleeding and rebleeding in patients with portal hypertension. Their efficacy has been demonstrated by numerous trials; however, there exist safety concerns in advanced disease, such as in patients with refractory ascites. Importantly, nonselective beta-blockers also exert nonhemodynamic beneficial effects that may contribute to a prolonged decompensation-free survival, as recently shown in the PREDESCI trial. This review summarizes the current evidence on nonselective beta-blocker therapy and proposes a tailored, patient-centered approach for the use of nonselective beta-blockers in patients with portal hypertension.

than either condition alone, may be overlooked. Lifestyle intervention aiming for moderate weight reduction can be offered to obese compensated cirrhotic patients, with diet consisting of reduced caloric intake, achieved by reduction of carbohydrate and fat intake, while maintaining high protein intake. Dietary and moderate exercise interventions in patients with cirrhosis are beneficial. Cirrhotic patients with malnutrition should have nutritional counseling, and all patients should be encouraged to avoid a sedentary lifestyle.

Hepatic encephalopathy (HE) is a severe complication of cirrhosis. The prevalence of overt HE (OHE) ranges from 30% to 45%, whereas the prevalence of minimal HE (MHE) is as high as 85% in some case series. Widespread use of transjugular intrahepatic portosystemic shunt to control complications related to portal hypertension is associated with an increase in HE incidence. If the diagnosis of OHE remains simple in most cases, then the diagnosis of MHE is less codified because of many differential diagnoses with different therapeutic implications. This review analyzes current knowledge about the pathophysiology, diagnosis, and different therapeutic options of HE.

Liver cirrhosis is a major healthcare problem. Acute decompensation, and in particular its interplay with dysfunction of other organs, is responsible for the majority of deaths in patients with cirrhosis. Acute decompensation has different courses, from stable decompensated cirrhosis over unstable decompensated cirrhosis to pre-acute-on-chronic liver failure and finally acute-on-chronic liver failure, a syndrome with high short-term mortality. This review focuses on the recent developments in the field of acute decompensation and acute-on-chronic liver failure.

Considering the poor prognosis, severe and refractory ascites is a milestone in cirrhotic patients. Liver transplantation must be considered first. In the case of contraindication to liver transplantation or when the waiting period is estimated to be more than 6 months, transjugular intrahepatic portosystemic shunt should be discussed in eligible patients. Regardless of the type of treatment, a careful selection of patients is crucial to avoid further decompensation and specific complications of each treatment.

Acute kidney injury (AKI) is a frequent complication in patients with cirrhosis. Patients with cirrhosis can develop AKI due to different causes.

Hepatorenal syndrome (HRS) is a unique cause of AKI occurring in patients with advanced cirrhosis and is associated with high short-term mortality. The differential diagnosis between different causes of AKI may be challenging. In this regard, new urine biomarkers may be helpful. Liver transplantation is the definitive treatment of patients with HRS-AKI. Vasoconstrictors and albumin represent the first-line pharmacologic treatment of HRS-AKI. This review summarizes current knowledge for the diagnosis and management of HRS in cirrhosis.

The aim on of this article is to provide an update on the coagulation disturbances of patients with cirrhosis. It summarizes basic concepts of coagulation in cirrhosis, available tests used to predict bleeding, procedures and risk of bleeding, and the rationale and expert-based recommendations of prophylactic measures for patients with cirrhosis who undergo invasive procedures.

 Video content accompanies this article at http://www.liver.theclinics.com.

Cirrhotic cardiomyopathy (CCM) connotes systolic and/or diastolic dysfunction in patients with end-stage liver disease in the absence of prior heart disease. Its prevalence is variable across different studies but recent data suggest that CCM may affect up to one third of liver transplant candidates. The etiology of CCM is multifactorial. CCM defining features were recently revised to improve the diagnostic and prognostic yield of CCM criteria and inform candidate selection for liver transplantation. CCM appears to increase the risk for unfavorable outcomes pre- and post-transplant. Close clinical and echocardiographic follow-up of patients with CCM may mitigate adverse cardiac outcomes.

CLINICS IN LIVER DISEASE

THE CLINICS ARE AVAILABLE ONLINE!
Access your subscription at:
www.theclinics.com

Preface

Complications of Cirrhosis

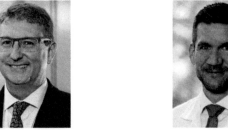

Andres Cardenas, MD, MMSc, PhD, AGAF, FAASLD   Thomas Reiberger, MD
Editors

Cirrhosis ranks among the most common global causes of morbidity and mortality. While effective therapies for some liver diseases, such as direct-acting antivirals against hepatitis C, have profoundly changed the landscape, an increasing number of patients with cirrhosis due to fatty liver disease, alcoholic liver disease, and autoimmune disease need to be evaluated for liver transplantation in the absence of effective treatment options. The knowledge gained from recent trials and the important results obtained from landmark research studies continuously inform our clinical practice. Thus, it is important to stay up-to-date with the current level of evidence underlying the recommendations for the management of patients at risk for developing various complications of cirrhosis. A thorough understanding of the diagnosis and management of cirrhosis and its complications is mandatory for the practicing physician.

In this special issue, we have gathered a unique group of experts that have contributed up-to-date articles on key aspects in the clinical management of complications of cirrhosis. We would like to thank them for their exceptional contributions that summarize the currently available management options and review increasingly important topics surrounding delivery of care to patients with cirrhosis. We hope that you enjoy reading this special issue of *Clinics in Liver Disease*, which should ultimately help to

Clin Liver Dis 25 (2021) xiii–xiv
https://doi.org/10.1016/j.cld.2021.02.002
1089-3261/21/© 2021 Published by Elsevier Inc.

liver.theclinics.com

guide you in your daily decision making while caring for your patients with advanced chronic liver disease.

Andres Cardenas, MD, MMSc, PhD, AGAF, FAASLD
Hospital Clinic of Barcelona
Villarroel 170, Esc 3-2
08036 Barcelona, Spain

Thomas Reiberger, MD
Universitätsklinikum AKH Wien
Gastroenterology Office 7I Red Tower
Währinger Gürtel 18-20
A-1090 Vienna, Austria

E-mail addresses:
acardena@clinic.cat (A. Cardenas)
thomas.reiberger@meduniwien.ac.at (T. Reiberger)

Noninvasive Detection of Clinically Significant Portal Hypertension in Compensated Advanced Chronic Liver Disease

Élise Vuille-Lessard, MD, MSc[a,b], Susana G. Rodrigues, MD[a,b],
Annalisa Berzigotti, MD, PhD[a,b],*

KEYWORDS

• Elastography • Cirrhosis • Varices • Spleen • Decompensation

KEY POINTS

- Clinically significant portal hypertension can be identified noninvasively (liver stiffness >21 kPa; portosystemic collaterals on imaging), but cannot be ruled out with confidence.
- Endoscopic screening of varices can be safely avoided if liver stiffness is less than 20 kPa and platelet count is greater than 150 g/L, because varices needing treatment are rare in these patients.
- Spleen stiffness is a novel promising parameter for the noninvasive assessment of portal hypertension.

INTRODUCTION

The natural history of chronic liver disease is characterized by a long asymptomatic or compensated phase. During this long phase, fibrosis progresses eventually leading to cirrhosis, which is histologically defined by marked anatomic changes encompassing septae formation, hepatocyte extinction and regeneration, and angiogenesis. Portal pressure increases progressively as well, and in patients with bridging fibrosis and cirrhosis the hepatic venous pressure gradient (HVPG; the best method to assess portal hypertension in cirrhosis) is over the normal threshold of 5 mm Hg.[1] Once the HVPG doubles its normal values, namely, once it exceeds 10 mm Hg, portosystemic collateralization becomes relevant, gastroesophageal varices can develop, and patients are

Funding: Élise Vuille-Lessard is supported by a Clinical Hepatology Fellowship of the Canadian Association for the Study of the Liver - Canadian Liver Foundation (CASL-CLF 2020-2021).
[a] Hepatology, University Clinic for Visceral Surgery and Medicine (UVCM), Inselspital, University Hospital of Bern, Freiburgstrasse, 3010 Bern, Switzerland; [b] Department of Biomedical Research, University of Bern, Switzerland
* Corresponding author. MEM F807, Maurice Müller Haus, Murtenstrasse 35, Bern 3008, Switzerland.
E-mail address: Annalisa.berzigotti@insel.ch

prone to experience clinical decompensation, including ascites, bleeding from portal hypertensive sources, and hepatic encephalopathy. This is why an HVPG of 10 mm Hg or higher is as defined clinically significant portal hypertension (CSPH). As discussed, liver fibrosis progression is a slow, dynamic process, often not completely homogenous within the liver, and distinguishing between severe fibrosis and cirrhosis in a compensated patients is not trivial. This led to propose the term compensated advanced chronic liver disease (cACLD).[2,3] The HVPG measurement remains the reference standard to identify CSPH and to further stratify the risk of complications in cACLD, but is relatively expensive, not point of care, is available only in specialized centers with personnel with adequate training, and can be (rarely) associated with complications.[1]

Given the strong prognostic value of CSPH and owing to its therapeutic implications, noninvasive tests to detect this hemodynamic threshold in a simple and accurate manner have been object of an increasing number of studies in the last 20 years. Ideally, noninvasive tests should reflect exactly the HVPG, or should at least correctly classify patients as having or not CSPH, and as having or not varices needing treatment.

From a logical point of view, noninvasive tests should be used stepwise to identify CSPH first, and then to identify patients who require endoscopy owing to a negligible risk of varices needing treatment. Within the compensated stage, the presence of gastroesophageal varices identify patients at further risk of complications[4–7] (**Fig. 1**). It is very important to underline that the field of action of noninvasive tests for the detection of CSPH and varices is restricted to patients with compensated ACLD, who can have or not have these conditions and are object of the present review. In patients with decompensated cirrhosis, portal hypertension is per definition present,[1] and screening of CSPH is therefore superfluous.

Noninvasive tests investigated in this field include laboratory tests, imaging tests, and elastography. These modalities complement the clinical history and physical examination of patients, and have different costs and complexities.

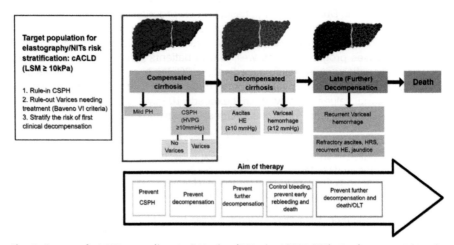

Fig. 1. Stages of cACLD according to D'Amico (D'Amico, 2014 #62). As shown, noninvasive tests (NITs) play a role in the compensated stage of the disease, when the patient is asymptomatic but at risk of carrying CSPH and varices. HE, hepatic encephalopathy; HRS, hepatorenal syndrome; OLT, orthotopic liver transplantation.

LABORATORY TESTS AND PHYSICAL SIGNS

The physical examination can reveal signs of CSPH, including ascites (sometimes associated with abdominal hernias), splenomegaly, spider nevi, visible abdominal portosystemic collaterals, pleural effusions, and lower limb edema. However, their absence cannot rule out CSPH. Of note, the presence of subclinical ascites (ascites sole detected by ultrasound examination) has been shown to be associated with similar HVPG values than clinical ascites, and to an intermediary survival compared with patients without ascites and with clinical ascites,[6] suggesting a subclinical decompensated stage.

In terms of laboratory data, serum biomarkers have initially been introduced to detect liver fibrosis and cirrhosis noninvasively and are classified as direct when reflecting matrix deposition and as indirect when reflecting liver dysfunction. A subset of them has been correlated to portal hypertension and its complications.[8] The advantages of using laboratory tests to noninvasively assess portal hypertension include their high applicability, good interlaboratory reproducibility, and availability.[9]

However, serum biomarkers need to be interpreted critically because some of their individual components can be affected by a variety of comorbidities. Overall, their diagnostic accuracy to detect CSPH and gastroesophageal varices, when used alone, remains modest. Moreover, none of them has been validated to monitor portal pressure and HVPG changes with or without treatment, limiting further their clinical usefulness.[10]

A low platelet count, the most common hematologic abnormality in cirrhosis,[11] has been consistently shown to correlate with HVPG[12] and a platelet count of less than 100×10^9/L strongly suggests CSPH. Von Willebrand factor antigen, produced by activated endothelial cells, also correlates with HVPG and was shown to be an independent predictor of CSPH (area under the receiver operating characteristic curve [AUROC] 0.85 using a cut-off value of $\geq 241\%$).[13] The derived VITRO score (Von Willebrand factor antigen/thrombocyte ratio) had an AUROC of 0.86 to detect CSPH in one study[14] and a VITRO score 2.5 or higher was recently associated with a higher 1-year probability of decompensation (9% vs 0%).[15]

A variety of biomarkers based on a combination of routine liver blood tests including aspartate aminotransferase (AST)-to-alanine aminotransferase ratio, AST to platelet ratio index, Fibrosis index, Fibrosis 4 index, Forns index, King's score, and the Lok index (Table 1) have shown a moderate diagnostic accuracy in predicting CSPH. A recent study showed that King's score, AST to platelet ratio index, and the Lok index had the best diagnostic accuracy, but that the latter was modest, with AUROCs of 0.755 and 0.742, 0.740 and 0.742, and 0.722 and 0.717, for CSPH, and severe portal hypertension, respectively.[16]

Some scores combining direct and indirect biomarkers with the use of patented formulas were also shown to be able to detect CSPH. For instance, the FibroTest (Biopredictive, Paris, France) had in 1 study an AUROC of 0.79 for severe portal hypertension; however, it correlated weakly with the HVPG in patients with cirrhosis.[17]

Numerous other individual biomarkers have shown a correlation with CSPH, such as the prothrombin index (Pearson correlation coefficient, -0.72; AUROC 0.89 with a cut-off value of 82.5%),[18] soluble CD163 (alone or combined with the Enhanced Liver Fibrosis test),[19,20] inflammatory markers such as IL-1β and its receptor IL-1Rα, Fas-R, serum VCAM-1[21] and osteopontin,[22] serum bile acids,[23] chemerin,[24] apelin,[25] hyaluronic acid and laminin,[26,27] and fragments of extracellular matrix,[28] as well as the indocyanine green retention test.[29] Despite some interesting data, the evidence is currently not strong enough to recommend the use of these markers in clinical practice.

Table 1
Available serum biomarkers for the noninvasive evaluation of portal hypertension

Score	Formula
AST to platelet ratio index	(AST/ULN)/PLT(10^9/L) × 100
AST-to-ALT ratio	AST/ALT
Fibrosis 4 index	(age × AST)/(PLT × ALT$^{1/2}$)
FibroIndex	1.738–0.064 × PLT + 0.005 × AST + 0.463 × gamma globulin
Fibrosis index	8–0.01 × PLT– ALB
Forns index	7.811–3.131 × ln(PLT) + 0.781 × ln(GGT) + 3.467 × ln(age) – 0.014 × (cholesterol)
King's score	Age × AST × INR/PLT
Lok index	−5.56–0.0089 × PLT + 1.26 × AST/ALT + 5.27 × INR

Abbreviations: ALB, albumin; ALT, alanine aminotransferase; AST, aspartate aminotransferase; GGT, gamma glutamyl transpeptidase; INR, international normalized ratio; PLT, platelet count; ULN, upper limit of normal.

Looking specifically at the diagnosis of gastroesophageal varices, the platelet count is usually lower in patients with gastroesophageal varices, but no absolute cut-off value used alone has a satisfactory performance to detect them, with AUROCs in the 0.60 to 0.75 range.[30,31] A systematic review and meta-analysis concluded that AST to platelet ratio index, AST-to-alanine aminotransferase ratio, Fibrosis 4 index, and Lok and Forns scores had low to moderate diagnostic accuracy in predicting the presence of varices and large varices in cirrhosis, with AUROCs of 0.65 to 0.79 overall and summary sensitivities and specificities of 0.60 to 0.78 and 0.56 to 0.68, respectively.[32] The FibroTest was shown to be a good predictor of large esophageal varices (AUROC, 0.77) and had an 86% negative predictive value at a cut-off of 0.80.[33] The prothrombin index,[18] indocyanine green retention test,[34] and soluble CD163[35] have also been showed to predict the presence of gastroesophageal varices, contrary to hyaluronic acid, laminin, amino-terminal propeptide of type III procollagen, and collagen IV.[36]

Despite data showing that individual laboratory tests have a moderate performance in detecting CSPH and gastroesophageal varices, their use alone cannot currently be recommended. Nevertheless, their combination with other noninvasive methods has shown promising results.

IMAGING

Imaging methods used for portal hypertension include ultrasound (complemented by color, power, and pulsed Doppler, and contrast-enhanced techniques), computed tomography (CT) scan and magnetic resonance (MR). All these methods are able to depict the macroscopic changes occurring in the liver, spleen, and vessels of the portal venous system as a consequence of the progression of liver disease and portal hypertension. Some recent studies reported that the nodularity of the liver surface (as quantified by using a specific software) by ultrasound examination[37] and by CT scan (Liver Surface Nodularity Score)[38] is able to detect the presence of cirrhosis confidently and correlates with the HVPG, so allowing the identification of patients with likely CSPH

(AUROC, 0.88; cut-off, 2.8; positive predictive value, 88%). The advantage of this simple method is that it could be implemented automatically in CT scans.

The portal vein, splenic vein, and superior mesenteric vein progressively dilate, splenomegaly often appears, and portosystemic collaterals (**Fig. 2**) can be evident. Particular attention should be paid to portosystemic collaterals, because they are pathognomonic signs of portal hypertension in cACLD,[3] and are associated with higher HVPG[39] and poorer outcomes;[40,41] in addition, large gastroesophageal varices can be detected on CT scans with about 90% accuracy.[42]

Doppler measurements are not sufficiently accurate for CSPH; however, a very low velocity of flow in the portal vein (<12 cm/s) has been associated consistently to the presence of gastroesophageal varices, and is a risk factor for developing portal vein thrombosis.

Several new MR techniques are being tested in patients with portal hypertension and include diffusion-weighted imaging, hepatocellular contrast-enhanced MRI, T1 relaxometry, T1ρ imaging, textural analysis, susceptibility-weighted imaging, and perfusion imaging.[43] They are highly promising, but need further evaluation and clinical validation.

Among the emerging methods, contrast-enhanced ultrasound examination, taking advantage of the physical properties of the inert gas contained in the microbubbles, has been shown to provide information on portal hypertension. In particular, it has been observed that the amplitude of the subharmonic ultrasound waves decreases in parallel (linearly) to the pressure of the liquid surrounding the microbubbles. Hence, by measuring the subharmonic signal amplitude in the liver veins and in the hepatic veins by contrast-enhanced ultrasound examination, a subharmonic gradient reflecting the HVPG can be measured through adequate mathematical modeling. This approach subharmonic aided pressure estimation (SHAPE) has proven successful and allowed an excellent correlation between the SHAPE HVPG and the HVPG

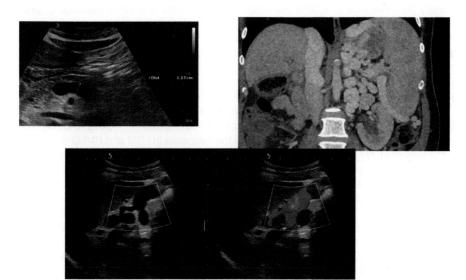

Fig. 2. Imaging signs of portal hypertension. (*Upper left panel*) Dilatation of the splenic vein by ultrasound examination. (*Upper right panel*) Large splenomegaly and numerous large splenorenal collaterals. (*Lower panel*) Large splenorenal collaterals on conventional ultrasound examination (*left*) and color Doppler ultrasound examination (*right*).

measured invasively ($R^2 = 0.82$); the proposed cut-off was greater than 90% accurate for CSPH.[44,45]

Imaging methods, and ultrasound examination in particular, are routinely used to follow-up patients with cACLD. Signs suggesting worsening of portal hypertension in compensated patients include enlargement of the portal venous system, further enlargement of spleen size,[46] and the onset of new portosystemic collaterals.[47]

LIVER ELASTOGRAPHY FOR THE ASSESSMENT OF CLINICALLY SIGNIFICANT PORTAL HYPERTENSION
Transient Elastography

Liver stiffness measurement (LSM) by transient elastography (TE) has been demonstrated to detect CSPH in patients with cACLD owing to different causes, although the majority of data is linked to viral hepatitis (**Table 2**). LSM obtained by TE correlates significantly with the HVPG in patients with cACLD, showing a correlation coefficient ranging between 0.55 to 0.86.[48] As mentioned elsewhere in this article, the correlation between the HVPG and LSM is excellent below the threshold of 10 mm Hg, although it decreases in patients with an HVPG above the threshold for CSPH, likely owing to a flow-dependent increase in portal pressure, not reflected in LSM.[49] Thus, LSM does not provide an accurate estimation of the HVPG value.[50,51] However, LSM is a reliable noninvasive tool to accurately identify patients with CSPH, showing an AUROC ranging between 0.74 and 0.94.[48] A meta-analysis confirmed the diagnostic capability of this method, reporting an AUROC of 0.93 with a sensitivity of 87.5% (95% confidence interval [CI], 75.8%–93.9%) and a specificity of 85.3% (95% CI, 76.9%–90.9%). The summary correlation coefficient was 0.783 (95% CI, 0.737–0.823).[48]

The cut-off of 21 kPa to identify the presence of CSPH demonstrated a high specificity (>90%) for an HVPG of more than 10 mm Hg.[18,49,52] Based on these data, the Baveno VI consensus stated that an LSM greater than 20 to 25 kPa can be used to identify the presence of CSPH (varices) in patients with untreated hepatitis C virus (HCV) or hepatitis B virus cACLD.[3] The specificity of this cut-off was more than 90% in the meta-analysis by You and colleagues.[48] In another recent meta-analysis[53] performed exclusively in patients with chronic viral hepatitis, it was suggested that 2 cut-offs can be used, namely, less than 13.6 kPa to rule out CSPH (pooled sensitivity 96%; CI 95% 93%–97%), and greater than 22 kPa to rule in CSPH (pooled specificity, 94%; 95% CI, 86%–97%), thus confirming Baveno VI consensus recommendations.[53]

After achieving a sustained virological response (SVR) in patients with chronic hepatitis C, LSM quickly and sometimes dramatically decreases.[54–58] Despite being statistically significant, the correlation between the decrease in LSM and HVPG was weak in the largest study published thus far.[57] Consequently, the 13.6 kPa cut-off to rule out CSPH performed poorly after achieving a SVR, because almost one-half of patients with an LSM less than 13.6 kPa still showed an HVPG of 10 mm Hg or greater. In contrast, an LSM of greater than 21 kPa showed to accurately rule in CSPH even after achieving a SVR.[57] Nevertheless, current evidence does indicate an LSM cut-off that could be used to safely rule out persistence of CSPH, in patients with SVR after HCV therapy.

Because the etiology of the underlying liver disease influences LSM, the application of previous described cut-offs, it has been postulated that LSM accuracy may be limited in patients with nonviral cACLD.[59] LSM correlated well with the HVPG in patients with alcohol-related liver disease (ArLD) in a recent retrospective study (correlation coefficient, 0.753; AUROC, 0.925).[60] The cut-off of 30.6 kPa showed the best capacity to rule in CSPH (sensitivity, 81%; specificity, 94%).[60] In a recent meta-

Table 2
Accuracy of LSM for the diagnosis of CSPH

Study, Year	Study Design	Population	Correlation Coefficient Between LSM and HVPG	AUROC for CSPH	Cut-off for CSPH	Sensitivity (%)	Specificity (%)
TE (only studies with ≥100 patients selected)							
Bureau et al,[18] 2008	Prospective	144 patients with HCV or alcoholic cirrhosis	0.858	0.945	21 kPa	89.9	93.2
Colecchia et al,[106] 2012	Prospective	100 patients with HCV cirrhosis	0.836	0.836	24.2 kPa	52.3	97.1
Reiberger et al,[143] 2012	Retrospective	502 patients with/without cirrhosis, some decompensated (mixed etiologies)	0.794	0.871	18 kPa	82.2	83.4
Schwabl et al,[144] 2015	Retrospective	188 patients with chronic liver disease	0.846	0.957	16.1 kPa	94.8	86.9
Cho et al,[145] 2015	Retrospective	219 patients with alcoholic cirrhosis (some decompensated)	n. a.	0.85	n. a.	n. a.	n. a.
Zykus et al,[146] 2015	Prospective	107 patients with cirrhosis (mixed etiologies)	0.750	0.949	17.4 kPa	88	87.5
Hametner et al,[147] 2015	Retrospective	236 patients with cirrhosis (mixed etiologies)	n. a.	0.92	24.8 kPa	81	93
Kumar et al,[148] 2017	Retrospective	326 patients with cirrhosis (mixed etiologies)	n. a.	0.74	21.46 kPa	79	67
Salavrakos et al,[60] 2018	Retrospective	118 patients with alcoholic liver disease	0.753	0.925	30.6 kPa	81	94
Point shear wave elastography							
Salzl et al,[63] 2014	Prospective	88 patients with liver cirrhosis	0.646	0.855	2.58 m/s	71.4	87.5
Attia et al,[64] 2015	Prospective	78 patients with chronic liver disease	0.650	0.93	2.17 m/s	97	89
Takuma et al,[65] 2016	Prospective	60 patients with liver cirrhosis	0.609	0.83	n. a.	n. a.	n. a.
2D-SWE (only studies with >100 patients)							
Jansen et al,[71] 2017	Prospective	158 patients with cirrhosis (mixed etiologies)	0.626	24.6 kPa < 16 kPa rule out > 29.5 kPa rule in	0.86	68.3	80.4

(continued on next page)

Table 2
(continued)

Study, Year	Study Design	Population	Correlation Coefficient Between LSM and HVPG	AUROC for CSPH	Cut-off for CSPH	Sensitivity (%)	Specificity (%)
Elkrief et al,[72] 2017	Prospective	191 patients with liver cirrhosis (mixed etiologies) 77 included in a previous study[71]	n. a.	n. a.	0.80	n. a.	n. a.
Zhu et al,[69] 2019	Retrospective	104 hepatitis B-related patients with cirrhosis	0.607	16.1 kPa < 13.2 kPa rule out > 24.9 kPa rule in	0.72	81	83
Thiele et al,[68] 2020	Meta-analysis	328 patients with compensated and decompensated cirrhosis (alcohol and viral etiology)	n.a.	Rule out <14 kPa 0.88 (85-91)	0.88	91	37

Abbreviations: ACLD, advanced chronic liver disease; AUROC, area under receiver operator curve; HCC, hepatocellular carcinoma; HCV, hepatitis C virus.

analysis focused on ArLD including 9 studies, the authors identified a cut-off value of 21.8 kPa for CSPH.[61] Despite a good pooled sensitivity (0.89; 95% CI, 0.83–0.93), both the specificity (0.71; 95% CI, 0.64–0.78) and positive likelihood ratio (3.1; 95% CI, 2.4–4 were modest.[61] Therefore, the cut-off value of 21.8 kPa has a good performance in ruling out CSPH, but it is not satisfactory in ruling in CSPH (similarly to what described for the 13.6 kPa cut-off in viral ACLD).[53,61] According to these data, the cut-off value to be used to rule in CSPH in ArLD seems to be higher than that for viral ACLD. In a recent meeting, a multicenter study with 786 patients showed that LSM was accurate in diagnosing CSPH in most etiologies, including nonalcoholic steatohepatitis, but not in obese patients with nonalcoholic steatohepatitis.[62] Data on the accuracy of LSM for CSPH in cholestatic liver disease (in which a presinusoidal component of portal hypertension is invariably present) and autoimmune hepatitis are lacking and require targeted studies.

Point Shear Wave Elastography

Similar to TE, point shear wave elastography (pSWE) (acoustic radiation force impulse imaging; Acuson Siemens 2000, Germany) based LSM showed a significant correlation with HVPG (r = 0.609–0.650) and a good diagnostic accuracy for CSPH (AUROC, 0.83–0.93).[63–65] Nevertheless, the data are lacking to establish an accurate cut-off value to rule in and rule out CSPH. The current cut-offs are highly variable (ranging from 2.17 to 2.58 m/s), likely owing to the population. Owing to these limitations, pSWE is not recommended for the diagnosis of CSPH.[50]

Two-Dimensional Shear Wave Elastography

Two-dimensional shear wave elastography (2D-SWE) demonstrated a good discriminative capacity (AUROC, 0.80–0.87), with sensitivity and specificity ranging between 80% and 90% in most of the studies. In a meta-analysis, Suh and colleagues[66] confirmed a good diagnostic performance (AUROC, 0.88; 95% CI, 0.85–0.91). The summary sensitivity and summary specificity were 85% (95% CI 75%–91%) and 85% (95% CI, 77%–90%), respectively. The correlation between LSM by 2D-SWE and HVPG was high with a summary correlation coefficient of 0.741 (95% CI, 0.658–0.825).[66]

In a recent study, 2D-SWE correlated with HVPG (r = 0.704; P<.0001), especially if the HVPG was less than 10 mm Hg and was significantly higher in patients with CSPH (15.52 vs 8.14 kPa; P<.0001) and not inferior to LSM-TE (0.92; P = .79). Furthermore, in the subgroup of compensated patients with ArLD, 2D-SWE classified CSPH better than TE (93.33% vs 85.71%; P = .039).[67]

A recent individual patient meta-analysis including 328 patients, 27% with cACLD, showed that LSM using a 2D-SWE of less than 14 kPa may be used to rule out CSPH in patients with cirrhosis.[68]

In the context of hepatitis B virus–related cACLD, a cut-off of less than 13.2 kPa ruled out CSPH with a sensitivity of greater than 90%, and a cut-off greater than 24.9 kPa ruled in CSPH with a specificity of greater than 90%.[69] Jansen and colleagues[70,71] developed 2 algorithms to noninvasively rule in and rule out CSPH using 2D-SWE using LSM followed by spleen stiffness measurement (SSM). An LSM of less than 16 kPa and an SSM of less than 26.6 were able to rule out CSPH with a sensitivity of 98.6%.[70] An LSM of greater than 38 kPa correctly ruled in CSPH in all patients. In patients with an LSM of less than 38 kPa, an SSM of greater than 27.9 kPa was able to rule in CSPH with a specificity of 91.4%. Combining both algorithms, patients were correctly classified as having or not CSPH in 91.6% of cases with a sensitivity of

98.3% and a specificity of 96.3%.[71] A large cohort of 191 patients showed that their accuracy was insufficient for the application in clinical practice.[72]

Overall, LSM performance using 2D-SWE for CSPH is likely consistent with that of TE.[48] However, the heterogeneity of cut-offs (2D-SWE, 16–38 kPa), possibly underlines a lack of standardization. Although currently not implemented in clinical practice, the method seems promising and further data are awaited.[50] **Fig. 3** summarizes the advantages and disadvantages of LSM and SSM using the different available ultrasound elastography techniques.

LIVER ELASTOGRAPHY FOR THE ASSESSMENT OF GASTROESOPHAGEAL VARICES

Screening endoscopy for esophageal varices in patients with a diagnosis of ACLD is a crucial part of the management, because it can precisely identify varices needing treatment aimed at decreasing the risk of bleeding.[73] LSM has been proven extensively to predict varices needing treatment. This section includes more recent studies in this field published after the Baveno VI workshop (**Table 3**).

Transient Elastography

Although it is not as accurate as for defining the presence of CSPH, it is the single best noninvasive method for varices detection.[74] A recent meta-analysis with a total of 3644 patients reported a correct diagnosis of esophageal varices or varices needing treatment after a positive measurement of LSM (with variable cut-offs) did not exceed 70%.[74] The majority of studies including LSM by TE after the publication of the Baveno VI consensus report have been focused on combination tests (see **Table 3**).

Point Shear Wave Elastography

pSWE has been widely evaluated for the prediction of esophageal varices, with varied results. A 2014 cohort study reported an AUROC of 0.743 for the prediction of esophageal varices using pSWE (vs TE with an AUROC of 0.802).[63] Later, a Japanese study showed an AUROC of 0.789 for any varices and an AUROC of 0.788 for varices

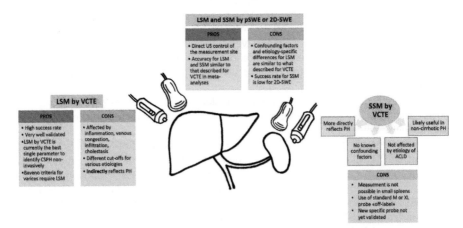

Fig. 3. Advantages and disadvantages of LSM and spleen stiffness measurement (SSM) for portal hypertension using the different available ultrasound elastography techniques. 2D-SWE, 2-dimensional shear wave elastography; ACLD, advanced chronic liver disease; PH, portal hypertension; US, ultrasound examination.

Table 3
Accuracy of LSM using ultrasound elastography techniques (TE, pSWE, and 2D-SWE) for the diagnosis of gastroesophageal varices in the post-Baveno VI era

Study, Year	Design	Type of Ultrasound Elastography Method ± Other Combined	Patient Population; Number of Esophageal Varices, Number Varices Needing Treatment	TE-Cut-offs and AUC Esophageal Varices/ Varices Needing Treatment	Conclusions
TE (studies included ≥ 200 patients)					
Maurice et al,[149] 2016	Retrospective	TE + platelet count	310 mixed	LSM: 20 kPa, AUC 0.686 LSM (20 kPa) and PLT (150 G/L): AUC 0.746	SENS. 67%, SPEC. 55%, PPV 7%, NPV 97%; SENS.87%, SPEC. 34%, PPV 6%, NPV 98%
Abraldes et al,[150] 2016	Retrospective	TE + platelet count ± spleen size; LSPS score and platelet-spleen ratio [PSR]	518 mixed	LSM: 14.0 kPa (AUC 0.67) LSM (20 kPa) and PLT (150 G/L): AUC 0.76	LSPS and a model with TE and platelet count identified patients with very low risk (<5%) risk of varices needing treatment
Marot et al,[140] 2017	Meta-analysis	TE ± platelet count or TE alone	3364 mixed	<20 kPa; PLT>150 G/L	LSM + PLT (150 G/L): SENS. 89%, SPEC. 38%, PPV: 43%, NPV: 86% SENS. 93%, SPEC. 30%, PPV 14%, NPV 97%
Pu et al,[151] 2017	Meta-analysis	TE alone	2697 mixed	LSM (pooled): 20 kPa, AUC 0.83; 30 kPa, AUC: 0.83	LSM: Pooled: SENS. 84%, SPEC. 62%, Cut-off 20 kPa: SENS. 83%, SPEC. 68%; Pooled: SENS. 78%, SPEC. 76%, Cut-off 30 kPa: SENS. 73%, SPEC. 74%

(continued on next page)

Table 3
(continued)

Study, Year	Design	Type of Ultrasound Elastography Method ± Other Combined	Patient Population; Number of Esophageal Varices, Number Varices Needing Treatment	TE-Cut-offs and AUC Esophageal Varices/ Varices Needing Treatment	Conclusions
Jangouk et al,[142] 2017	Retrospective	Baveno VI (LSM 20 kPa, PLT>150 G/L), PLT >150, MELD = 6	262 mixed	LSM (20 kPa) and PLT >150 G/L; MELD = 6 (150 G/L)	Baveno criteria 26% (US) and 16% (Italy) spared. SENS. and NPV were 100%. PLT >150 G/L and MELD = 6, increased the number of endoscopies avoided to 54% (US) while maintaining a SENS. and NPV of 100%.
Agustin et al,[125] 2017	Retrospective	TE ± PLT, expanded Baveno	925 mixed	LSM (25 kPa) and PLT >110 G/L	Expanded-Baveno VI: spare 40%; missing varices needing treatment of 1.6%
Petta et al,[152] 2018	Retrospective analysis of prospective data	Baveno VI and expanded Baveno VI (TE ± PLT)	790 NAFLD/NASH	LSM: 20 kPa + PLT 150 G/L LSM 25 kPa + Plt 110 G/L LSM 30 kPa + Plt 110 G/L	Best cut-offs to rule out varices needing treatment: PLT>110 G/L + LSM <30 kPa (M probe), PLT>110 G/L + LSM <25 kPa (XL probe)

Manatsathit et al,[123] 2018	Meta-analysis 45 studies	LSM alone vs SSM alone vs LSPS	4337 Mixed	AUC SSM and LSPS vs LSM: 0.899 and 0.851 vs 0.817	For esophageal varices detection: SSM and LSPS vs LSM (0.90 and 0.91 vs 0.85), specificity (0.73 and 0.76 vs 0.64) For varices needing treatment: SSM (0.87) > LSM (0.85) > LSPS (0.82); LSM, SSM, and LSPS cannot be recommended for detection of varices needing treatment
Bae et al,[153] 2018	Cross-sectional	TE	282 mixed (60% HBV)	LSM (20 kPa) and PLT >150 G/L LSM (25 kPa) and PLT >110 G/L	Expanded Baveno VI criteria spare more (51.7%) than (27.6%). expanded missed varices needing treatment (6.8%) than the original criteria (3.8%). Baveno VI: NPV HBV: 0.92, HCV: 1.00, ARLD: 1.00, NAFLD:1.00
Lee et al,[154] 2018	Retrospective	Baveno VI and expanded Baveno VI (TE ± PLT)	1218 (40% HBV)	LSM (20 kPa) and PLT >150 G/L; LSM (25 kPa) and PLT >110 G/L AUC LSPS: 0.780 (95% CI: 0.774–0.820)	Baveno VI: 25.7% saved endoscopy; varices needing treatment miss rate: 1.9%. Expanded Baveno VI: saved endoscopy: 39.1%; varices needing treatment miss rate <5%

(continued on next page)

Table 3
(continued)

Study, Year	Design	Type of Ultrasound Elastography Method ± Other Combined	Patient Population; Number of Esophageal Varices, Number Varices Needing Treatment	TE-Cut-offs and AUC Esophageal Varices/ Varices Needing Treatment	Conclusions
Moctezuma-Velazquez et al,[155] 2018	Cross-sectional	TE ± PLT Baveno VI and expanded Baveno VI	227 cholestatic PBC (n = 147) PSC (n = 80)		Baveno-VI criteria 0% False negative rate in PBC and PSC, saving 39% and 30% of endoscopies. In PBC the other LSM-TE: FNRs >5%. In PSC the expanded Baveno: adequate performance. In both conditions.
Thabut et al,[101] 2019	Prospective ancillary study ANRS CO12 CirVir cohort	TE ± PLT (Baveno VI)	200 HBV- (n = 98) or HCV- (n = 94) or both (n = 8) with SVR to antivirals		Baveno VI valid patients with compensated viral cirrhosis, even SVR. Endoscopy is no longer necessary in the subgroup of low-risk patients
Point shear wave elastography					
Salzl et al,[63] 2014	Cross-sectional	pSWE; Acuson S2000	88 mixed	L-SWE: 2.74 m/s (0.743)	For esophageal varices: 62.5%/89.5 %/PPV: 91.5%/NPV: 56.9%
Takuma et al,[65] 2016	Cross-sectional	pSWE; Acuson S2000	340 mixed	For esophageal varices: AUC: 0.789; varices needing treatment: AUC 0.788	

Study	Design	Technique; Device	N	Results	Sensitivity/Specificity
Attia et al,[64] 2015	Cross-sectional	pSWE; Acuson S2000	78 mixed		LSM in both groups of patients (SSM: 0.90 and 0.93 vs LSM: 0.84 and 0.88, respectively).
Lucchina et al,[156] 2018	Cross-sectional	pSWE; iU22	42 mixed	L-SWE: 12.27 kPa AUC: 0.913	SENS: 100%/SPEC: 66.67%
2D-SWE (only studies with > 100 patients selected)					
Cassinotto et al,[75] 2015	Prospective	2D-SWE, Aixplorer	401 mixed	L-SWE: AUC 0.80 LSM: AUC 0.73	L-SWE: SENS. 92%/SPEC. 36%
Kasai et al,[77] 2015	Retrospective	2D-SWE, Aixplorer	273 mixed	0.807	
Kim et al,[78] 2016	Retrospective	2D-SWE, Aixplorer	103 mixed	For esophageal varices: L-SWE: 13.9 kPa AUC 0.887 varices needing treatment cut-off 16.1 kPa; AUC 0.887 for any esophageal varices and 0.880 varices needing treatment; L-SWE: All patients: 26.3 kPa; AUC:0.683 cACLD:14.2 kPa (0.925)	Esophageal varices: SENS 75%/SPEC 88.9%/ Varices needing treatment: 84.6%/ 85.6%

(continued on next page)

Table 3
(continued)

Study, Year	Design	Type of Ultrasound Elastography Method ± Other Combined	Patient Population; Number of Esophageal Varices, Number Varices Needing Treatment	TE-Cut-offs and AUC Esophageal Varices/ Varices Needing Treatment	Conclusions
Jansen et al.[71] 2017	Prospective	2D-SWE; Aixplorer SSI	158 mixed		Rule-out for esophageal varices SENS: 0.98; SPEC: 0.50; PPV: 0.80; NPV: 0.93; Diagnostic accuracy: 0.83 Rule-in for esophageal varices SENS: 0.90; SPEC: 0.60; PPV: 0.83; NPV: 0.73; Diagnostic accuracy: 0.81
Petzold G et al,[157] 2019	Prospective	2D-SWE; GE Logiq E9	100 mixed	L-SWE: AUC: 0.781	L-SWE combined with gallbladder wall thickness (GBWT) for esophageal varices: SENS: 86.3% SPEC: 71.4%; At L-SWE >9 kPa or GBWT >4 mm: SENS 100% (NPV 1.0)

Abbreviations: 2D-SWE, bidimensional shear wave elastography; AUC, area under the curve; kPa, kilopascal; LSPS, liver stiffness to spleen/platelet score; L-SWE, liver stiffness by Shear wave elastography; MELD, Model for End-stage Liver Disease; NASH, nonalcoholic steatohepatitis; NPV, negative predictive value; PBC, primary biliary sclerosis; pSWE, point shear wave elastography; SENS, sensibility; SPEC, specificity; SSI, supersonic imaging.

needing treatment, respectively.[65] Currently, evidence is not strong enough to recommend pSWE to rule in or rule out varices needing treatment.

Two-Dimensional Shear Wave Elastography

Three studies showed an AUROC around 0.80 for LSM in patients with cACLD for esophageal varices.[75–77] LSM yielded an AUROC of 0.887 for any esophageal varices and 0.880 (cut-off of 16.1 kPa) for varices needing treatment,[78] which was not confirmed in another study including 79 patients revealing no difference between LSM and SSM values (L-2D-SWE and by TE) between patients for varices needing treatment.[79] Stefanescu and colleagues[80] demonstrated that, with a stepwise approach combining LSM at a cut-off less than 19 kPa with a cut-off of PLT greater than 100 G/L, esophageal varices were ruled out with 83% accuracy. Another cohort study of patients with cACLD supported these data.[71] More recently, diagnostic performance of 2D-SWE was shown to be similar to that of TE for predicting the presence of esophageal varices. The AUROCs for predicting varices needing treatment for 2D-SWE and a modified Liver Stiffness-Spleen Size-To-Platelet Ratio Risk Score were 0.712 (95% CI, 0.621–0.738) and 0.834 (95% CI, 0.785–0.875), respectively.[81] The diagnostic performance of 2D-SWE is similar to that of TE for predicting the presence of esophageal varices.

Overall, larger scale studies are needed to overcome significant discrepancies between among reported cut-offs for both pSWE and 2D-SWE–based LSM. There is solid evidence to support the use of LSM and platelet count, but the future implementation of SSM and other tests to further enhance esophageal varices screening strategies in cACLD is promising.

Liver Stiffness Measurement for the Follow-up of Portal Hypertension

CSPH is a key predictor of risk of clinical decompensation in patients with cACLD.[82] Robic and colleagues[83] showed that LSM and HVPG were similarly accurate in predicting a first episode of decompensation in patients with cACLD. All of the clinical events occurred in patients with an LSM of 21.1 kPa or higher.

Different studies[83–88] have shown that in patients with cACLD, LSM holds prognostic value for liver-related events and death. Recently, this finding was confirmed in a systematic review and meta-analysis[89] of 17 prospective studies, including 7058 patients. In 1 study, an increase of more than 1.5 kPa per year in LSM seemed to add prognostic value to baseline LSM in both primary biliary sclerosis[90] and HCV.[91]

As for the combination of LSM with other noninvasive tests, the liver stiffness to spleen/platelet score predicted first decompensation in an hepatitis B virus cohort better than LSM alone cACLD.[92] Our group recently reported that the liver stiffness to spleen/platelet score was superior to LSM (using an XL probe) and portal hypertension risk score to predict the first clinical decompensation in obese/overweight patients with nonalcoholic steatohepatitis.[93] Furthermore, Wong and colleagues[94] followed 548 patients with cACLD for 3 years and showed that an LSM/SSM–guided screening strategy for varices had a similar low risk of variceal hemorrhage as compared with universal screening endoscopy.

As far as prediction of hepatocellular carcinoma is concerned, a number of prospective studies have identified that LSM in patients with viral cirrhosis is associated with the risk of incidence of hepatocellular carcinoma.[95–99]

Regarding nonselective beta-blockers (NSBB) response, LSM changes in patients with portal hypertension undergoing therapy do not correlate with changes in HVPG.[100]

As for patients with cACLD who did not undergo variceal screening being within the Baveno criteria, LSM should be repeated yearly, and an increase of LSM or more than 10 kPa indicates the need of starting variceal screening.[3] This recommendation has been validated in a recent study from France.[101]

SPLEEN ELASTOGRAPHY

In patients with portal hypertension, the elevated portal pressure is transmitted to the splenic vein and leads to passive congestion in the spleen. Combined with an increased arterial inflow from splanchnic vasodilation, hyperactivation of splenic lymphoid tissue, fibrogenesis and angiogenesis, this causes an increase in spleen stiffness.[102]

The advantages of SSM in comparison with LSM to assess portal hypertension are multiple (see **Fig. 3**). First, SSM is devoid of some of the confounding factors that may affect LSM reliability, such as liver congestion, inflammation, infiltration or cholestasis, although a recent study suggested that liver inflammation could potentially increase SSM.[103] Moreover, SSM takes into account the dynamic component of portal hypertension that is not reflected by LSM and hence correlates better with portal pressure in later stages of liver disease.[104] SSM can also be useful to differentiate between cirrhotic and noncirrhotic (prehepatic, idiopathic, and presinusoidal) portal hypertension, where there is a mismatch between the LSM and the SSM.[105]

However, 2 main disadvantages have made SSM difficult to implement in clinical practice to date. The first is the high failure rate ($\leq15\%$–30%) that has been observed with SSM, mostly with TE and 2D-SWE (supersonic imaging) compared with pSWE, which is feasible most of the time (**Table 4**). The absence of splenomegaly, ascites, and obesity, as well as movements caused by the heart beating in the case of 2D-SWE, negatively affect the success rate.[75] SSM by TE was improved significantly with the use of ultrasound examination to localize the spleen[106,107] and with a novel, spleen-dedicated TE examination (SSM at 100 Hz, where the shear wave frequency is set at 100 Hz instead of 50 Hz) (6%–13% and 7.5% failure rate, respectively).[67] All 3 techniques have an excellent reproducibility.[106,108,109]

The second disadvantage of SSM is the ceiling effect at 75 kPa, specific to TE. The spleen is a stiffer organ than the liver, even in normal subjects, and the use of the same probes and software than for LSM may not be appropriate. To overcome this effect, some authors have proposed to use a modified software, where the SSM can be reflected up to 150 kPa[110] and others, as discussed elsewhere in this article, suggested a novel, spleen-dedicated TE examination (SSM at 100 Hz) with values up to 100 kPa.[67]

Spleen Elastography for the Assessment of Portal Hypertension

A number of studies have evaluated the ability of SSM to predict portal hypertension (see **Table 4**). A recent meta-analysis of 9 studies concluded that SSM strongly correlates with HVPG (summary R = 0.72; 95% CI, 0.63–0.80) and has a good accuracy for predicting CSPH (AUROC, summary sensitivity and specificity of 0.92 [95% CI, 0.89–0.94], 0.88 [95% CI, 0.70–0.96], and 0.84 [95% CI, 0.72–0.92], respectively),[111] comparable with LSM,[48] although the heterogeneity of studies included limits the interpretation of these results. Another recent meta-analysis including only studies evaluating 2D-SWE (supersonic imaging) showed a moderate diagnostic accuracy for CSPH.[112] Studies that reported a poor performance of SS to detect CSPH (AUROCs in the 0.60 range) included patients with more advanced CLD.[79,113]

Table 4
Accuracy of SSM using ultrasound elastography techniques for CSPH and esophageal varices in ACLD

Study, Year	Method Used	N Included and Etiology	Failure Rate (%)	End Point	AUROC for the Selected Endpoint	Chosen Cut-off for the Selected Endpoint	Sensitivity (%)	Specificity (%)
Stefanescu et al,[158] 2011	TE	174, mixed	14, 4	Esophageal varices	0.781	46.4 kPa	83.6	71.4
Colecchia et al,[106] 2012	TE	113, HCV, compensated	11.5	CSPH Esophageal varices	0.966 0.941	40.0 kPa (rule out) 52.8 kPa (rule in) 41.3 kPa (rule out) 55.0 kPa (rule in)	98.5 76.9 98.1 71.7	74.3 97.1 66.0 95.7
Sharma et al,[113] 2013	TE	200, mixed	13	Esophageal varices	0.898	40.8 kPa	94	76
Calvaruso et al,[110] 2013	TE (modified range)	112, HCV, compensated	14.3	Esophageal varices Large esophageal varices	0.701 0.820	50.0 kPa 54.0 kPa	65 80	61 70
Zykus et al,[146] 2015	TE	107, mixed, most compensated	7.5	CSPH	0.846	47.6 kPa	77.3	79.2
Stefanescu et al,[159] 2015	TE	136, mixed	N/A	High-risk esophageal varices	0.742	53 kPa	89	54
Wong et al,[130] 2016	TE	176, HBV	15.9	Esophageal varices	0.685	21.4 kPa (rule out) 50.5 kPa (rule in)	90.3 45.2	43.4 90.3
Arribas Anta et al,[160] 2019	TE	66, mixed	9.1	Esophageal varices	0.800	48 kPa	87	69
Stefanescu et al,[67] 2020	TE (spleen-dedicated, 100 Hz)	260, mixed	7.5 (vs. 24for 50 Hz)	CSPH Esophageal varices High-risk esophageal varices	0.811 0.728 0.756	34.15 kPa 33.3 kPa (rule out) 70 kPa (rule in) 40 kPa (rule out) 79.9 kPa (rule in)	N/A 90.3 29.1 91.3 26.1	N/A 33.7 90.5 40.8 90.1
Rifai et al,[161] 2011	pSWE (VTQ)	100, mixed	22	CSPH	0.680	3.29 m/s	47	73

(continued on next page)

Table 4
(continued)

Study, Year	Method Used	N Included and Etiology	Failure Rate (%)	End Point	AUROC for the Selected Endpoint	Chosen Cut-off for the Selected Endpoint	Sensitivity (%)	Specificity (%)
Bota et al,[162] 2012	pSWE (VTQ)	145, mixed	2.1	Large esophageal varices	0.578	2.55 m/s	96.7	21.0
Ye et al,[163] 2012	pSWE (VTQ)	204, HBV	N/A	Esophageal varices Large esophageal varices	0.830 0.839	3.16 m/s 3.39 m/s	84.1 78.9	81 78.3
Vermehren et al,[164] 2012	pSWE (VTQ)	166, mixed	0	Large esophageal varices	0.580	3.04 m/s	90	25
Takuma et al,[165] 2013	pSWE (VTQ)	340, mixed	4.5	Esophageal varices High-risk esophageal varices	0.937 (viral) 0.923 (others) 0.930 (all)	3.18 m/s 3.24 m/s 3.30 m/s	98.9 97.7 98.9	59.9 65.2 62.9
Rizzo et al,[166] 2014	pSWE (VTQ)	54, HCV	N/A	Esophageal varices	0.959	3.10 m/s	96.4	88.5
Attia et al,[64] 2015	pSWE (VTQ)	78, mixed, some decompensated, 90CSPH, 76% esophageal varices	0	CSPH	0.968	2.32 m/s	96	89
Kim et al,[167] 2015	pSWE (VTQ)	132, mixed	4.5	Esophageal varices Large esophageal varices	0.785 0.786	3.16 m/s 3.40 m/s	87.0 78.9	60.4 63.0
Park et al,[168] 2016	pSWE (ElastPQ)	366, viral and alcohol	24	Esophageal varices	0.859	29.9 kPa	85.1 kPa	79.1 kPa
Takuma et al,[65] 2016	pSWE (VTQ)	62, mixed, most compensated	3.2	CSPH HVPG $\geq$12 mm Hg Esophageal varices Large esophageal varices	0.943 0.963 0.937 0.955	3.10 m/s 3.15 m/s 3.36 m/s 3.51 m/s	97.1 96.6 95.8 93.8	57.7 61.3 77.8 84.1

Study	Technique	Population		Outcome	AUC	Cutoff		
Lucchina et al,[156] 2018	pSWE (ElastPQ)	54, mixed (only patients without esophageal varices or with small esophageal varices were included)	22	Esophageal varices	0.675	23.9 kPa	73.8	59.5
Fierbinteanu-Braticevici et al,[169] 2019	pSWE (VTQ)	135, mixed	0	Esophageal varices High-risk esophageal varices	0.776 0.972	2.5 m/s (rule out) 3.5 m/s (rule in) 3.2 m/s (rule out) 3.8 m/s (rule in)	92 47 97 55	22 96 69 98
Peagu et al,[170] 2019	pSWE (VTQ)	178, viral	N/A	Esophageal varices Large esophageal varices	0.872 0.969	2.89 m/s 3.30 m/s	91.4 96.4	67.7 88.5
Darweesh et al,[171] 2019	pSWE (VTQ)	200, HCV	1	Esophageal varices	0.760	3.25 m/s	85	58
Giuffrè et al,[103] 2020	pSWE (ElastPQ)	210, mixed, compensated	4.5	Esophageal varices High-risk esophageal varices	0.95 N/A	31 kPa (rule out) 69 kPa (rule in) 46 kPa (rule out)	100 14 100	60 100 84
Elkrief et al,[79] 2015	2D-SWE (SSI)	79, mixed, most decompensated, 89 CSPH, 69% Child-Pugh B-C	3	CSPH Large esophageal varices	0.640 0.580	34.7 kPa 32.3 kPa	40 48	100 71
	TE		58	CSPH Large esophageal varices	0.630 0.650	56.3 kPa 73.5 kPa	73 54	67 78
Procopet et al,[109] 2015	2D-SWE (SSI)	55, mixed, most compensated	34	CSPH	0.725	22.7 kPa (rule out) 40 kPa (rule in)	90 N/A	N/A 90
Cassinotto et al,[75] 2015	2D-SWE (SSI)	401, mixed, some decompensated	29.2	Esophageal varices High-risk esophageal varices	0.80 0.78 (all) 0.75 (compensated)	N/A N/A 25.6 kPa (with NPV >90%)	N/A N/A 94	N/A N/A 36

(continued on next page)

Table 4
(continued)

Study, Year	Method Used	N Included and Etiology	Failure Rate (%)	End Point	AUROC for the Selected Endpoint	Chosen Cut-off for the Selected Endpoint	Sensitivity (%)	Specificity (%)
Grgurevic et al,[118] 2015	2D-SWE (SSI)	126, mixed	29.4	Esophageal varices	0.790	30.3 kPa	79.6	75.8
Jansen et al,[71] 2017	2D-SWE (SSI)	158, mixed, some decompensated	18.8	CSPH	0.840	26.3 kPa 21.7 kPa (rule out) 35.6 kPa (rule in)	79.7 91.9 51.4	84.2 50 92
Zhu et al,[69] 2019	2D-SWE (SSI)	104, HBV, most compensated	24.6	CSPH	0.810	23.2 kPa (rule out) 34.2 kPa (rule in)	>90 N/A	N/A >90
Karagiannakis et al,[124] 2019	2D-SWE (SSI)	64, mixed, compensated	9.8	High-risk esophageal varices	0.792 (all) 0.854 (excluding cholestatic liver disease)	33.7 kPa (rule out) 35.8 kPa (rule out)	91.7 88.9	60.0 72.4

Abbreviations: HBV, hepatitis B virus; HCV, hepatitis C virus; N/A, not applicable; NPV, negative predictive value; PPV, positive predictive value; pSWE, point shear wave elastography; SS, spleen stiffness; SSI, supersonic imagine; SWE, shear wave elastography; VTQ, virtual touch quantification.

As for the prediction of severe portal hypertension, a recent study confirms that the correlation between SSM and HVPG decreases with increasing HVPG, especially greater than 16 mm Hg,[104] where SS is more dependent on the chronic spleen parenchymal remodeling rather than reflecting passive congestion. Thus, SSM is likely not a good tool to identify patients with severe portal hypertension.

Determining the optimal SSM cut-off values to predict CSPH is challenging, as highlighted by the multiple cut-off values proposed in various studies, which depend on the population included (the etiology of liver disease and compensated or decompensated stage) (see **Table 4**). The use of a single cut-off value is usually associated with suboptimal sensitivity and specificity, whereas the use of 2 values (one rule out with high sensitivity and one rule in with high specificity) has the disadvantage of leading to a large number of unclassified patients. As with LSM, the use of specific cut-offs for each etiology of CLD has been proposed,[61] but its importance is probably less than for LSM.

SSM has also been shown to be able to predict clinical decompensation and mortality,[114–118] as well as late hepatocellular carcinoma recurrence.[119] As for the ability of SSM to predict liver failure after hepatectomy, the data are inconclusive.[120,121]

MR elastography (MRE) of the spleen has recently emerged as a potential tool to evaluate portal hypertension. A recent systematic review and meta-analysis of 14 studies (8 studies including spleen MRE) concluded that MRE had a good diagnostic accuracy in detecting portal hypertension with a summary AUROC, sensitivity, and specificity of 0.92 (95% CI, 0.89–0.94), 0.79 (95% CI, 0.61–0.90), and 0.90 (95% CI, 0.80–0.95), respectively.[122] The major inconvenient of MRE remains its limited availability and cost.

Spleen Elastography for the Assessment of Gastroesophageal Varices

Because the development of gastroesophageal varices depends on CSPH, it is not surprising that SSM can predict their presence (see **Table 4**). A recent systematic review and meta-analysis of 45 studies (17 evaluating SS with various techniques) concluded that SSM was superior to LSM in predicting esophageal varices in CLD with AUROC, summary sensitivity, and summary specificity of 0.899, 0.90 (95% CI, 0.87–0.94), and 0.73 (95% CI, 0.65–0.80), respectively, compared with 0.817, 0.85 (95% CI, 0.81–0.89), and 0.64 (95% CI, 0.56–0.71) for LSM.[123] This result is likely attributable to the better performance of SSM compared with LSM in more severe portal hypertension because it reflects better the hemodynamic component of portal hypertension. The diagnostic accuracy was not as good for high-risk esophageal varices (AUROC, 0.807). A study published after showed a slightly better performance for high-risk esophageal varices (AUROC, 0.847).[107] The results of this meta-analysis, however, need to be interpreted carefully given the heterogeneity of the population included, with both compensated and decompensated patients.

As discussed elsewhere in this article, some studies have evaluated new technologies to improve further the diagnostic capacity of SSM. In a recent study, prediction of large esophageal varices was improved with the use of a novel, spleen-dedicated TE with higher shear wave frequency (100 Hz, compared with the traditional 50 Hz).[67] In this study, the use of SSM at 100 Hz alone (with a cut-off of 41.3 kPa) could spare 37.8% esophagogastroduodenoscopy compared with Baveno VI alone (8.1%), with a 4.7% rate of missed high-risk esophageal varices (with the total number of high-risk esophageal varices as denominator). Colecchia and associates[107] with regular TE and Karagiannakis and colleagues[124] with 2D-SWE showed similar rates of spared endoscopy with SSM alone, so did studies on expanded Baveno VI criteria.[125]

As with CSPH, once again, determining optimal rule out and rule in cut-off values is challenging. For SSM by TE, a value of 46 kPa has been accepted as an adequate rule out cut-off, whereas for pSWE and 2D-SWE, no single values can currently be recommended, although they probably are in the range of 2.5 to 3.5 m/s and 21 to 33 kPa, respectively. The Spleen Stiffness Probability Index was recently proposed by Giuffrè and coworkers[103] to establish, instead of cut-offs, a probability of high-risk esophageal varices for each SSM value, supporting the clinician in deciding whom to screen or not and avoiding the issue of false negatives and false positives that occur with cut-offs.

SSM was also found to be a good predictor of esophageal variceal bleeding (cumulative incidence 7.4%), with an AUROC of 0.857 (0.911 in compensated patients) in a prospective study by Takuma and colleagues,[126] where patients were followed for a median duration of 32.7 months. In this study, the SSM with the maximal negative predictive value was 3.64 m/s (3.48 m/s in compensated cirrhosis). A retrospective study using TE showed similar results with a 100% negative predictive value at a cut-off SSM value of 42.6 kPa.[127]

Spleen Elastography for the Follow-up of Portal Hypertension

Given the rationale behind SSM, it can be expected that the most efficient treatment for portal hypertension, liver transplantation, causes a net decline in SSM.[128] Whether SSM could be a useful tool to assess response to other treatments for portal hypertension is a topic of interest. A recent study showed a good performance (AUROC, 0.848) of a model based on dynamic changes in SSM (by pSWE) in predicting the hemodynamic response to NSBB prophylaxis in patients with high-risk esophageal varices.[129] Of note, beta-blockers were previously shown not to affect the diagnostic accuracy of SSM.[130] SSM has also been repeatedly shown to decrease after transjugular intrahepatic portosystemic shunt and, therefore, could be a reliable tool to monitor transjugular intrahepatic portosystemic shunt function,[131–135] except when there is concurrent embolization or thrombosis of competitive shunts, where SSM may increase after transjugular intrahepatic portosystemic shunting.[136] In a recent study by Takuma and colleagues,[137] SSM by virtual touch quantification increased after balloon-occluded retrograde transvenous obliteration and was a predictor of exacerbation of esophageal varices. Studies done in the post-direct-acting antiviral era showed that SSM also decreases after HCV eradication[54,138]

In conclusion, there are now enough solid data to include SSM in the list of standard, noninvasive tools available to assess CSPH. A number of studies have also proven its good performance in detecting the presence of esophageal varices, justifying its integration in algorithms to select patients for screening endoscopy for varices.

COMBINATION TESTS

Strategies combining other noninvasive markers of portal hypertension have been implemented to improve diagnostic accuracy of LSM. In a recent meta-analysis, esophageal varices detection for the liver stiffness to spleen/platelet score and SSM was superior to LSM.[123] Furthermore, in a prospective cohort of patients with cACLD, the liver stiffness to spleen/platelet score correctly classified esophageal varices in around 80% of patients.[139] Subsequently, the Baveno VI Consensus suggested that a platelet count of more than 150 g/L and a LSM of less than 20 kPa could identify patients with cACLD, with a very low risk (<5%) of varices needing treatment.[3]

A meta-analysis concluded that varices needing treatment are found in no more than 4% of patients when the LSM is less than 20 kPa with a normal platelet count.[140]

Moreover, another study tested earlier noninvasive test-based algorithms and Baveno VI and found that esophageal varices misdiagnosed when using platelets in 3.1%, TE in 3.7%, the liver stiffness to spleen/platelet score in 10%, variceal risk index in 11.3%, Baveno VI in 1.8%, and Augustin algorithm in 3.7% of patients. The rate of unnecessary gastroscopies was 46% for platelet count, 25% for TE, 13% for the liver stiffness to spleen/platelet score, 6% for the variceal risk index, 53% for Baveno VI, and 39.1% for the Augustin algorithm.[141]

In an attempt to reduce the number of unnecessary endoscopies, Jangouk and colleagues[142] reported that a strategy using platelet count or more than 150 G/L and a Model for End-stage Liver Disease of 6 without LSM, substantially increased the number of endoscopies avoided to 54%, with a very low rate of missing varices needing treatment. These findings without LSM were not validated because of an unacceptable high rate of missed varices needing treatment.[125] The Expanded Baveno VI criteria used a platelet count or more than 110 G/L and a LSM of less than 25 kPa potentially spared 40% of endoscopies (21% with Baveno VI criteria) with a risk of missing varices needing treatment of 1.6%.[125]

More recently, combined approaches have included SSM. The combination of SSM with Baveno VI criteria could spare 43.8% of endoscopies. The combined Baveno VI/SSM of 46 or less model would have safely spared 37.4% of endoscopies (0 high-risk esophageal varices missed), compared with 16.5% without SSM.[107]

Fig. 4 summarizes the existing strategies combining noninvasive tests to optimize the selection of patients for endoscopy in the context of cACLD.

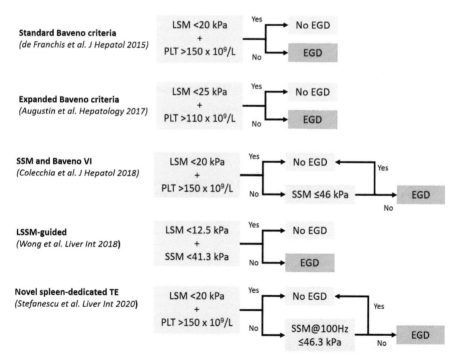

Fig. 4. Existing strategies based on noninvasive tests to decrease the need of screening for varices treatment (VNT). EGD, esophagogastroduodenoscopy; PLT, platelet count; SSM, spleen stiffness measurement; TE, transient elastography.

SUMMARY

Noninvasive tests, and in particular liver elastography, have represented a major advantage in the assessment of patients with cACLD in the last years. Although a perfect method to quantify noninvasively the HVPG is still lacking, novel techniques such as MR-based techniques and SHAPE by contrast-enhanced ultrasound examination have a large potential to become game-changers in this field within the next 5 years. The authors expect also radiomics to expand and become a novel strategy integrating the existing imaging data into robust algorithms allowing better identifying in a completely automated way the presence of CSPH and varices. Given the new data regarding a protective role of NSBB on the onset of decompensation (and not just variceal bleeding), a quick and accurate way of diagnosing CSPH noninvasively will become the standard of care. Awaiting for the validation of these methods, LSM and SSM used in combination, and combined to unrelated methods such as spleen size by imaging and platelet count, already allow to rule in CSPH with an accuracy exceeding 90%.

Recent data showing that the hemodynamic response to NSBB can be mirrored by changes in SSM by pSWE are awaiting validation and, if confirmed, would represent a major advantage in the management of patients with portal hypertension. The HVPG measurement remains the reference standard and it should be used whenever noninvasive tests provide inconsistent results or whenever the clinical decision based on the result implies possible risks for patients (eg, selection of candidates to liver resection for hepatocellular carcinoma; identification of patients nonresponding to medical therapy of portal hypertension after variceal bleeding, potential candidate to transjugular intrahepatic portosystemic shunt).

CLINICS CARE POINTS

- CSPH can be diagnosed noninvasively in patients with cACLD by the following findings: portosystemic collaterals on imaging and a LSM of more than 20 to 25 kPa.
- Splenomegaly, thrombocytopenia, and a SSM of more than 46 kPa further increase the likelihood of CSPH.
- Patients presenting any of the signs discussed in this article while compensated should undergo endoscopy for screening of varices requiring treatment according to the existing guidelines.
- In the future, patients with signs of CSPH on noninvasive tests might be started on carvedilol straight away to decrease the risk of a first clinical decompensation.

DISCLOSURE

The authors have nothing to disclose.

REFERENCES

1. Bosch J, Abraldes JG, Berzigotti A, et al. The clinical use of HVPG measurements in chronic liver disease. Nat Rev Gastroenterol Hepatol 2009;6:573–82.
2. Rosselli M, MacNaughtan J, Jalan R, et al. Beyond scoring: a modern interpretation of disease progression in chronic liver disease. Gut 2013;62:1234–41.

3. de Franchis R, Baveno VIF. Expanding consensus in portal hypertension: report of the Baveno VI Consensus Workshop: stratifying risk and individualizing care for portal hypertension. J Hepatol 2015;63:743–52.
4. Garcia-Tsao G, Abraldes JG, Berzigotti A, et al. Portal hypertensive bleeding in cirrhosis: risk stratification, diagnosis, and management: 2016 practice guidance by the American Association for the study of liver diseases. Hepatology 2017;65:310–35.
5. Bruno S, Zuin M, Crosignani A, et al. Predicting mortality risk in patients with compensated HCV-induced cirrhosis: a long-term prospective study. Am J Gastroenterol 2009;104:1147–58.
6. Zipprich A, Garcia-Tsao G, Rogowski S, et al. Prognostic indicators of survival in patients with compensated and decompensated cirrhosis. Liver Int 2012;32: 1407–14.
7. D'Amico G, Pasta L, Morabito A, et al. Competing risks and prognostic stages of cirrhosis: a 25-year inception cohort study of 494 patients. Aliment Pharmacol Ther 2014;39:1180–93.
8. Colecchia A, Marasco G, Taddia M, et al. Liver and spleen stiffness and other noninvasive methods to assess portal hypertension in cirrhotic patients: a review of the literature. Eur J Gastroenterol Hepatol 2015;27:992–1001.
9. European Association for Study of Liver, Asociacion Latinoamericana para el Estudio del H. EASL-ALEH clinical practice guidelines: non-invasive tests for evaluation of liver disease severity and prognosis. J Hepatol 2015;63:237–64.
10. Qi X, Berzigotti A, Cardenas A, et al. Emerging non-invasive approaches for diagnosis and monitoring of portal hypertension. Lancet Gastroenterol Hepatol 2018;3:708–19.
11. Qamar AA, Grace ND, Groszmann RJ, et al. Incidence, prevalence, and clinical significance of abnormal hematologic indices in compensated cirrhosis. Clin Gastroenterol Hepatol 2009;7:689–95.
12. Berzigotti A, Seijo S, Arena U, et al. Elastography, spleen size, and platelet count identify portal hypertension in patients with compensated cirrhosis. Gastroenterology 2013;144:102–11.e101.
13. Ferlitsch M, Reiberger T, Hoke M, et al. von Willebrand factor as new noninvasive predictor of portal hypertension, decompensation and mortality in patients with liver cirrhosis. Hepatology 2012;56:1439–47.
14. Hametner S, Ferlitsch A, Ferlitsch M, et al. The VITRO Score (Von Willebrand Factor Antigen/Thrombocyte Ratio) as a new marker for clinically significant portal hypertension in comparison to other non-invasive parameters of fibrosis including ELF test. PLoS One 2016;11:e0149230.
15. Schwarzer R, Reiberger T, Mandorfer M, et al. The von Willebrand Factor antigen to platelet ratio (VITRO) score predicts hepatic decompensation and mortality in cirrhosis. J Gastroenterol 2020;55(5):533–42.
16. Wang L, Feng Y, Ma X, et al. Diagnostic efficacy of noninvasive liver fibrosis indexes in predicting portal hypertension in patients with cirrhosis. PLoS One 2017;12:e0182969.
17. Thabut D, Imbert-Bismut F, Cazals-Hatem D, et al. Relationship between the Fibrotest and portal hypertension in patients with liver disease. Aliment Pharmacol Ther 2007;26:359–68.
18. Bureau C, Metivier S, Peron JM, et al. Transient elastography accurately predicts presence of significant portal hypertension in patients with chronic liver disease. Aliment Pharmacol Ther 2008;27:1261–8.

19. Waidmann O, Brunner F, Herrmann E, et al. Macrophage activation is a prognostic parameter for variceal bleeding and overall survival in patients with liver cirrhosis. J Hepatol 2013;58:956–61.
20. Sandahl TD, McGrail R, Moller HJ, et al. The macrophage activation marker sCD163 combined with markers of the Enhanced Liver Fibrosis (ELF) score predicts clinically significant portal hypertension in patients with cirrhosis. Aliment Pharmacol Ther 2016;43:1222–31.
21. Buck M, Garcia-Tsao G, Groszmann RJ, et al. Novel inflammatory biomarkers of portal pressure in compensated cirrhosis patients. Hepatology 2014;59:1052–9.
22. Bruha R, Jachymova M, Petrtyl J, et al. Osteopontin: a non-invasive parameter of portal hypertension and prognostic marker of cirrhosis. World J Gastroenterol 2016;22:3441–50.
23. Horvatits T, Drolz A, Roedl K, et al. Serum bile acids as marker for acute decompensation and acute-on-chronic liver failure in patients with non-cholestatic cirrhosis. Liver Int 2017;37:224–31.
24. Horn P, von Loeffelholz C, Forkert F, et al. Low circulating chemerin levels correlate with hepatic dysfunction and increased mortality in decompensated liver cirrhosis. Sci Rep 2018;8:9242.
25. Lim YL, Choi E, Jang YO, et al. Clinical implications of the serum apelin level on portal hypertension and prognosis of liver cirrhosis. Gut Liver 2016;10:109–16.
26. Kondo M, Miszputen SJ, Leite-mor MM, et al. The predictive value of serum laminin for the risk of variceal bleeding related to portal pressure levels. Hepatogastroenterology 1995;42:542–5.
27. Kropf J, Gressner AM, Tittor W. Logistic-regression model for assessing portal hypertension by measuring hyaluronic acid (hyaluronan) and laminin in serum. Clin Chem 1991;37:30–5.
28. Leeming DJ, Karsdal MA, Byrjalsen I, et al. Novel serological neo-epitope markers of extracellular matrix proteins for the detection of portal hypertension. Aliment Pharmacol Ther 2013;38:1086–96.
29. Moller S, la Cour Sibbesen E, Madsen JL, et al. Indocyanine green retention test in cirrhosis and portal hypertension: accuracy and relation to severity of disease. J Gastroenterol Hepatol 2019;34:1093–9.
30. Qamar AA, Grace ND, Groszmann RJ, et al. Platelet count is not a predictor of the presence or development of gastroesophageal varices in cirrhosis. Hepatology 2008;47:153–9.
31. Sebastiani G, Tempesta D, Fattovich G, et al. Prediction of oesophageal varices in hepatic cirrhosis by simple serum non-invasive markers: results of a multicenter, large-scale study. J Hepatol 2010;53:630–8.
32. Deng H, Qi X, Guo X. Diagnostic accuracy of APRI, AAR, FIB-4, FI, King, Lok, Forns, and FibroIndex scores in predicting the presence of esophageal varices in liver cirrhosis: a systematic review and meta-analysis. Medicine (Baltimore) 2015;94:e1795.
33. Thabut D, Trabut JB, Massard J, et al. Non-invasive diagnosis of large oesophageal varices with FibroTest in patients with cirrhosis: a preliminary retrospective study. Liver Int 2006;26:271–8.
34. Pind ML, Bendtsen F, Kallemose T, et al. Indocyanine green retention test (ICG-r15) as a noninvasive predictor of portal hypertension in patients with different severity of cirrhosis. Eur J Gastroenterol Hepatol 2016;28:948–54.
35. Fouad R, Hamza I, Khairy M, et al. Role of serum soluble CD163 in the diagnosis, risk of bleeding, and prognosis of gastro-esophageal varices in cirrhotic patients. J Interferon Cytokine Res 2017;37:112–8.

36. Qi X, Li H, Chen J, et al. Serum liver fibrosis markers for predicting the presence of gastroesophageal varices in liver cirrhosis: a retrospective cross-sectional study. Gastroenterol Res Pract 2015;2015:274534.
37. Berzigotti A, Abraldes JG, Tandon P, et al. Ultrasonographic evaluation of liver surface and transient elastography in clinically doubtful cirrhosis. J Hepatol 2010;52:846–53.
38. Sartoris R, Rautou PE, Elkrief L, et al. Quantification of liver surface nodularity at CT: utility for detection of portal hypertension. Radiology 2018;289:698–707.
39. Berzigotti A, Rossi V, Tiani C, et al. Prognostic value of a single HVPG measurement and Doppler-ultrasound evaluation in patients with cirrhosis and portal hypertension. J Gastroenterol 2011;46:687–95.
40. Praktiknjo M, Simon-Talero M, Romer J, et al. Total area of spontaneous portosystemic shunts independently predicts hepatic encephalopathy and mortality in liver cirrhosis. J Hepatol 2020;72:1140–50.
41. Simon-Talero M, Roccarina D, Martinez J, et al. Association between portosystemic shunts and increased complications and mortality in patients with cirrhosis. Gastroenterology 2018;154:1694–705.e1694.
42. Deng H, Qi X, Guo X. Computed tomography for the diagnosis of varices in liver cirrhosis: a systematic review and meta-analysis of observational studies. Postgrad Med 2017;129:318–28.
43. Palaniyappan N, Cox E, Bradley C, et al. Non-invasive assessment of portal hypertension using quantitative magnetic resonance imaging. J Hepatol 2016;65:1131–9.
44. Halldorsdottir VG, Dave JK, Leodore LM, et al. Subharmonic contrast microbubble signals for noninvasive pressure estimation under static and dynamic flow conditions. Ultrason Imaging 2011;33:153–64.
45. Eisenbrey JR, Dave JK, Halldorsdottir VG, et al. Chronic liver disease: noninvasive subharmonic aided pressure estimation of hepatic venous pressure gradient. Radiology 2013;268:581–8.
46. Berzigotti A, Zappoli P, Magalotti D, et al. Spleen enlargement on follow-up evaluation: a noninvasive predictor of complications of portal hypertension in cirrhosis. Clin Gastroenterol Hepatol 2008;6:1129–34.
47. Berzigotti A, Merkel C, Magalotti D, et al. New abdominal collaterals at ultrasound: a clue of progression of portal hypertension. Dig Liver Dis 2008;40:62–7.
48. You MW, Kim KW, Pyo J, et al. A meta-analysis for the diagnostic performance of transient elastography for clinically significant portal hypertension. Ultrasound Med Biol 2017;43:59–68.
49. Vizzutti F, Arena U, Romanelli RG, et al. Liver stiffness measurement predicts severe portal hypertension in patients with HCV-related cirrhosis. Hepatology 2007;45:1290–7.
50. Ferraioli G, Wong VW, Castera L, et al. Liver ultrasound elastography: an update to the world federation for ultrasound in medicine and biology guidelines and recommendations. Ultrasound Med Biol 2018;44:2419–40.
51. Berzigotti A. Non-invasive evaluation of portal hypertension using ultrasound elastography. J Hepatol 2017;67:399–411.
52. Llop E, Berzigotti A, Reig M, et al. Assessment of portal hypertension by transient elastography in patients with compensated cirrhosis and potentially resectable liver tumors. J Hepatol 2012;56:103–8.
53. Song J, Ma Z, Huang J, et al. Comparison of three cut-offs to diagnose clinically significant portal hypertension by liver stiffness in chronic viral liver diseases: a meta-analysis. Eur Radiol 2018;28:5221–30.

54. Pons M, Santos B, Simon-Talero M, et al. Rapid liver and spleen stiffness improvement in compensated advanced chronic liver disease patients treated with oral antivirals. Therap Adv Gastroenterol 2017;10:619–29.

55. Mandorfer M, Kozbial K, Schwabl P, et al. Sustained virologic response to interferon-free therapies ameliorates HCV-induced portal hypertension. J Hepatol 2016;65:692–9.

56. Rincon D, Ripoll C, Lo Iacono O, et al. Antiviral therapy decreases hepatic venous pressure gradient in patients with chronic hepatitis C and advanced fibrosis. Am J Gastroenterol 2006;101:2269–74.

57. Lens S, Alvarado-Tapias E, Marino Z, et al. Effects of all-oral anti-viral therapy on HVPG and systemic hemodynamics in patients with hepatitis C virus-associated cirrhosis. Gastroenterology 2017;153:1273–83.e1.

58. Radu C, Stancu O, Sav R, et al. Liver stiffness better predicts portal hypertension after HCV eradication. J Gastrointestin Liver Dis 2018;27:204.

59. Dietrich CF, Bamber J, Berzigotti A, et al. EFSUMB guidelines and recommendations on the clinical use of liver ultrasound elastography, update 2017 (long version). Ultraschall Med 2017;38:e48.

60. Salavrakos M, Piessevaux H, Komuta M, et al. Fibroscan reliably rules out advanced liver fibrosis and significant portal hypertension in alcoholic patients. J Clin Gastroenterol 2019;53(10):772–8.

61. Song J, Ma Z, Huang J, et al. Reliability of transient elastography-based liver stiffness for diagnosing portal hypertension in patients with alcoholic liver disease: a diagnostic meta-analysis with specific cut-off values. Ultraschall Med 2020;41(1):60–8.

62. Pons M, Augustin S, Scheiner B, et al. Validation of the Baveno VI criteria for noninvasive diagnosis of cACld and clinically significant portal hypertension by transient elastography. Hepatology 2018;68:610–611A.

63. Salzl P, Reiberger T, Ferlitsch M, et al. Evaluation of portal hypertension and varices by acoustic radiation force impulse imaging of the liver compared to transient elastography and AST to platelet ratio index. Ultraschall Med 2014;35:528–33.

64. Attia D, Schoenemeier B, Rodt T, et al. Evaluation of liver and spleen stiffness with acoustic radiation force impulse quantification elastography for diagnosing clinically significant portal hypertension. Ultraschall Med 2015;36:603–10.

65. Takuma Y, Nouso K, Morimoto Y, et al. Portal hypertension in patients with liver cirrhosis: diagnostic accuracy of spleen stiffness. Radiology 2016;279:609–19.

66. Suh CH, Kim KW, Park SH, et al. Shear wave elastography as a quantitative biomarker of clinically significant portal hypertension: a systematic review and meta-analysis. AJR Am J Roentgenol 2018;210:W185–95.

67. Stefanescu H, Marasco G, Cales P, et al. A novel spleen-dedicated stiffness measurement by FibroScan(R) improves the screening of high-risk oesophageal varices. Liver Int 2020;40:175–85.

68. Thiele M, Hugger MB, Kim Y, et al. 2D shear wave liver elastography by Aixplorer to detect portal hypertension in cirrhosis: an individual patient data meta-analysis. Liver Int 2020;40:1435–46.

69. Zhu YL, Ding H, Fu TT, et al. Portal hypertension in hepatitis B-related cirrhosis: diagnostic accuracy of liver and spleen stiffness by 2-D shear-wave elastography. Hepatol Res 2019;49(5):540–9.

70. Jansen C, Bogs C, Verlinden W, et al. Algorithm to rule out clinically significant portal hypertension combining Shear-wave elastography of liver and spleen: a prospective multicentre study. Gut 2016;65:1057–8.

71. Jansen C, Bogs C, Verlinden W, et al. Shear-wave elastography of the liver and spleen identifies clinically significant portal hypertension: a prospective multi-centre study. Liver Int 2017;37:396–405.

72. Elkrief L, Ronot M, Andrade F, et al. Non-invasive evaluation of portal hypertension using shear-wave elastography: analysis of two algorithms combining liver and spleen stiffness in 191 patients with cirrhosis. Aliment Pharmacol Ther 2018; 47:621–30.

73. European Association for the Study of the Liver, Electronic address eee, European Association for the Study of the L. EASL Clinical practice guidelines for the management of patients with decompensated cirrhosis. J Hepatol 2018; 69:406–60.

74. Shi KQ, Fan YC, Pan ZZ, et al. Transient elastography: a meta-analysis of diagnostic accuracy in evaluation of portal hypertension in chronic liver disease. Liver Int 2013;33:62–71.

75. Cassinotto C, Charrie A, Mouries A, et al. Liver and spleen elastography using supersonic shear imaging for the non-invasive diagnosis of cirrhosis severity and oesophageal varices. Dig Liver Dis 2015;47:695–701.

76. Grgurevic I, Bokun T, Mustapic S, et al. Real-time two-dimensional shear wave ultrasound elastography of the liver is a reliable predictor of clinical outcomes and the presence of esophageal varices in patients with compensated liver cirrhosis. Croat Med J 2015;56:470–81.

77. Kasai Y, Moriyasu F, Saito K, et al. Value of shear wave elastography for predicting hepatocellular carcinoma and esophagogastric varices in patients with chronic liver disease. J Med Ultrason (2001) 2015;42:349–55.

78. Kim TY, Kim TY, Kim Y, et al. Diagnostic performance of shear wave elastography for predicting esophageal varices in patients with compensated liver cirrhosis. J Ultrasound Med 2016;35:1373–81.

79. Elkrief L, Rautou PE, Ronot M, et al. Prospective comparison of spleen and liver stiffness by using shear-wave and transient elastography for detection of portal hypertension in cirrhosis. Radiology 2015;275:589–98.

80. Stefanescu H, Allegretti G, Salvatore V, et al. Bidimensional shear wave ultrasound elastography with supersonic imaging to predict presence of oesophageal varices in cirrhosis. Liver Int 2017;37:1405.

81. Yoo HW, Kim YS, Kim SG, et al. Usefulness of noninvasive methods including assessment of liver stiffness by 2-dimensional shear wave elastography for predicting esophageal varices. Dig Liver Dis 2019;51:1706–12.

82. Ripoll C, Groszmann R, Garcia-Tsao G, et al. Hepatic venous pressure gradient predicts clinical decompensation in patients with compensated cirrhosis. Gastroenterology 2007;133:481–8.

83. Robic MA, Procopet B, Metivier S, et al. Liver stiffness accurately predicts portal hypertension related complications in patients with chronic liver disease: a prospective study. J Hepatol 2011;55:1017–24.

84. Merchante N, Rivero-Juárez A, Téllez F, et al. Liver stiffness predicts clinical outcome in human immunodeficiency virus/hepatitis C virus-coinfected patients with compensated liver cirrhosis. Hepatology 2012;56:228–38.

85. Macías J, Camacho A, Von Wichmann MA, et al. Liver stiffness measurement versus liver biopsy to predict survival and decompensations of cirrhosis among HIV/hepatitis C virus-coinfected patients. AIDS 2013;27:2541–9.

86. Wang JH, Chuah SK, Lu SN, et al. Baseline and serial liver stiffness measurement in prediction of portal hypertension progression for patients with compensated cirrhosis. Liver Int 2014;34:1340–8.

87. Kitson MT, Roberts SK, Colman JC, et al. Liver stiffness and the prediction of clinically significant portal hypertension and portal hypertensive complications. Scand J Gastroenterol 2015;50:462–9.

88. Merchante N, Rivero-Juárez A, Téllez F, et al. Liver stiffness predicts variceal bleeding in HIV/HCV-coinfected patients with compensated cirrhosis. AIDS 2017;31:493–500.

89. Singh S, Fujii LL, Murad MH, et al. Liver stiffness is associated with risk of decompensation, liver cancer, and death in patients with chronic liver diseases: a systematic review and meta-analysis. Clin Gastroenterol Hepatol 2013;11: 1573–84.e1571-2 [quiz: e1588–9].

90. Corpechot C, Gaouar F, El Naggar A, et al. Baseline values and changes in liver stiffness measured by transient elastography are associated with severity of fibrosis and outcomes of patients with primary sclerosing cholangitis. Gastroenterology 2014;146:970–9 [quiz: e915–76].

91. Vergniol J, Boursier J, Coutzac C, et al. Evolution of noninvasive tests of liver fibrosis is associated with prognosis in patients with chronic hepatitis C. Hepatology 2014;60:65–76.

92. Kim BK, Park YN, Kim DY, et al. Risk assessment of development of hepatic decompensation in histologically proven hepatitis B viral cirrhosis using liver stiffness measurement. Digestion 2012;85:219–27.

93. Mendoza Y, CS, Murgia G, et al. Simple non-invasive surrogates of portal hypertension predict clinical decompensation in overweight/obese patients with cACLD. 2019;70:e664.

94. Wong GL, Liang LY, Kwok R, et al. Low risk of variceal bleeding in patients with cirrhosis after variceal screening stratified by liver/spleen stiffness. Hepatology 2019;70(3):971–81.

95. Masuzaki R, Tateishi R, Yoshida H, et al. Prospective risk assessment for hepatocellular carcinoma development in patients with chronic hepatitis C by transient elastography. Hepatology 2009;49:1954–61.

96. Narita Y, Genda T, Tsuzura H, et al. Prediction of liver stiffness hepatocellular carcinoma in chronic hepatitis C patients on interferon-based anti-viral therapy. J Gastroenterol Hepatol 2014;29:137–43.

97. Wang HM, Hung CH, Lu SN, et al. Liver stiffness measurement as an alternative to fibrotic stage in risk assessment of hepatocellular carcinoma incidence for chronic hepatitis C patients. Liver Int 2013;33:756–61.

98. Kim DY, Song KJ, Kim SU, et al. Transient elastography-based risk estimation of hepatitis B virus-related occurrence of hepatocellular carcinoma: development and validation of a predictive model. Onco Targets Ther 2013;6:1463–9.

99. Jung KS, Kim SU, Ahn SH, et al. Risk assessment of hepatitis B virus-related hepatocellular carcinoma development using liver stiffness measurement (FibroScan). Hepatology 2011;53:885–94.

100. Reiberger T, Ferlitsch A, Payer BA, et al, Vienna Hepatic Hemodynamic L. Nonselective beta-blockers improve the correlation of liver stiffness and portal pressure in advanced cirrhosis. J Gastroenterol 2012;47:561–8.

101. Thabut D, Bureau C, Layese R, et al. Validation of Baveno VI criteria for screening and surveillance of esophageal varices in patients with compensated cirrhosis and a sustained response to antiviral therapy. Gastroenterology 2019; 156:997–1009.e1005.

102. Mejias M, Garcia-Pras E, Gallego J, et al. Relevance of the mTOR signaling pathway in the pathophysiology of splenomegaly in rats with chronic portal hypertension. J Hepatol 2010;52:529–39.

103. Giuffre M, Macor D, Masutti F, et al. Spleen Stiffness Probability Index (SSPI): a simple and accurate method to detect esophageal varices in patients with compensated liver cirrhosis. Ann Hepatol 2020;19:53–61.
104. Tseng Y, Li F, Wang J, et al. Spleen and liver stiffness for noninvasive assessment of portal hypertension in cirrhotic patients with large esophageal varices. J Clin Ultrasound 2018;46:442–9.
105. Seijo S, Reverter E, Miquel R, et al. Role of hepatic vein catheterisation and transient elastography in the diagnosis of idiopathic portal hypertension. Dig Liver Dis 2012;44:855–60.
106. Colecchia A, Montrone L, Scaioli E, et al. Measurement of spleen stiffness to evaluate portal hypertension and the presence of esophageal varices in patients with HCV-related cirrhosis. Gastroenterology 2012;143:646–54.
107. Colecchia A, Ravaioli F, Marasco G, et al. A combined model based on spleen stiffness measurement and Baveno VI criteria to rule out high-risk varices in advanced chronic liver disease. J Hepatol 2018;69:308–17.
108. Balakrishnan M, Souza F, Munoz C, et al. Liver and spleen stiffness measurements by point shear wave elastography via acoustic radiation force impulse: intraobserver and interobserver variability and predictors of variability in a US population. J Ultrasound Med 2016;35:2373–80.
109. Procopet B, Berzigotti A, Abraldes JG, et al. Real-time shear-wave elastography: applicability, reliability and accuracy for clinically significant portal hypertension. J Hepatol 2015;62:1068–75.
110. Calvaruso V, Bronte F, Conte E, et al. Modified spleen stiffness measurement by transient elastography is associated with presence of large oesophageal varices in patients with compensated hepatitis C virus cirrhosis. J Viral Hepat 2013;20:867–74.
111. Song J, Huang J, Huang H, et al. Performance of spleen stiffness measurement in prediction of clinical significant portal hypertension: a meta-analysis. Clin Res Hepatol Gastroenterol 2018;42:216–26.
112. Deng H, Qi X, Zhang T, et al. Supersonic shear imaging for the diagnosis of liver fibrosis and portal hypertension in liver diseases: a meta-analysis. Expert Rev Gastroenterol Hepatol 2018;12:91–8.
113. Sharma P, Kirnake V, Tyagi P, et al. Spleen stiffness in patients with cirrhosis in predicting esophageal varices. Am J Gastroenterol 2013;108:1101–7.
114. Meister P, Dechêne A, Büchter M, et al. Spleen stiffness differentiates between acute and chronic liver damage and predicts hepatic decompensation. J Clin Gastroenterol 2019;53(6):457–63.
115. Takuma Y, Morimoto Y, Takabatake H, et al. Measurement of spleen stiffness with acoustic radiation force impulse imaging predicts mortality and hepatic decompensation in patients with liver cirrhosis. Clin Gastroenterol Hepatol 2017;15:1782–90.e1784.
116. Zhang Y, Mao DF, Zhang MW, et al. Clinical value of liver and spleen shear wave velocity in predicting the prognosis of patients with portal hypertension. World J Gastroenterol 2017;23:8044–52.
117. Colecchia A, Colli A, Casazza G, et al. Spleen stiffness measurement can predict clinical complications in compensated HCV-related cirrhosis: a prospective study. J Hepatol 2014;60:1158–64.
118. Grgurević I, Bokun T, Mustapić S, et al. Real-time two-dimensional shear wave ultrasound elastography of the liver is a reliable predictor of clinical outcomes and the presence of esophageal varices in patients with compensated liver cirrhosis. Croat Med J 2015;56:470–81.

119. Marasco G, Colecchia A, Colli A, et al. Role of liver and spleen stiffness in predicting the recurrence of hepatocellular carcinoma after resection. J Hepatol 2019;70:440–8.

120. Wu D, Chen E, Liang T, et al. Predicting the risk of postoperative liver failure and overall survival using liver and spleen stiffness measurements in patients with hepatocellular carcinoma. Medicine (Baltimore) 2017;96:e7864.

121. Peng W, Li JW, Zhang XY, et al. A novel model for predicting posthepatectomy liver failure in patients with hepatocellular carcinoma. PLoS One 2019;14: e0219219.

122. Singh R, Wilson MP, Katlariwala P, et al. Accuracy of liver and spleen stiffness on magnetic resonance elastography for detecting portal hypertension: a systematic review and meta-analysis. Eur J Gastroenterol Hepatol 2021;32(2):237–45.

123. Manatsathit W, Samant H, Kapur S, et al. Accuracy of liver stiffness, spleen stiffness, and LS-spleen diameter to platelet ratio score in detection of esophageal varices: systemic review and meta-analysis. J Gastroenterol Hepatol 2018;33: 1696–706.

124. Karagiannakis DS, Voulgaris T, Koureta E, et al. Role of spleen stiffness measurement by 2D-shear wave elastography in ruling out the presence of high-risk varices in cirrhotic patients. Dig Dis Sci 2019;64:2653–60.

125. Augustin S, Pons M, Maurice JB, et al. Expanding the Baveno VI criteria for the screening of varices in patients with compensated advanced chronic liver disease. Hepatology 2017;66:1980–8.

126. Takuma Y, Nouso K, Morimoto Y, et al. Prediction of oesophageal variceal bleeding by measuring spleen stiffness in patients with liver cirrhosis. Gut 2016;65:354–5.

127. Buechter M, Kahraman A, Manka P, et al. Spleen and liver stiffness is positively correlated with the risk of esophageal variceal bleeding. Digestion 2016;94: 138–44.

128. Chin JL, Chan G, Ryan JD, et al. Spleen stiffness can non-invasively assess resolution of portal hypertension after liver transplantation. Liver Int 2015;35: 518–23.

129. Kim HY, So YH, Kim W, et al. Non-invasive response prediction in prophylactic carvedilol therapy for cirrhotic patients with esophageal varices. J Hepatol 2019; 70:412–22.

130. Wong GL, Kwok R, Chan HL, et al. Measuring spleen stiffness to predict varices in chronic hepatitis B cirrhotic patients with or without receiving non-selective beta-blockers. J Dig Dis 2016;17:538–46.

131. Ran HT, Ye XP, Zheng YY, et al. Spleen stiffness and splenoportal venous flow: assessment before and after transjugular intrahepatic portosystemic shunt placement. J Ultrasound Med 2013;32:221–8.

132. Gao J, Zheng X, Zheng YY, et al. Shear wave elastography of the spleen for monitoring transjugular intrahepatic portosystemic shunt function: a pilot study. J Ultrasound Med 2016;35:951–8.

133. De Santis A, Nardelli S, Bassanelli C, et al. Modification of splenic stiffness on acoustic radiation force impulse parallels the variation of portal pressure induced by transjugular intrahepatic portosystemic shunt. J Gastroenterol Hepatol 2018;33:704–9.

134. Buechter M, Manka P, Theysohn JM, et al. Spleen stiffness is positively correlated with HVPG and decreases significantly after TIPS implantation. Dig Liver Dis 2018;50:54–60.

135. Attia D, Rodt T, Marquardt S, et al. Shear wave elastography prior to transjugular intrahepatic portosystemic shunt may predict the decrease in hepatic vein pressure gradient. Abdom Radiol (NY) 2019;44:1127–34.

136. Novelli PM, Cho K, Rubin JM. Sonographic assessment of spleen stiffness before and after transjugular intrahepatic portosystemic shunt placement with or without concurrent embolization of portal systemic collateral veins in patients with cirrhosis and portal hypertension: a feasibility study. J Ultrasound Med 2015;34:443–9.

137. Takuma Y, Morimoto Y, Takabatake H, et al. Changes in liver and spleen stiffness by virtual touch quantification technique after balloon-occluded retrograde transvenous obliteration of gastric varices and exacerbation of esophageal varices: a preliminary study. Ultraschall Med 2020;41:157–66.

138. Ravaioli F, Colecchia A, Dajti E, et al. Spleen stiffness mirrors changes in portal hypertension after successful interferon-free therapy in chronic-hepatitis C virus patients. World J Hepatol 2018;10:731–42.

139. Berzigotti A, Seijo S, Arena U, et al. Elastography, spleen size, and platelet count identify portal hypertension in patients with compensated cirrhosis. Gastroenterology 2013;144:102–11.e1.

140. Marot A, Trepo E, Doerig C, et al. Liver stiffness and platelet count for identifying patients with compensated liver disease at low risk of variceal bleeding. Liver Int 2017;37:707–16.

141. Llop E, Lopez M, de la Revilla J, et al. Validation of noninvasive methods to predict the presence of gastroesophageal varices in a cohort of patients with compensated advanced chronic liver disease. J Gastroenterol Hepatol 2017;32:1867–72.

142. Jangouk P, Turco L, De Oliveira A, et al. Validating, deconstructing and refining Baveno criteria for ruling out high-risk varices in patients with compensated cirrhosis. Liver Int 2017;37:1177–83.

143. Reiberger T, Ferlitsch A, Payer BA, et al. Noninvasive screening for liver fibrosis and portal hypertension by transient elastography–a large single center experience. Wien Klin Wochenschr 2012;124:395–402.

144. Schwabl P, Bota S, Salzl P, et al. New reliability criteria for transient elastography increase the number of accurate measurements for screening of cirrhosis and portal hypertension. Liver Int 2015;35:381–90.

145. Cho EJ, Kim MY, Lee JH, et al. Diagnostic and prognostic values of noninvasive predictors of portal hypertension in patients with alcoholic cirrhosis. PLoS One 2015;10:e0133935.

146. Zykus R, Jonaitis L, Petrenkiene V, et al. Liver and spleen transient elastography predicts portal hypertension in patients with chronic liver disease: a prospective cohort study. BMC Gastroenterol 2015;15:183.

147. Hametner S, Ferlitsch A, Ferlitsch M, et al. The VITRO Score (Von Willebrand Factor Antigen/Thrombocyte Ratio) as a new marker for clinically significant portal hypertension in comparison to other non-invasive parameters of fibrosis including ELF test. PLoS One 2016;11:e0149230.

148. Kumar A, Khan NM, Anikhindi SA, et al. Correlation of transient elastography with hepatic venous pressure gradient in patients with cirrhotic portal hypertension: a study of 326 patients from India. World J Gastroenterol 2017;23:687–96.

149. Maurice JB, Brodkin E, Arnold F, et al. Validation of the Baveno VI criteria to identify low risk cirrhotic patients not requiring endoscopic surveillance for varices. J Hepatol 2016;65:899–905.

150. Abraldes JG, Bureau C, Stefanescu H, et al. Noninvasive tools and risk of clinically significant portal hypertension and varices in compensated cirrhosis: the "Anticipate" study. Hepatology 2016;64:2173–84.
151. Pu K, Shi JH, Wang X, et al. Diagnostic accuracy of transient elastography (FibroScan) in detection of esophageal varices in patients with cirrhosis: a meta-analysis. World J Gastroenterol 2017;23:345–56.
152. Petta S, Sebastiani G, Bugianesi E, et al. Non-invasive prediction of esophageal varices by stiffness and platelet in non-alcoholic fatty liver disease cirrhosis. J Hepatol 2018;69:878–85.
153. Bae J, Sinn DH, Kang W, et al. Validation of the Baveno VI and the expanded Baveno VI criteria to identify patients who could avoid screening endoscopy. Liver Int 2018;38:1442–8.
154. Lee HA, Kim SU, Seo YS, et al. Prediction of the varices needing treatment with non-invasive tests in patients with compensated advanced chronic liver disease. Liver Int 2019;39(6):1071–9.
155. Moctezuma-Velazquez C, Saffioti F, Tasayco-Huaman S, et al. Non-invasive prediction of high-risk varices in patients with primary biliary cholangitis and primary sclerosing cholangitis. Am J Gastroenterol 2019;114:446–52.
156. Lucchina N, Recaldini C, Macchi M, et al. Point shear wave elastography of the spleen: its role in patients with portal hypertension. Ultrasound Med Biol 2018;44:771–8.
157. Petzold G, Tsaknakis B, Bremer SCB, et al. Evaluation of liver stiffness by 2D-SWE in combination with non-invasive parameters as predictors for esophageal varices in patients with advanced chronic liver disease. Scand J Gastroenterol 2019;1–8.
158. Stefanescu H, Grigorescu M, Lupsor M, et al. Spleen stiffness measurement using Fibroscan for the noninvasive assessment of esophageal varices in liver cirrhosis patients. J Gastroenterol Hepatol 2011;26:164–70.
159. Stefanescu H, Radu C, Procopet B, et al. Non-invasive ménage à trois for the prediction of high-risk varices: stepwise algorithm using lok score, liver and spleen stiffness. Liver Int 2015;35:317–25.
160. Arribas Anta J, Garcia Gonzalez M, Torres Guerrero ME, et al. Prediction of the presence of esophageal varices using spleen stiffness measurement by transient elastography in cirrhotic patients. Acta Gastroenterol Belg 2018;81:496–501.
161. Rifai K, Cornberg J, Bahr M, et al. ARFI elastography of the spleen is inferior to liver elastography for the detection of portal hypertension. Ultraschall Med 2011;32(Suppl 2):E24–30.
162. Bota S, Sporea I, Sirli R, et al. Can ARFI elastography predict the presence of significant esophageal varices in newly diagnosed cirrhotic patients? Ann Hepatol 2012;11:519–25.
163. Ye XP, Ran HT, Cheng J, et al. Liver and spleen stiffness measured by acoustic radiation force impulse elastography for noninvasive assessment of liver fibrosis and esophageal varices in patients with chronic hepatitis B. J Ultrasound Med 2012;31:1245–53.
164. Vermehren J, Polta A, Zimmermann O, et al. Comparison of acoustic radiation force impulse imaging with transient elastography for the detection of complications in patients with cirrhosis. Liver Int 2012;32:852–8.
165. Takuma Y, Nouso K, Morimoto Y, et al. Measurement of spleen stiffness by acoustic radiation force impulse imaging identifies cirrhotic patients with esophageal varices. Gastroenterology 2013;144:92–101.e102.

166. Rizzo L, Attanasio M, Pinzone MR, et al. A new sampling method for spleen stiffness measurement based on quantitative acoustic radiation force impulse elastography for noninvasive assessment of esophageal varices in newly diagnosed HCV-related cirrhosis. Biomed Res Int 2014;2014:365982.
167. Kim HY, Jin EH, Kim W, et al. The role of spleen stiffness in determining the severity and bleeding risk of esophageal varices in cirrhotic patients. Medicine (Baltimore) 2015;94:e1031.
168. Park J, Kwon H, Cho J, et al. Is the spleen stiffness value acquired using acoustic radiation force impulse (ARFI) technology predictive of the presence of esophageal varices in patients with cirrhosis of various etiologies? Med Ultrason 2016;18:11–7.
169. Fierbinteanu-Braticevici C, Tribus L, Peagu R, et al. Spleen stiffness as predictor of esophageal varices in cirrhosis of different etiologies. Sci Rep 2019;9:16190.
170. Peagu R, Sararu R, Necula A, et al. The role of spleen stiffness using ARFI in predicting esophageal varices in patients with Hepatitis B and C virus-related cirrhosis. Rom J Intern Med 2019;57:334–40.
171. Darweesh SK, Yosry A, Salah M, et al. Acoustic radiation forced impulse-based splenic prediction model using data mining for the noninvasive prediction of esophageal varices in hepatitis C virus advanced fibrosis. Eur J Gastroenterol Hepatol 2019;31:1533–9.

Prevention of First Decompensation in Advanced Chronic Liver Disease

Mattias Mandorfer, MD, PhD[a,b,*], Benedikt Simbrunner, MD[a,b]

KEYWORDS

- ACLD • Cirrhosis • Ascites • Variceal bleeding • Hepatic encephalopathy • Fibrosis
- Portal hypertension • Inflammation

KEY POINTS

- The first occurrence of decompensation constitutes a watershed moment in the natural history of advanced chronic liver disease; it denotes a point of no return in a relevant proportion of patients.
- Cirrhosis-related morbidity and mortality are profoundly decreased by delaying or even preventing first decompensation.
- The magnitude of the effect of etiologic therapies is particularly high if a single causative factor is entirely removed.
- In patients who have progressed to clinically significant portal hypertension, etiologic therapies are far from being universally effective in inducing regression and preventing decompensation.
- Besides the removal of cofactors, etiology-unspecific treatments that target decisive pathomechanisms driving decompensation are already applied in clinical practice or being evaluated in randomized clinical trials.

IMPORTANCE OF PREVENTING FIRST DECOMPENSATION

The progression of chronic liver disease (CLD) to compensated advanced CLD (cACLD; a term that subsumes bridging fibrosis and cirrhosis, which can also be diagnosed noninvasively) is paralleled by an increase in the hepatic venous pressure gradient (HVPG). At values of 10 mmHg or more, which define clinically significant portal hypertension (CSPH),[1] patients may develop gastroesophageal varices or/and other portosystemic collaterals, but even more important, decompensation.[2] First decompensation (see **Fig. 1**; most commonly, the development of ascites, and less

[a] Division of Gastroenterology and Hepatology, Department of Internal Medicine III, Medical University of Vienna, Waehringer Guertel 18-20, Vienna 1090, Austria; [b] Vienna Hepatic Hemodynamic Lab, Medical University of Vienna, Vienna, Austria
* Corresponding author. Division of Gastroenterology and Hepatology, Department of Internal Medicine III, Medical University of Vienna, Waehringer Guertel 18-20, Vienna 1090, Austria.
E-mail address: mattias.mandorfer@meduniwien.ac.at

Clin Liver Dis 25 (2021) 291–310
https://doi.org/10.1016/j.cld.2021.01.003
1089-3261/21/© 2021 The Authors. Published by Elsevier Inc. This is an open access article under the CC BY license (http://creativecommons.org/licenses/by/4.0/).

liver.theclinics.com

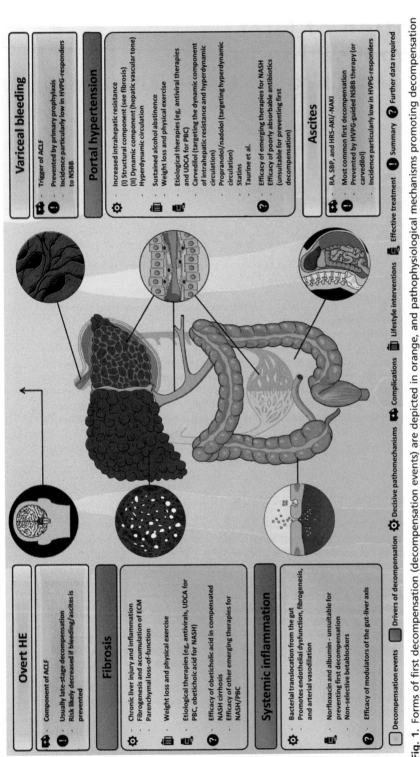

Fig. 1. Forms of first decompensation (decompensation events) are depicted in orange, and pathophysiological mechanisms promoting decompensation (drivers of decompensation) are depicted in gray. For each form of first decompensation, complications (ie, forms of further decompensation that may be direct sequelae of the initial decompensation event) and a summary of the clinical context are provided. Important drivers of decompensation are reported together with their decisive pathomechanisms, lifestyle interventions, as well as medical treatments that effectively target this pathomechanism. Finally, in relationship to all pathomechanisms, important areas of uncertainty (further data required are highlighted). ACLF, acute-on-chronic liver failure; ECM, extracellular matrix; HE, hepatic encephalopathy; HRS-AKI, hepatorenal syndrome type of acute kidney injury (formerly HRS type 1); HRS-NAKI, hepatorenal syndrome type of non-acute kidney injury (formerly HRS type 2); HVPG, hepatic venous pressure gradient; NASH, nonalcoholic steatohepatitis; NSBB, nonselective beta-blockers; PBC, primary biliary cholangitis; RA, refractory ascites; SBP, spontaneous bacterial peritonitis; UDCA, ursodeoxycholic acid.

commonly acute variceal bleeding [AVB] and overt hepatic encephalopathy [HE][3]) de-notes the transition from the compensated ACLD to decompensated cirrhosis, which confers a dramatic increase in mortality risk, in particular when the concept of competing risks is considered (incidence increasing from 14% to 93% at 20 years[4]). The latter concept is particularly important in this context, because it acknowledges that decompensation usually precedes death in a patient with compensated ACLD, a fact that has largely been neglected by previous studies. Thus, although the risk of death at 20 years of follow-up was 63% in a cohort of patients with compensated cirrhosis at baseline,[4] the mortality risk of a patients who remain compensated is dramatically lower.

Once decompensation has occurred, treatments aim at decreasing the risk of mortal-ity by preventing further decompensation and acute-on-chronic liver failure,[5] however, all currently investigated disease-modifying treatments (eg, nonselective beta-blockers [NSBB],[6,7] statins,[8] anticoagulation,[9] interventions targeting the gut–liver axis,[10,11] including poorly absorbable antibiotics[12] and microbiota transplantation,[13] long-term al-bumin administration,[14] and transjugular intrahepatic portosystemic shunt[15]) were—if at all—of limited effectiveness. Thus, despite the important advances regarding disease-modifying treatments for decompensated cirrhosis in recent years, which are summa-rized and discussed in a dedicated article of this issue, no one-size-fits-all treatment that prevents further decompensation is on the horizon, likely owing to the even higher complexity of decompensated (as compared with compensated) disease. Finally, although etiologic cure (ie, removal of the primary etiologic factor) may lead to hepatic recompensation in previously decompensated patients, a considerable proportion re-mains decompensated despite effective intervention (eg, cure of hepatitis C [HCV] infec-tion), because the mechanisms that initially triggered decompensation commonly perpetuate liver injury, thereby hindering liver disease regression. Accordingly, the first occurrence of decompensation constitutes a watershed moment in the natural history of ACLD as it denotes a point of no return in the natural history of CLD in a relevant pro-portion of patients.

Conclusively, cirrhosis-related morbidity and mortality can be profoundly decreased by delaying or even preventing a first decompensation.

ETIOLOGIC THERAPIES
Hepatitis B

In the seminal randomized controlled trial (RCT) by Liaw and colleagues,[16] viral sup-pression with lamivudine decreased the incidence of a composite end point of an $\geq$ 2-point increase in the Child–Turcotte–Pugh (CTP) score, spontaneous bacterial peri-tonitis with proven sepsis, renal insufficiency, AVB, the development of hepatocellular carcinoma, or liver-related death in cACLD patients with chronic hepatitis B with a hazard ratio of 0.45. Increases in the CTP score and the development of hepatocellular carcinoma were the most common events. The use of current antiviral therapies with a high barrier to resistance may even lead to a more profound effect, because the emer-gence of the YMDD-motif variants was linked to worse outcomes. Since the RCT by Liaw and coworkers,[16] several studies of varying quality have reported similar results; these and other studies are summarized in a systematic review with meta-analysis by the Baveno VII faculty.

The findings of studies on direct clinical outcomes are complemented by short-term hemodynamic data[17] and studies with protocol biopsies after long-term treatment.[18] After 12 months of lamivudine treatment, the HVPG decreased from 14.4 to 12.4 mmHg in 19 patients with chronic hepatitis B who underwent paired HVPG measurements; of note, an increase in the HVPG was observed only in a single patient.[17] Moreover, 74% of patients with chronic hepatitis B with pretreatment compensated cirrhosis showed a regression to noncirrhotic stages after a treatment duration of more than 5 years, whereas only 1% of patients without cirrhosis at treatment initiation progressed to cirrhosis. Importantly, the patients with cirrhosis at the end of long-term treatment had a considerably higher body mass index and a 4-fold increased prevalence of obesity, highlighting the importance of cofactors in this context.

Hepatitis C

Since highly effective interferon (IFN)-free direct-acting antiviral–based combination therapies for chronic HCV became available in 2014 (ie, approval of simeprevir and daclatasvir as combination partner for sofosbuvir), most long-term follow-up studies in patients with cACLD still used IFN-based regimens. Prominent examples include an Italian multicenter retrospective analysis by Bruno and colleagues,[19] which included 920 patients with biopsy-proven cirrhosis of whom—owing to the poor efficacy of IFN monotherapy—only 124 (13.5%) achieved a sustained virologic response (SVR). In this highly selected subgroup of patients, no patient developed decompensation (of note, patients were censored at the time of the development of hepatocellular carcinoma) during a mean follow-up of 8.6 years. In contrast, in the non-SVR group, 107 patients had a decompensation event, which resulted in 1.88 events per 100 person-years. Other retrospective cohort studies with a shorter duration of follow-up confirmed the beneficial effects of SVR on decompensation in patients with bridging fibrosis or cirrhosis; however, they also observed decompensation events despite achieving SVR.[20,21] In addition, the prospective HALT-C trial,[22] which included patients with cACLD found a decreased risk of decompensation at year 7.5 after enrollment in patients who achieved a SVR (0.9% vs breakthrough/relapse, 4.7% vs nonresponse, 11.7%; adjusted hazard ratio for SVR vs nonresponse, 0.13), even after adjusting for differences in baseline characteristics (platelet count and serum albumin). However, IFN-based regimens displayed limited virologic efficacy in patients with cACLD, in particular in patients with CSPH, who were found to be at the highest risk for treatment failure.[23] Accordingly, the probability of achieving SVR was directly dependent on the severity of underlying (baseline) liver disease and portal hypertension, which is also a central determinant of post-treatment decompensation.[24] Thus, these studies were at substantial risk of bias, because patients were usually poorly characterized in regard to the severity of their underlying portal hypertension. More recently, Di Marco and colleagues[25] prospectively investigated long-term outcomes in a cohort of patients with biopsy-proven compensated cirrhosis or small varices treated with pegylated IFN and ribavirin, who were further stratified by the presence (ruling-in CSPH) or absence (ie, patients with CSPH, or without) of small varices. SVR was protective of developing decompensation in both strata; however, although patients without varices seemed to be at negligible risk (0/67 patients), decompensation events occurred at a rate of 1.7 per 100 person-years in patients with small varices (ie, patients with CSPH) who achieved a SVR. In conclusion, findings of studies using IFN-based regimens suggested that achieving SVR decrease the risk of decompensation in patients with or without pretreatment varices and that the risk of decompensation is negligible in patients who are successfully treated before CSPH becomes evident. The latter conclusion is also supported by studies performing paired HVPG measurements that indicated that the resolution of subclinical PH is common and that progression to CSPH did not occur,[26] an observation that was also confirmed recently in a study using IFN-free regimens.[27,28]

IFN-free regimens combining several direct-acting antivirals uncoupled the severity of underlying liver disease/portal hypertension and the likelihood of SVR[29] in patients with cACLD, thereby raising the opportunity of comparing SVR and non-SVR patients in a less biased way. McDonald and colleagues[30] linked patients with chronic HCV and compensated cirrhosis who were included in a Scottish registry to hospital admissions and confirmed that achieving SVR by IFN-free treatments drastically decreased the risk of decompensation (0.188/100 patient-years vs 1.215/100 patient-years).[30] However, in another study based on the Veterans Affairs health care data, the impact of SVR on AVB analyzed as an individual end point seemed to be less pronounced in adjusted analysis (adjusted hazard ratio, 0.68) and did not attain statistical significance in the subgroups of patients with prior varices. This finding may be explained by hemodynamic studies, which indicate that the severity of portal hypertension at baseline determines the probability of (persisting) CSPH despite HCV cure, as well as the development of clinical events during follow-up.[31] CSPH—and thus, the risk of decompensation—persisted in 76% to 78% of patients during short-term follow-up (ie, at a median of 4.15 and 6.00 months after the end of treatment). The initial 2 studies also providing information on long-term changes of HVPG drew a very promising picture,[28,32] because they reported substantial HVPG decreases on the long term; however, the proportions of patients undergoing another HVPG measurement at later time points were very small, introducing the possibility of selection bias. In the 2 more recently published prospective studies reassessing HVPG during long-term follow-up (48 weeks[33] and 96 weeks[31]), persistence of CSPH was observed in 78%[33] and 53 to 65%,[31] respectively—that is, in the majority of patients. However, these studies included a variable proportion of patients with decompensated cirrhosis, in whom CSPH regression was found to be less likely. Accordingly, late decreases of HVPG could be less common than previously expected because the rates of CSPH resolution at this late timepoint were quite similar to those observed in short-term studies.

Of note, even in the IFN-free era, the comparability of treated and untreated patients or responders or nonresponders may be limited by factors that are hard to account for, for example, linkage to care, patient compliance, and concomitant alcohol use. Nevertheless, despite concerns about the appropriateness of comparing SVR and non-SVR patients, in patients with cACLD achieving SVR, the rates of decompensation are low (0.34/100 patient-years).[34]

Nevertheless, it is evident that a considerable proportion of patients with cACLD will develop decompensation despite HCV cure, underlining the need for further etiology-independent treatment strategies in this patient population.

Alcoholic Liver Disease

Although alcoholic liver disease (ALD) is the most common etiology of cirrhosis in Europe[35] and other parts of the world, robust data regarding the impact of abstinence on the development of decompensation in patients with cACLD are limited. This lack may be explained by patients with ALD presenting about 14 times more often with decompensated disease (ie, after the development of first decompensation), as compared with patients with HCV.[36] Accordingly, most studies focused on the outcome of alcoholic hepatitis, which commonly overlaps with ACLD, or decompensated cirrhosis owing to ALD. For instance, a meta-analyses confirming the impact of abstinence from alcohol on survival in patients with ALD with cirrhosis published in 2014 included only 68 patients with cACLD.[37] Masson and colleagues[38] demonstrated that, in a cohort of mostly compensated patients with biopsy-proven ACLD owing to ALD, persistent drinking is the key factor determining long-term mortality (odds ratio, 5.56), whereas the presence of alcoholic hepatitis or cirrhosis at the time of the index biopsy was not predictive. Recently, Lackner and colleagues[39] provided information on the composite end point of decompensation or liver-related death in 60 patients with biopsy-proven ALD (also including patients without ACLD). In addition to alcoholic steatohepatitis and grade F3/F4 fibrosis, abstinence was associated with a nearly 90% decreased risk of developing the composite end point in univariate analysis. However, it was not predictive in the multivariate analysis, in which grade F3/F4 fibrosis (ie, having ACLD) was the only factor determining the outcome—possibly owing to the limited duration of follow-up (a median of 4.1 years throughout all investigated subgroups) and low sample size. Additional evidence comes from long-term outcome data of survivors in the STOPAH trial[40,41] and another series of patients with severe alcoholic hepatitis treated with corticosteroids.[42] However, these studies have to be interpreted with caution because they included both compensated and decompensated cirrhosis, as well as also noncirrhotic patients. Both studies reported a dose-dependent association between alcohol consumption and long-term mortality; however, information on decompensation was not provided.[40–42]

These findings are supported by the impact of alcohol intake versus alcohol abstinence on portal hypertension. Alcohol intake acutely aggravates portal hypertension in patients with cirrhosis owing to ALD[43] and portal hypertension is most severe in patients who have alcohol-related acute decompensation or acute-on-chronic liver failure.[44] Moreover, comparatively high HVPG values were reported in patients with alcoholic hepatitis.[45] Patients with alcoholic hepatitis or active drinkers with cirrhosis owing to ALD who did not return to harmful drinking had a 45% probability of achieving an HVPG decrease of 20% or more after a median of 100 days, whereas such decreases did not occur in patients who returned to harmful drinking. In line with these observations, in a study by Vorobioff and colleagues[46] investigating patients with cirrhosis owing ALD, a baseline of 12 mm Hg or higher, and varices, the HVPG decreased by 15.9% in abstinent patients, whereas it increased by 18.4% in nonabstinent patients after 1 year of follow-up. Interestingly, both having achieved an HVPG decrease of 15% or more and alcohol abstinence at 1 year of follow-up were independently linked to a decreased risk of AVB, suggesting that the impact of alcohol abstinence reaches even beyond what is captured by a single follow-up HVPG measurement.[46] Additional evidence for the close link between alcohol intake and hemodynamic changes is provided by studies investigating HVPG response to NSBB treatment,[47] which observed higher rates of (maintained) HVPG response in patients with alcoholic etiology,[48] particularly in those who continued to abstain from alcohol.[49,50]

Nonalcoholic Fatty Liver Disease

Only a limited number of studies investigated the impact of etiologic therapies in patients with nonalcoholic steatohepatitis (NASH), who have already progressed to ACLD. Although weight loss via lifestyle modification improves fibrosis—the main histologic determinant for decompensation in NASH—in noncirrhotic patients,[51] its impact in F4 patients has yet to be systematically investigated. Two phase 2 RCT[52] investigated 2 different dosing regimens of simtuzumab (anti-lysyl oxidase homolog 2) in compensated patients with F3 (GS-US-321–0105; n = 219)/F4 (GS-US-321–0106; n = 258) fibrosis, obtaining liver biopsies, and in F4 patients, also HVPG-measurements at weeks 48 and 96. The primary efficacy end points were changes in morphometrically quantified hepatic collagen in the F3 and HVPG-changes in the F4 study. However, both studies also investigated primary clinical efficacy end points, that is, progression to cirrhosis (histologically or decompensation) and event-free survival (the absence of decompensation, newly diagnosed varices, or worsening of CTP or model of end-stage liver disease scores) in the F3 and F4 studies, respectively.

There was no evidence of treatment efficacy in regard to liver histology, HVPG, or composite outcomes, indicating that simtuzumab is ineffective.

Another compound that has been intensively studied in cACLD is the apoptosis signal-regulating kinase 1 (ASK1)-inhibitor selonsertib. The STELLAR-3 (F3; n = 802) and −4 (F4; n = 877) RCT[53] assigned patients to different doses of selonsertib and assessed ≥1-stage improvement in fibrosis without worsening of NASH as the main histologic outcome; the investigated composite end points for F3 and F4 patients were similar to those of the above-described phase 2 studies on simtuzumab. Importantly, selonsertib had no impact on the end points assessed after/during a 48-week period.

Moreover, 24 weeks of emricasan (a pan-caspase inhibitor targeting apoptosis) failed to reduce HVPG as compared with placebo in a study comprising 263 mostly compensated patients with a baseline HVPG ≥12 mm Hg. In accordance with this observation, emricasan did not improve clinical outcomes over a 48-week period. However, there were some signs of efficacy, particularly in compensated patients with HVPG ≥16 mm Hg,[54] which is in line with the findings of a small short-term observation in patients with portal hypertension of diverse etiologies.[55] Since emricasan failed to improve liver fibrosis in noncirrhotic patients and even worsened some histologic features,[56] emricasan—if at all—could be of value for treating severe portal hypertension to prevent decompensation, but not as an etiologic treatment for NASH.

Another compound with some evidence of efficacy in regard to lowering HVPG is belapectin (a galectin-3 inhibitor). Belapectin has been evaluated in an RCT comprising 162 patients with portal hypertension owing to NASH.[57] While being ineffective in improving HVPG, histology, and clinical outcomes in the overall study population, among patients without varices, treatment with the lower dose of 2 mg was associated with a statistically significantly more pronounced absolute decrease in HVPG, which was also accompanied by a lower probability of developing varices.

These mostly negative findings regarding monotherapies in compensated F3/F4 patients—despite some of them showing signs of efficacy at earlier stages of the disease—indicate that this is a particularly difficult-to-treat population. This has led to studies investigating regimens combining different modes of action such as the phase 2 ATLAS study,[58] which evaluated different combinations of selonsertib (ie, a presumably ineffective agent), cilofexor (a selective nonsteroidal farnesoid X receptor FXR-agonist), and firsocostat (an acetyl coenzyme A carboxylase-inhibitor). Based on a press release,[59] none of the tested combinations statistically significantly increased the rate of a ≥1-stage improvement in fibrosis without worsening of NASH. However, cilofexor/firsocostat combination therapy led to improvements in some histologic components as well as surrogate markers of liver fibrosis. Of note, this study was not designed to evaluate, and thus, did not provide information on clinical end points.

Finally, the results of phase 3 studies on other compounds (eg, RESOLVE-IT and AURORA) that also include patients with F3 fibrosis, as well as the REVERSE study, focusing on obeticholic acid—a steroidal FXR-agonist which has proven effective in a phase 3 study in noncirrhotic patients[60]—in F4[61] have yet to become available.

Despite several major setbacks in the clinical development of effective treatments for patients with cACLD owing to NASH, these clinical trials have undoubtedly provided important insights in the natural history of NASH which will guide the design of future studies.

Cholestatic and Autoimmune Liver Disease

Ursodeoxycholic acid (UCDA) ameliorates the progression of portal hypertension in primary biliary cholangitis (PBC), as evaluated by measurement of the portal pressure gradient (PPG, ie, direct measurement of the portohepatic gradient),[62] thereby avoiding the underestimation of the severity of portal hypertension owing to the pre-hepatic component of increased intrahepatic resistance in cholestatic liver disease.[63] In the 30 compensated PBC patients randomized 1:1 to UDCA or placebo for 2 years, PPG increased in untreated patients during the first 2 years, while it did not change significantly in treated patients. Following the initiation of UDCA treatment, PPG decreased to baseline values in patients who were initially treated with placebo. In the 101 PBC patients with paired PPG measurements in the overall study population, stable (as defined by no change or an PPG-increase ≤20%) or decreasing PPG-values after 2 years of UDCA treatment translated into a survival benefit (hazard ratio, 4.64). However, this study included a considerable proportion of patients who only had sub-clinical portal hypertension at study inclusion (ie, patients who were unlikely to have had ACLD at baseline and therefore had a low risk of liver-related events) and decom-pensation was not evaluated as an end point. Nevertheless, the study provides impor-tant insights into the impact of UDCA treatment on the evolution of PBC, suggesting that UDCA treatment may halt disease progression but is less effective in promoting liver disease regression than other etiologic therapies, which is possibly related to inadequate responses to UDCA. In line with the observations on PPG, UDCA treat-ment prevents/delays disease progression to CSPH as evidenced by the decreased risk of developing varices[64] and ultimately improves transplant-free survival.[65] In addi-tion, the prognosis of PBC may further improve with emerging treatment options such as obeticholic acid[66–69] and fibrates,[70,71] owing to further improvements in biochem-ical response. However, based on the available evidence, it is difficult to assess the impact of current and emerging therapies on the development of first decompensation in patients who have already progressed to ACLD.

The efficacy of UDCA treatment for PSC is controversial[72] and novel therapeutic op-tions are currently under evaluation[73–76]; however, long-term results on direct clinical end points have yet to become available.

Although response to immunosuppressive therapy is linked to long-term outcomes in autoimmune hepatitis,[77] there are insufficient data to draw firm conclusions on its impact decompensation in patients with ACLD owing to autoimmune hepatitis.

Summary of the Impact of Etiologic Therapies and Outlook

In conclusion, there is a body of evidence indicating that etiologic therapies decrease the risk of first decompensation (see **Fig. 1**). The magnitude of the effect seemed to be particularly high in etiologies in which a (theoretically) single causative factor (ie, HBV replication, HCV infection, or alcohol consumption) is entirely removed. However, in patients who have already progressed to CSPH, even 'perfect' etiologic therapies are far from being universally effective in inducing CSPH regression and preventing decompensation. Although the underlying pathophysiological mechanisms have yet to be fully elucidated, the gut-liver-axis[10] could be of great relevance for the long-term evolution of liver disease in these patients, as bacterial translocation-induced he-patic[78] and systemic inflammation may perpetuate liver injury despite the cure of the primary etiologic factor or even directly trigger decompensation. Interestingly, markers of bacterial translocation (ie, lipopolysaccharide binding protein[28,33]) as well as associated endothelial dysfunction[79] (ie, von Willebrand factor [VWF][80]) decreased in patients achieving SVR and the observed changes were unrelated to the dynamics of HVPG.[28]

Patients who underwent etiologic therapies are less likely to require liver trans-plantation or die from liver-related causes, indicating that they will remain in the same disease state/need to be followed for a longer time period, as compared with patients with progressive disease. Considering that current surveillance/

treatment strategies have primarily been developed based on/extrapolated from patients with progressive disease, their application may result in unnecessary interventions in patients who underwent etiologic treatment, and thus, have a more favorable prognosis. The high interindividual variability in the impact of etiologic therapies on the course of ACLD is a major challenge in this context, which highlights the need for surrogate markers that reflect the risk of decompensation after etiologic therapies to monitor the evolution of liver disease after etiologic treatments in an individual patient. We have recently demonstrated that post-treatment HVPG/relative changes in HVPG (ie, HVPG-response, as defined by a decrease ≥10%) predict decompensation after HCV-cure,[28] in particular first decompensation patients with compensated CSPH. In contrast, in another study by Lens and coworkers[34] that included a considerably higher proportion of patients with decompensated cirrhosis, there was only an association between post-treatment HVPG and decompensation during follow-up in univariate analysis, which did not attain statistical significance in multivariate analysis. In addition, changes in HVPG have also been linked to outcomes in patients with ALD with HVPG ≥12 mm Hg who were advised to abstain from alcohol (HVPG-decrease cut-off: ≥15%),[46] or patients with compensated cirrhosis owing to nonalcoholic steatohepatitis (NASH) treated with simtuzumab or placebo (HVPG-decrease cut-off: ≥20%).[81] However, it is clear that HVPG-measurement—although being highly informative—cannot be applied for risk stratification on a broad scale, as it is not available at most centers. This indicates the need for development and validation of noninvasive methods for this specific clinical scenario.[82] In the post-SVR setting, Baveno VI criteria[83] as well as combinations of liver stiffness measurement (LSM) by vibration-controlled elastography (VCTE) and albumin[80] or VWF to platelet count ratio[80] have shown a high prognostic ability for decompensation, thereby facilitating risk stratification, individualization of surveillance, and possibly, selection of patients who may benefit from additional strategies to prevent first decompensation.

REMOVAL OF COFACTORS

Concomitant alcohol consumption modulates the impact of the removal of the primary etiologic factor on outcomes. For instance, in (mostly compensated) ACLD patients who achieved HCV-cure, alcohol consumption above the sex-specific thresholds for NAFLD (ie, >30 g/d and >20 g/d for males and females, respectively[84]) was substantially more prevalent (50% vs 9.1%) in patients who developed post-treatment decompensation and was also independently predictive of the outcome of interest.

In addition, the impact of obesity and associated metabolic disturbances on portal hypertension owing to etiologies other than NAFLD is increasingly recognized. For instance, a 16-week lifestyle intervention comprising diet and physical exercise has been shown to lead to 'clinically meaningful' HVPG-decreases ≥10% in 42% of obese patients with portal hypertension, with particularly profound decreases in those who achieve ≥10% of weight loss.[85]

Accordingly, cessation of alcohol consumption and weight loss (in obese patients) should be strongly advised to prevent decompensation.

PATHOPHYSIOLOGY-ORIENTED THERAPIES
Drivers of Decompensation

As outlined in the introduction section, sinusoidal portal hypertension (as defined by portal pressure gradient (PPG)/HVPG ≥6 mm Hg) is initiated by intrahepatic microcirculatory disturbances manifesting as increases in intrahepatic resistance, which comprises tightly interrelated structural (fibrosis, microvascular occlusion, and sinusoidal capillarization) and functional (hepatic vascular tone; regulated mainly by liver sinusoidal endothelial cells and hepatic stellate cells) components.[86] The functional component (ie, hepatic vascular tone) is directly impacted by bacterial translocation from the gut which leads to hepatic and systemic inflammation—highlighting the central role of the 'gut-liver axis'[10,11] for disease progression. Systemic inflammation also promotes arterial vasodilation leading to compensatory increases in cardiac output, and thus, hyperdynamic circulation.[87] Hyperdynamic circulation further aggravates portal hypertension, which, at this point, exceeds the threshold defining CSPH.[1] At the same time, vasodilation results in effective hypovolemia which induces compensatory responses leading to sodium and fluid retention and ascites formation.[88]

These mechanisms that are summarized in **Fig. 1** are targeted by several medical therapies, of which NSBB and statins are supported by a broad body of clinical evidence.

Nonselective Beta-Blockers

Current guidelines[89,90] recommend NSBB treatment in patients with (medium to) large varices as well as high-risk small varices to prevent AVB. According to Baveno VI[89] and American Association for the Study of the Liver recommendations, CTP stage C (usually conferring to decompensated cirrhosis) or the presence of red wale marks define high-risk varices. Alternatively, endoscopic variceal ligation (EVL) may be used for primary prophylaxis in patients with (medium to) large varices. Although a meta-analysis[91] showed that EVL decreased AVB when compared with NSBB treatment (relative risk, 0.69), the beneficial effect of EVL was not confirmed in a subsequent analysis restricted to high-quality trials. Moreover, EVL—in contrast to NSBB—acts exclusively downstream of the pathophysiologic cascade of portal hypertension.

Although primary prophylaxis with NSBB therapy is well-established for these indications, early studies did not find a benefit in patients with cACLD who did not meet those criteria. In a study by Groszmann and colleagues,[92] patients with cirrhosis, with an HVPG of 6 mmHg or higher, but without varices were randomly assigned to the NSBB timolol or placebo. After a median follow-up of nearly 5 years, about 40% of patients in both groups met the composite primary end point of the development of varices or AVB. Importantly, patients who had a relative HVPG decrease of more than 10% after 1 year showed a lower incidence of the primary end point, but such decreases were only slightly more common in timolol-treated patients (53% vs 38%), which may be explained by the inclusion of a high proportion of patients with only subclinical portal hypertension (59%). Conventional NSBB such as timolol or propranolol/nadolol decrease the HVPG by decreasing cardiac output (anti-β1) and ameliorating splanchnic vasodilation (anti-β2). Accordingly, the absence of or less pronounced hyperdynamic circulation in patients with subclinical portal hypertension attenuates their antiportal hypertensive effect. This hypothesis is supported by the findings of a study by Villanueva and colleagues,[1] in which patients with subclinical portal hypertension—who had lower cardiac index and higher systemic vascular resistance—achieved a relative HVPG decrease of only 8% to intravenous (IV) propranolol, whereas the relative HVPG decrease was 16% in patients with CSPH.

Moving to patients with low-risk small varices, there is no conclusive evidence for a decrease in AVB with NSBB treatment.[6] Of note, an absence of evidence is not evidence of absence, particularly because the trials were not sufficiently powered to detect favorable treatment effects—as discussed elsewhere in this article, sample size requirements for studies evaluating preventive strategies in low-risk patients are tremendously high.[5] To overcome this limitation, several trials investigated the efficacy of NSBB treatment to prevent the more common surrogate end point variceal growth; however, the findings were mixed.[93] Finally, it is unclear whether a decrease in variceal growth translates into a clinically meaningful benefit.

In contrast, the benefit of preventing decompensation is well-established, and findings in patients with HVPG response to NSBB treatment indicated, that NSBB-induced decreases in HVPG decrease the risk of decompensation, in particular the incidence of AVB (the decompensation event that is most directly driven by portal hypertension) and ascites.[47] Some studies also suggested a decrease in overt HE; however, it may be argued that the decreased incidence in overt HE could also be secondary to decreases in the latter 2 forms of decompensation, because AVB and the use of diuretics may precipitate overt HE. Findings of studies investigating the predictive values of acute changes in HVPG to IV propranolol provided the most convincing evidence for the preventive effect of HVPG-response to NSBB treatment, because chronic changes in HVPG are also affected by the evolution of underlying liver disease.[47] Of note, in addition to the effects that are directly related to HVPG decreases, NSBBs decrease bacterial translocation and systemic inflammation in an HVPG response-independent manner,[94] which may further add to its disease-modifying properties (see **Fig. 1**).

In their seminal PREDESCI trial, Villanueva and colleagues[95] assigned 201 compensated patients with CSPH with no or small low-risk varices to propranolol (in case of HVPG decrease of $\geq$10% to IV propranolol)/carvedilol (hemodynamic nonresponders to IV propranolol) treatment or placebo. Propranolol/carvedilol decreased the risks of decompensation or liver-related death, mostly by decreasing the incidence of ascites.[95] Although improvements in patients selection such as the exclusion of patients without CSPH and the use of HVPG-guided therapy may have been instrumental for demonstrating the ability of NSBB treatment to prevent decompensation in patients with no or only low-risk small varices, this HVPG-centric approach hampers the applicability of these findings in clinical practice. Until more evidence becomes available, this limitation could be overcome by a more pragmatic approach using noninvasive methods for ruling-in CSPH[82] and a target dose of 12.5 mg of carvedilol per day[96] in all patients, because—owing to its additional anti–alpha-adrenergic activity—carvedilol reduces HVPG more potently as compared to propranolol[97] and achieves an HVPG response in a relevant proportion of nonresponders to propranolol.[98]

Importantly, another RCT (the BOPPP trial[99]) that is adequately powered (1200 patients) to detect a potential benefit in direct clinical end points (ie, AVB; other forms of decompensation are assessed as secondary end points) in patients with small low-risk varices who have not bled (the subpopulation that benefited the most in the PREDESCI trial[95]) is currently on the way and will provide further evidence regarding the use of carvedilol in this context.

Statins

Until recently, CLD—in particular if advanced—was considered a relative contraindication for statin prescription, mainly driven by concerns regarding hepatotoxicity.[100] However, an increasing number of studies reported potential beneficial effects of statins in patients with CLD[101] (see **Fig. 1**), although the risk of severe hepatic injury seems to be comparable with that in the general population (only high-dose atorvastatin was associated with hepatotoxicity).[102] Importantly, the pharmacokinetics of statins display alterations that depend on disease stage,[8] as underlined by the observation of dose-dependent toxicity (rhabdomyolysis) upon treatment with

40 mg/d in CTP C, whereas a rescue dose of 20 mg/d seemed to yield an acceptable safety profile.[103]

By now, experimental studies demonstrated that statins exert beneficial effects on ACLD, which may be explained by an amelioration of hepatic inflammation as well as endothelial dysfunction, thus improving liver function and portal hypertension, and preventing acute-on-chronic liver failure.[8] To this end, an RCT in 59 patients with portal hypertension (HVPG of $\geq$12 mm Hg; n = 55 eligible for efficacy analysis; 38% compensated cirrhosis) reported a significant decrease in the HVPG after 1 month of therapy in both compensated and decompensated patients with or without concomitant NSBB therapy who were treated with simvastatin 40 mg/d.[104] Similarly, patients receiving simvastatin 40 mg/d for 3 months displayed a trend toward an HVPG reduction in an RCT including 34 patients, of whom only 24 patients were eligible for per-protocol analysis.[105] Finally, another RCT including 23 patients displayed that atorvastatin 20 mg/d plus propranolol led to a more pronounced HVPG decrease after 30 days of treatment, as compared with propranolol alone,[106] confirming that the effects of statins add to those of propranolol therapy.

Although these studies support the use of statins for the treatment of portal hypertension, it has yet to be demonstrated that statins prevent first decompensation. A systematic review and meta-analysis of available studies indicated a decrease in the incidence of decompensation and mortality by statin treatment, however, also highlighted the need for an RCT to draw firm conclusions.[101] Of note, the BLEPS trial including 158 patients requiring secondary prophylaxis for variceal bleeding investigated whether simvastatin 40 mg/d decreases the risk of rebleeding or death.[103] Although simvastatin displayed no benefit toward the primary (composite) end point, it was associated with a substantial decrease in the risk of death (hazard ratio, 0.39)[103] in the context of decompensated cirrhosis; however, it is unclear whether these findings can be extrapolated to patients with cACLD. The SACRED trial[107] randomly assigns patients with cACLD and (evidence of) CSPH (among other criteria, liver stiffness of $\geq$25 kPa, platelet counts of <70 G/L, or the presence of varices) to investigate to the efficacy of simvastatin 40 mg/d toward the prevention of decompensation as a primary outcome; liver-related death is assessed as a secondary outcome. Of note, this study is complemented by the LIVERHOPE efficacy trial[108] investigating whether the combination of simvastatin 20 to 40 mg/d and rifaximin (which, similarly to norfloxacin, ameliorates bacterial translocation-induced systemic inflammation[109]) prevents acute-on-chronic liver failure in patients with decompensated cirrhosis—a combination that could also be suitable to prevent first decompensation based on pathophysiologic considerations. The results of these trials will provide further important evidence regarding the use of simvastatin in ACLD.

Other Potential Therapeutic Targets

In addition to all the previously discussed measures, several additional medical therapies have the potential to prevent first decompensation (see **Fig. 1**), mostly by ameliorating portal hypertension and/or systemic inflammation. However, we abstained from discussing them in detail because they have recently been reviewed elsewhere[5,10] and only proof-of-concept clinical studies are available.

DESIGN OF TRIALS ON THE PREVENTION OF FIRST DECOMPENSATION

Future trials should analyze a composite of all forms of decompensation—rather than an individual complication such as AVB—as a primary end point. This approach decreases the sample size requirements by increasing the number of events and ensures clinically meaningful results. Moreover, selection of patients at risk is key to obtain a sufficient number of events; in this regard, only patients with CSPH (which may be diagnosed noninvasively) should be considered, because the risk in patients with subclinical portal hypertension patients is negligible. Still, the required sample size is high: When assuming a hazard ratio of 0.7 and a 2-year rate of first decompensation of 20% (corresponding with a median HVPG of about 14 mm Hg) in the control group, 700 patients would be required.[5] Another approach to decrease sample size is to restrict the inclusion to patients who are most likely to benefit from the treatment (thereby decreasing the hazard ratio) because the pathomechanism that is, targeted by the study intervention is highly active in the individual patient. In this regard, pathophysiologically oriented biomarkers could be instrumental for study design and may facilitate personalized therapy. Such an approach may considerably decrease resource utilization; a decrease in the hazard ratio from 0.7 to 0.6 would nearly halve the required sample size (380 instead of 700).[5]

CLINICS CARE POINTS

- In patients with compensated advanced chronic liver disease, prevention of decompensation is the primary treatment goal to avoid the downward spiral of further decompensation and acute-on-chronic liver failure.

- Etiological therapies may improve liver function and fibrosis, as well as portal hypertension, thereby decreasing the risk of decompensation.

- Moreover, the effective management co-factors – in particular alcohol and overweight/obesity – is crucial.

- Hepatic venous pressure gradient (HVPG)-guided non-selective beta-blocker therapy prevents decompensation in those at risk, i.e., patients with clinically significant portal hypertension (CSPH; as defined by an HVPG ≥10 mmHg).

- Comparable effects may be achieved by ruling-in CSPH using non-invasive methods (e.g., liver stiffness measurement ≥20-25 kPa) and administering carvedilol (12.5 mg/d).

DISCLOSURE STATEMENT

M. Mandorfer served as a speaker and/or consultant and/or advisory board member for AbbVie, Bristol-Myers Squibb, Collective Acumen, Gilead, and W. L. Gore & Associates and received travel support from AbbVie, Bristol-Myers Squibb, and Gilead. B. Simbrunner received travel support from AbbVie and Gilead.

REFERENCES

1. Villanueva C, Albillos A, Genesca J, et al. Development of hyperdynamic circulation and response to beta-blockers in compensated cirrhosis with portal hypertension. Hepatology 2016;63(1):197–206.
2. Ripoll C, Groszmann R, Garcia-Tsao G, et al. Hepatic venous pressure gradient predicts clinical decompensation in patients with compensated cirrhosis. Gastroenterology 2007;133(2):481–8.
3. D'Amico G, Pasta L, Morabito A, et al. Competing risks and prognostic stages of cirrhosis: a 25-year inception cohort study of 494 patients. Aliment Pharmacol Ther 2014;39(10):1180–93.

4. D'Amico G, Morabito A, D'Amico M, et al. Clinical states of cirrhosis and competing risks. J Hepatol 2018;68(3):563–76.

5. Abraldes JG, Trebicka J, Chalasani N, et al. Prioritization of therapeutic targets and trial design in cirrhotic portal hypertension. Hepatology 2019;69(3): 1287–99.

6. Mandorfer M, Reiberger T. Beta blockers and cirrhosis, 2016. Dig Liver Dis 2017;49(1):3–10.

7. Reiberger T, Mandorfer M. Beta adrenergic blockade and decompensated cirrhosis. J Hepatol 2017;66(4):849–59.

8. Bosch J, Gracia-Sancho J, Abraldes JG. Cirrhosis as new indication for statins. Gut 2020;69(5):953–62.

9. Turco L, de Raucourt E, Valla DC, et al. Anticoagulation in the cirrhotic patient. JHEP Rep 2019;1(3):227–39.

10. Simbrunner B, Mandorfer M, Trauner M, et al. Gut-liver axis signaling in portal hypertension. World J Gastroenterol 2019;25(39):5897–917.

11. Albillos A, de Gottardi A, Rescigno M. The gut-liver axis in liver disease: pathophysiological basis for therapy. J Hepatol 2020;72(3):558–77.

12. Komolafe O, Roberts D, Freeman SC, et al. Antibiotic prophylaxis to prevent spontaneous bacterial peritonitis in people with liver cirrhosis: a network meta-analysis. Cochrane Database Syst Rev 2020;(1):CD013125.

13. Bajaj JS, Khoruts A. Microbiota changes and intestinal microbiota transplantation in liver diseases and cirrhosis. J Hepatol 2020;72(5):1003–27.

14. Bernardi M, Angeli P, Claria J, et al. Albumin in decompensated cirrhosis: new concepts and perspectives. Gut 2020;69(6):1127–38.

15. Garcia-Pagan JC, Saffo S, Mandorfer M, et al. Where does TIPS fit in the management of patients with cirrhosis? JHEP Rep 2020;2(4):100122.

16. Liaw YF, Sung JJ, Chow WC, et al. Lamivudine for patients with chronic hepatitis B and advanced liver disease. N Engl J Med 2004;351(15):1521–31.

17. Manolakopoulos S, Triantos C, Theodoropoulos J, et al. Antiviral therapy reduces portal pressure in patients with cirrhosis due to HBeAg-negative chronic hepatitis B and significant portal hypertension. J Hepatol 2009;51(3):468–74.

18. Marcellin P, Gane E, Buti M, et al. Regression of cirrhosis during treatment with tenofovir disoproxil fumarate for chronic hepatitis B: a 5-year open-label follow-up study. Lancet 2013;381(9865):468–75.

19. Bruno S, Stroffolini T, Colombo M, et al. Sustained virological response to interferon-alpha is associated with improved outcome in HCV-related cirrhosis: a retrospective study. Hepatology 2007;45(3):579–87.

20. Veldt BJ, Heathcote EJ, Wedemeyer H, et al. Sustained virologic response and clinical outcomes in patients with chronic hepatitis C and advanced fibrosis. Ann Intern Med 2007;147(10):677–84.

21. Cardoso AC, Moucari R, Figueiredo-Mendes C, et al. Impact of peginterferon and ribavirin therapy on hepatocellular carcinoma: incidence and survival in hepatitis C patients with advanced fibrosis. J Hepatol 2010;52(5):652–7.

22. Morgan TR, Ghany MG, Kim HY, et al. Outcome of sustained virological responders with histologically advanced chronic hepatitis C. Hepatology 2010; 52(3):833–44.

23. Reiberger T, Rutter K, Ferlitsch A, et al. Portal pressure predicts outcome and safety of antiviral therapy in cirrhotic patients with hepatitis C virus infection. Clin Gastroenterol Hepatol 2011;9(7):602–8.

24. Lens S, Rincon D, Garcia-Retortillo M, et al. Association between severe portal hypertension and risk of liver decompensation in patients with Hepatitis C,

regardless of response to antiviral therapy. Clin Gastroenterol Hepatol 2015; 13(10):1846–53.

25. Di Marco V, Calvaruso V, Ferraro D, et al. Effects of eradicating Hepatitis C virus infection in patients with cirrhosis differ with stage of portal hypertension. Gastroenterology 2016;151(1):130–9.

26. Reiberger T, Payer BA, Ferlitsch A, et al. A prospective evaluation of pulmonary, systemic and hepatic haemodynamics in HIV-HCV-coinfected patients before and after antiviral therapy with pegylated interferon and ribavirin. Antivir Ther 2012;17(7):1327–34.

27. Mandorfer M, Kozbial K, Schwabl P, et al. Sustained virologic response to interferon-free therapies ameliorates HCV-induced portal hypertension. J Hepatol 2016;65(4):692–9.

28. Mandorfer M, Kozbial K, Schwabl P, et al. Changes in hepatic venous pressure gradient predict hepatic decompensation in patients who achieved sustained virologic response to interferon-free therapy. Hepatology 2020;71(3):1023–36.

29. Mandorfer M, Kozbial K, Freissmuth C, et al. Interferon-free regimens for chronic hepatitis C overcome the effects of portal hypertension on virological responses. Aliment Pharmacol Ther 2015;42(6):707–18.

30. McDonald SA, Pollock KG, Barclay ST, et al. Real-world impact following initiation of interferon-free hepatitis C regimens on liver-related outcomes and all-cause mortality among patients with compensated cirrhosis. J Viral Hepat 2020;27(3):270–80.

31. Lens S, Baiges A, Alvarado E, et al. Clinical outcome and hemodynamic changes following HCV eradication with oral antiviral therapy in patients with clinically significant portal hypertension. J Hepatol 2020;73(6):1415–24.

32. Afdhal N, Everson GT, Calleja JL, et al. Effect of viral suppression on hepatic venous pressure gradient in hepatitis C with cirrhosis and portal hypertension. J Viral Hepat 2017;24(10):823–31.

33. Diez C, Berenguer J, Ibanez-Samaniego L, et al. Persistence of clinically significant portal hypertension after eradication of HCV in patients with advanced cirrhosis. Clin Infect Dis 2020, in press.

34. Pons M, Rodriguez-Tajes S, Esteban JI, et al. Non-invasive prediction of liver-related events in patients with HCV-associated compensated advanced chronic liver disease after oral antivirals. J Hepatol 2020;72(3):472–80.

35. Blachier M, Leleu H, Peck-Radosavljevic M, et al. The burden of liver disease in Europe: a review of available epidemiological data. J Hepatol 2013;58(3):593–608.

36. Shah ND, Ventura-Cots M, Abraldes JG, et al. Alcohol-related liver disease is rarely detected at early stages compared with liver diseases of other etiologies worldwide. Clin Gastroenterol Hepatol 2019;17(11):2320–9.

37. Xie YD, Feng B, Gao Y, et al. Effect of abstinence from alcohol on survival of patients with alcoholic cirrhosis: a systematic review and meta-analysis. Hepatol Res 2014;44(4):436–49.

38. Masson S, Emmerson I, Henderson E, et al. Clinical but not histological factors predict long-term prognosis in patients with histologically advanced non-decompensated alcoholic liver disease. Liver Int 2014;34(2):235–42.

39. Lackner C, Spindelboeck W, Haybaeck J, et al. Histological parameters and alcohol abstinence determine long-term prognosis in patients with alcoholic liver disease. J Hepatol 2017;66(3):610–8.

40. Atkinson SR, Way MJ, McQuillin A, et al. Homozygosity for rs738409:G in PNPLA3 is associated with increased mortality following an episode of severe alcoholic hepatitis. J Hepatol 2017;67(1):120–7.
41. Atkinson SR, McQuillin A, Morgan MY, et al. People who survive an episode of severe alcoholic hepatitis should be advised to maintain total abstinence from alcohol. Hepatology 2018;67(6):2479–80.
42. Louvet A, Labreuche J, Artru F, et al. Main drivers of outcome differ between short term and long term in severe alcoholic hepatitis: a prospective study. Hepatology 2017;66(5):1464–73.
43. Luca A, Garcia-Pagan JC, Bosch J, et al. Effects of ethanol consumption on hepatic hemodynamics in patients with alcoholic cirrhosis. Gastroenterology 1997;112(4):1284–9.
44. Mehta G, Mookerjee RP, Sharma V, et al. Systemic inflammation is associated with increased intrahepatic resistance and mortality in alcohol-related acute-on-chronic liver failure. Liver Int 2015;35(3):724–34.
45. Spahr L, Goossens N, Furrer F, et al. A return to harmful alcohol consumption impacts on portal hemodynamic changes following alcoholic hepatitis. Eur J Gastroenterol Hepatol 2018;30(8):967–74.
46. Vorobioff J, Groszmann RJ, Picabea E, et al. Prognostic value of hepatic venous pressure gradient measurements in alcoholic cirrhosis: a 10-year prospective study. Gastroenterology 1996;111(3):701–9.
47. Mandorfer M, Hernández-Gea V, Reiberger T, et al. Hepatic venous pressure gradient response in non-selective beta-blocker treatment—is it worth measuring? Curr Hepatol Rep 2019;18(2):174–86.
48. Groszmann RJ, Bosch J, Grace ND, et al. Hemodynamic events in a prospective randomized trial of propranolol versus placebo in the prevention of a first variceal hemorrhage. Gastroenterology 1990;99(5):1401–7.
49. Villanueva C, Lopez-Balaguer JM, Aracil C, et al. Maintenance of hemodynamic response to treatment for portal hypertension and influence on complications of cirrhosis. J Hepatol 2004;40(5):757–65.
50. Augustin S, Gonzalez A, Badia L, et al. Long-term follow-up of hemodynamic responders to pharmacological therapy after variceal bleeding. Hepatology 2012;56(2):706–14.
51. Vilar-Gomez E, Martinez-Perez Y, Calzadilla-Bertot L, et al. Weight loss through lifestyle modification significantly reduces features of nonalcoholic steatohepatitis. Gastroenterology 2015;149(2):367–78.
52. Harrison SA, Abdelmalek MF, Caldwell S, et al. Simtuzumab is ineffective for patients with bridging fibrosis or compensated cirrhosis caused by nonalcoholic steatohepatitis. Gastroenterology 2018;155(4):1140–53.
53. Harrison SA, Wong VW, Okanoue T, et al. Selonsertib for patients with bridging fibrosis or compensated cirrhosis due to NASH: results from randomized phase III STELLAR trials. J Hepatol 2020;73(1):26–39.
54. Garcia-Tsao G, Bosch J, Kayali Z, et al. Randomized placebo-controlled trial of emricasan for non-alcoholic steatohepatitis-related cirrhosis with severe portal hypertension. J Hepatol 2020;72(5):885–95.
55. Garcia-Tsao G, Fuchs M, Shiffman M, et al. Emricasan (IDN-6556) lowers portal pressure in patients with compensated cirrhosis and severe portal hypertension. Hepatology 2019;69(2):717–28.
56. Harrison SA, Goodman Z, Jabbar A, et al. A randomized, placebo-controlled trial of emricasan in patients with NASH and F1-F3 fibrosis. J Hepatol 2020;72(5):816–27.

57. Chalasani N, Abdelmalek MF, Garcia-Tsao G. Effects of Belapectin, an Inhibitor of Galectin-3, in Patients With Nonalcoholic Steatohepatitis With Cirrhosis and Portal Hypertension. Gastroenterology 2020;158(5):1334–45,,e5.

58. Safety and efficacy of selonsertib, firsocostat, cilofexor, and combinations in participants with bridging fibrosis or compensated cirrhosis due to nonalcoholic steatohepatitis (NASH) (ATLAS). Available at: https://clinicaltrials.gov/ct2/show/NCT03449446. Accessed February 10, 2021.

59. Gilead announces topline results from phase 2 ATLAS study in patients with bridging fibrosis (F3) and compensated cirrhosis (F4) due to nonalcoholic steatohepatitis (NASH). Available at: https://www.gilead.com/news-and-press/press-room/press-releases/2019/12/gilead-announces-topline-results-from-phase-2-atlas-study-in-patients-with-bridging-fibrosis-f3-and-compensated-cirrhosis-f4-due-to-nonalcoholic-s. Accessed February 10, 2021.

60. Younossi ZM, Ratziu V, Loomba R, et al. Obeticholic acid for the treatment of non-alcoholic steatohepatitis: interim analysis from a multicentre, randomised, placebo-controlled phase 3 trial. Lancet 2019;394(10215):2184–96.

61. Study evaluating the efficacy and safety of obeticholic acid in subjects with compensated cirrhosis due to nonalcoholic steatohepatitis (REVERSE). Available at: https://clinicaltrials.gov/ct2/show/NCT03439254. Accessed February 10, 2021.

62. Huet PM, Vincent C, Deslaurier J, et al. Portal hypertension and primary biliary cirrhosis: effect of long-term ursodeoxycholic acid treatment. Gastroenterology 2008;135(5):1552–60.

63. Navasa M, Pares A, Bruguera M, et al. Portal hypertension in primary biliary cirrhosis. Relationship with histological features. J Hepatol 1987;5(3):292–8.

64. Lindor KD, Jorgensen RA, Therneau TM, et al. Ursodeoxycholic acid delays the onset of esophageal varices in primary biliary cirrhosis. Mayo Clin Proc 1997;72(12):1137–40.

65. Harms MH, van Buuren HR, Corpechot C, et al. Ursodeoxycholic acid therapy and liver transplant-free survival in patients with primary biliary cholangitis. J Hepatol 2019;71(2):357–65.

66. Nevens F, Andreone P, Mazzella G, et al. A placebo-controlled trial of obeticholic acid in primary biliary cholangitis. N Engl J Med 2016;375(7):631–43.

67. Samur S, Klebanoff M, Banken R, et al. Long-term clinical impact and cost-effectiveness of obeticholic acid for the treatment of primary biliary cholangitis. Hepatology 2017;65(3):920–8.

68. Trauner M, Nevens F, Shiffman ML, et al. Long-term efficacy and safety of obeticholic acid for patients with primary biliary cholangitis: 3-year results of an international open-label extension study. Lancet Gastroenterol Hepatol 2019;4(6):445–53.

69. Bowlus CL, Pockros PJ, Kremer AE, et al. Long-term obeticholic acid therapy improves histological endpoints in patients with primary biliary cholangitis. Clin Gastroenterol Hepatol 2020;18(5):1170–8.

70. Cheung AC, Lapointe-Shaw L, Kowgier M, et al. Combined ursodeoxycholic acid (UDCA) and fenofibrate in primary biliary cholangitis patients with incomplete UDCA response may improve outcomes. Aliment Pharmacol Ther 2016;43(2):283–93.

71. Corpechot C, Chazouilleres O, Rousseau A, et al. A placebo-controlled trial of bezafibrate in primary biliary cholangitis. N Engl J Med 2018;378(23):2171–81.

72. Halilbasic E, Fuchs C, Hofer H, et al. Therapy of primary sclerosing cholangitis–today and tomorrow. Dig Dis 2015;33(Suppl 2):149–63.

73. Fickert P, Hirschfield GM, Denk G, et al. norUrsodeoxycholic acid improves cholestasis in primary sclerosing cholangitis. J Hepatol 2017;67(3):549–58.

74. Hirschfield GM, Chazouilleres O, Drenth JP, et al. Effect of NGM282, an FGF19 analogue, in primary sclerosing cholangitis: a multicenter, randomized, double-blind, placebo-controlled phase II trial. J Hepatol 2019;70(3):483–93.

75. Trauner M, Gulamhusein A, Hameed B, et al. The nonsteroidal farnesoid X receptor agonist cilofexor (GS-9674) improves markers of cholestasis and liver injury in patients with primary sclerosing cholangitis. Hepatology 2019;70(3): 788–801.

76. Kowdley KV, Vuppalanchi R, Levy C, et al. A randomized, placebo-controlled, phase II study of obeticholic acid for primary sclerosing cholangitis. J Hepatol 2020;73(1):94–101.

77. Hoeroldt B, McFarlane E, Dube A, et al. Long-term outcomes of patients with autoimmune hepatitis managed at a nontransplant center. Gastroenterology 2011;140(7):1980–9.

78. Schwabl P, Mandorfer M, Steiner S, et al. Interferon-free regimens improve portal hypertension and histological necroinflammation in HIV/HCV patients with advanced liver disease. Aliment Pharmacol Ther 2017;45(1):139–49.

79. Mandorfer M, Schwabl P, Paternostro R, et al. Von Willebrand factor indicates bacterial translocation, inflammation, and procoagulant imbalance and predicts complications independently of portal hypertension severity. Aliment Pharmacol Ther 2018;47(7):980–8.

80. Semmler G, Binter T, Kozbial K, et al. Non-invasive risk stratification after HCV-eradication in patients with advanced chronic liver disease. Hepatology 2020, in press.

81. Sanyal AJ, Harrison SA, Ratziu V, et al. The natural history of advanced fibrosis due to nonalcoholic steatohepatitis: data from the simtuzumab trials. Hepatology 2019;70(6):1913–27.

82. Mandorfer M, Hernandez-Gea V, Garcia-Pagan JC, et al. Noninvasive diagnostics for portal hypertension: a comprehensive review. Semin Liver Dis 2020; 40(3):240–55.

83. Thabut D, Bureau C, Layese R, et al. Validation of Baveno VI criteria for screening and surveillance of esophageal varices in patients with compensated cirrhosis and a sustained response to antiviral therapy. Gastroenterology 2019; 156(4):997–1009.

84. European Association for the Study of the Liver, European Association for the Study of Diabetes, European Association for the Study of Obesity. EASL-EASD-EASO clinical practice guidelines for the management of non-alcoholic fatty liver disease. J Hepatol 2016;64(6):1388–402.

85. Berzigotti A, Albillos A, Villanueva C, et al. Effects of an intensive lifestyle intervention program on portal hypertension in patients with cirrhosis and obesity: the SportDiet study. Hepatology 2017;65(4):1293–305.

86. Gracia-Sancho J, Marrone G, Fernandez-Iglesias A. Hepatic microcirculation and mechanisms of portal hypertension. Nat Rev Gastroenterol Hepatol 2019; 16(4):221–34.

87. Turco L, Garcia-Tsao G, Magnani I, et al. Cardiopulmonary hemodynamics and C-reactive protein as prognostic indicators in compensated and decompensated cirrhosis. J Hepatol 2018;68(5):949–58.

88. European Association for the Study of the Liver. EASL clinical practice guidelines for the management of patients with decompensated cirrhosis. J Hepatol 2018;69(2):406–60.

89. de Franchis R, Baveno VI Faculty. Expanding consensus in portal hypertension: report of the Baveno VI Consensus Workshop: stratifying risk and individualizing care for portal hypertension. J Hepatol 2015;63(3):743–52.
90. Garcia-Tsao G, Abraldes JG, Berzigotti A, et al. Portal hypertensive bleeding in cirrhosis: risk stratification, diagnosis, and management: 2016 practice guidance by the American Association for the study of liver diseases. Hepatology 2017;65(1):310–35.
91. Gluud LL, Krag A. Banding ligation versus beta-blockers for primary prevention in oesophageal varices in adults. Cochrane Database Syst Rev 2012;(8):CD004544.
92. Groszmann RJ, Garcia-Tsao G, Bosch J, et al. Beta-blockers to prevent gastroesophageal varices in patients with cirrhosis. N Engl J Med 2005;353(21):2254–61.
93. Mandorfer M, Peck-Radosavljevic M, Reiberger T. Prevention of progression from small to large varices: are we there yet? An updated meta-analysis. Gut 2017;66(7):1347–9.
94. Reiberger T, Ferlitsch A, Payer BA, et al. Non-selective betablocker therapy decreases intestinal permeability and serum levels of LBP and IL-6 in patients with cirrhosis. J Hepatol 2013;58(5):911–21.
95. Villanueva C, Albillos A, Genesca J, et al. Beta blockers to prevent decompensation of cirrhosis in patients with clinically significant portal hypertension (PREDESCI): a randomised, double-blind, placebo-controlled, multicentre trial. Lancet 2019;393(10181):1597–608.
96. Schwarzer R, Kivaranovic D, Paternostro R, et al. Carvedilol for reducing portal pressure in primary prophylaxis of variceal bleeding: a dose-response study. Aliment Pharmacol Ther 2018;47(8):1162–9.
97. Sinagra E, Perricone G, D'Amico M, et al. Systematic review with meta-analysis: the haemodynamic effects of carvedilol compared with propranolol for portal hypertension in cirrhosis. Aliment Pharmacol Ther 2014;39(6):557–68.
98. Reiberger T, Ulbrich G, Ferlitsch A, et al. Carvedilol for primary prophylaxis of variceal bleeding in cirrhotic patients with haemodynamic non-response to propranolol. Gut 2013;62(11):1634–41.
99. BOPPP trial synopsis. Available at: https://www.basl.org.uk/uploads/BOPPP_Summary_Feb2020.pdf. Accessed February 10, 2021.
100. Tolman KG. Defining patient risks from expanded preventive therapies. Am J Cardiol 2000;85(12a):15e–9e.
101. Kim RG, Loomba R, Prokop LJ, et al. Statin use and risk of cirrhosis and related complications in patients with chronic liver diseases: a systematic review and meta-analysis. Clin Gastroenterol Hepatol 2017;15(10):1521–30.
102. Chang CH, Chang YC, Lee YC, et al. Severe hepatic injury associated with different statins in patients with chronic liver disease: a nationwide population-based cohort study. J Gastroenterol Hepatol 2015;30(1):155–62.
103. Abraldes JG, Villanueva C, Aracil C, et al. Addition of simvastatin to standard therapy for the prevention of variceal rebleeding does not reduce rebleeding but increases survival in patients with cirrhosis. Gastroenterology 2016;150(5):1160–70.
104. Abraldes JG, Albillos A, Banares R, et al. Simvastatin lowers portal pressure in patients with cirrhosis and portal hypertension: a randomized controlled trial. Gastroenterology 2009;136(5):1651–8.

105. Pollo-Flores P, Soldan M, Santos UC, et al. Three months of simvastatin therapy vs. placebo for severe portal hypertension in cirrhosis: a randomized controlled trial. Dig Liver Dis 2015;47(11):957–63.
106. Bishnu S, Ahammed SM, Sarkar A, et al. Effects of atorvastatin on portal hemodynamics and clinical outcomes in patients with cirrhosis with portal hypertension: a proof-of-concept study. Eur J Gastroenterol Hepatol 2018;30(1):54–9.
107. Multi-center study of the effects of simvastatin on hepatic decompensation and death in subjects presenting with high-risk compensated cirrhosis (SACRED). Available at: https://clinicaltrials.gov/ct2/show/NCT03654053. Accessed February 10, 2021.
108. Efficacy of the Combination of Simvastatin Plus Rifaximin in Patients With Decompensated Cirrhosis to Prevent ACLF Development (2018-001698-25). Available at: https://clinicaltrials.gov/ct2/show/NCT03780673. Accessed February 10, 2021.
109. Mendoza YP, Rodrigues SG, Bosch J, et al. Effect of poorly absorbable antibiotics on hepatic venous pressure gradient in cirrhosis: a systematic review and meta-analysis. Dig Liver Dis 2020;52(9):958–65.

Prevention of Variceal Bleeding and Rebleeding by Nonselective Beta-Blockers
A Tailored Approach

Mathias Jachs, MD[a,b,c], Thomas Reiberger, MD[a,b,c],*

KEYWORDS

- Portal hypertension • Variceal bleeding • Adrenergic beta blockers

KEY POINTS

- Nonselective beta-blockers are the cornerstone of medical therapy for the prevention of variceal bleeding and rebleeding.
- Recent studies have shown that nonselective beta-blockers not only decrease bleeding rates, but also prolong decompensation-free survival in compensated cirrhosis.
- Hepatic venous pressure gradient-guided therapy is the gold standard for the prophylaxis of variceal bleeding. Endoscopy represents a widely available alternative for prestratification and prognostication of patients.
- A tailored, individualized approach to nonselective beta-blocker therapy in the prevention of first variceal bleeding and rebleeding based on hepatic venous pressure gradient availability or varix status is proposed.

BACKGROUND

Two major pathophysiologic factors contribute to elevated levels of portal pressure in patients with cirrhosis: increased intrahepatic (sinusoidal) vascular resistance and increased portal blood inflow. Over the natural course of advanced chronic liver disease (ACLD), portal pressure rises, eventually surpassing the threshold of 10 mmHg or greater that defines clinically significant portal hypertension (CSPH).[1] In the setting of CSPH, progressive peripheral and splanchnic vasodilation ultimately lead to increases in both heart rate and cardiac output, defining the hyperdynamic circulatory portal-hypertensive syndrome.[2] Endoscopic screening for gastroesophageal varices

[a] Division of Gastroenterology and Hepatology, Department of Medicine III, Medical University of Vienna, Waehringer Guertel 18-20, Vienna A-1090, Austria; [b] Vienna Hepatic Hemodynamic Lab, Medical University of Vienna, Vienna, Austria; [c] Christian Doppler Lab for Portal Hypertension and Liver Fibrosis, Medical University of Vienna, Vienna, Austria
* Corresponding author. Division of Gastroenterology and Hepatology, Department of Medicine III, Waehringer Guertel 18-20, Vienna A-1090, Austria.
E-mail address: thomas.reiberger@meduniwien.ac.at

Clin Liver Dis 25 (2021) 311–326
https://doi.org/10.1016/j.cld.2021.01.004
1089-3261/21/© 2021 The Authors. Published by Elsevier Inc. This is an open access article under the CC BY license (http://creativecommons.org/licenses/by/4.0/).

(GEV) is traditionally most commonly used in clinical practice to assess the presence of CSPH; however, the presence of other portosystemic collaterals on cross-sectional imaging[3] and measurement of hepatic venous pressure gradient (HVPG)[4] allow an early diagnosis of CSPH when GEVs may not yet be present. Importantly, portal pressure, that is, the HVPG, is the main determinant for the risk of GEVs to rupture and to cause acute variceal bleeding, which is still associated with considerable mortality of up to 20%.[5]

Hemodynamic changes in patients with portal hypertension are predominantly mediated through activation of the sympathetic nervous system, and in turn, beta-adrenergic blockade through nonselective beta-blockers (NSBBs) decreases the portal pressure, thereby decreasing the risk of variceal bleeding. Thus, NSBBs represent the medical treatment of choice both for primary[6–8] and secondary[9,10] prophylaxis of acute variceal bleeding. The therapeutic effect of carvedilol as an NSBB with additional anti-α1-adrenergic activity that has a stronger effect on portal pressure as well as on systemic vasodilation has been established in the setting of primary prophylaxis,[11–13] but the evidence for its role in secondary prophylaxis[12,14] and in the setting of advanced disease with ascites[15–17] is still limited. Despite the strong body of evidence for the efficacy of NSBBs in the prevention of bleeding and potential other complications of CSPH, clinicians sometimes face difficult decisions regarding NSBB therapy in individual patients owing to side effects and tolerability issues, as well as concerns about safety in certain patient cohorts. Therefore, this article aims to provide a comprehensive review of NSBB therapy in different stages of portal hypertension, arguing for a tailored and individualized approach for the use of NSBBs for the prevention of first variceal bleeding and rebleeding.

DIAGNOSIS OF CLINICALLY SIGNIFICANT PORTAL HYPERTENSION AND ASSESSING HEMODYNAMIC RESPONSE TO NONSELECTIVE BETA-BLOCKER THERAPY BY MEASUREMENT OF THE HEPATIC VENOUS PRESSURE GRADIENT

The measurement of the HVPG represents the current gold standard for the diagnosis and monitoring of portal hypertension.[4,18] Although the procedure is invasive and requires considerable expertise and specialized infrastructure, in trained hands the measurement of the HVPG is a safe and reproducible way to evaluate portal pressure and has indisputable advantages.[4] Importantly, compensated patients might have already developed CSPH, which is associated with an important prognostic implication,[19] whereas the clinical signs of CSPH such as varices, portosystemic collaterals, and ascites occur only subsequently after CSPH has devleoped.[20] Not all patients with ACLD will show a decrease in portal pressure with NSBB treatment[21] and the efficacy of NSBB is mostly evident after CSPH has developed, that is, when HVPG is 10 mmHg or greater and splanchnic vasodilation is present, as elegantly shown by Villanueva and colleagues[22] in a mechanistic study: In their study, the authors compared the effects of NSBBs in patients with subclinical portal hypertension, that is, an HVPG of 6 to 9 mmHg, versus patients with CSPH (HVPG $\geq$10 mmHg). It was found that mean relative decreases were significantly higher (−16%) in patients with CSPH, as compared with patients with subclinical portal hypertension (−8%). This result explains why NSBBs were shown to be generally ineffective in the setting of preprimary prophylaxis, that is, in patients subclinical portal hypertension who have not yet developed varices.[23]

Sequential HVPG measurements before and after NSBB treatment initiation represent the only validated means to monitor the chronic hemodynamic effects of NSBBs, that is, to assess the hemodynamic HVPG response. The HVPG response is defined as a decrease to absolute values of 12 mmHg or less or a relative decrease of 10% or more (primary prophylaxis)[13] or of 20% or more (secondary prophylaxis).[20] The achievement of an HVPG response is an excellent predictor of a negligible risk of variceal bleeding and a low risk for mortality in the setting of secondary prophylaxis.[24] However, the evaluation of chronic HVPG response by sequential HVPG measurements is resource intensive and, thus, is mostly performed only in specialized centers and/or within an academic or trial setting. Additionally, the predictive value of sequential HVPG measurements is limited by the potential loss of the HVPG response during follow-up that can be related to modifications of the NSBB dose, alcohol intake,[25] and worsening of liver function as by natural history of the underlying etiology of ACLD.[26] However, as of this writing, no other biomarker has shown comparable predictive quality in comparison with the invasive assessment of HVPG response. Although the achievement of an acute hemodynamic response to intravenous propranolol yielded prognostic value, it may not essentially correlate with a chronic HVPG response,[27] especially when oral carvedilol is used later,[11] however, only a single procedure of liver vein catheterization is required.[24,27]

NONINVASIVE DIAGNOSIS OF CLINICALLY SIGNIFICANT PORTAL HYPERTENSION AND DYNAMIC SURROGATES OF HEMODYNAMIC RESPONSE TO NONSELECTIVE BETA-BLOCKERS

Among potential noninvasive markers for CSPH, the measurement of liver[28] and spleen stiffness[29] by different ultrasound-based elastography methods, spleen diameter,[30,31] platelet count and von Willebrand factor[32] have been widely assessed and have been integrated into composite scores for prediction of CSPH or ruling out varices needing treatment.[30,33] Numerous other noninvasive and largely imaging-based methods have been assessed as dynamic surrogates for an HVPG response; changes in liver stiffness correlated well with changes in HVPG in a small cohort (n = 23) of patients, but have not yet been validated in a larger prospective study.[34] In contrast, changes in spleen stiffness—which at least in theory better reflects the portal venous inflow component—as estimated by transient elastography[29] and shear wave elastography[35] showed promising results. Last, it was shown that MRI-based estimated liver perfusion showed a strong positive correlation with HVPG; however, it remains to be explored in future prospective trials whether MRI perfusion studies are able to predict clinical outcomes.[36]

Further studies on non–imaging-based HVPG response surrogates have demonstrated that Ras homolog family member A (RhoA) and RhoA-kinase 2 transcription in the antrum mucosa[37] as well as serum levels of a phosphatidylcholine and a free fatty acid[38] correlated well with acute HVPG-response to intravenous propranolol and, thus, these surrogates warrant further investigation. Importantly, potential predictors that might support clinicians in the evaluation of benefits of NSBB therapy do not solely comprise hemodynamic markers, because beneficial nonhemodynamic effects of NSBB treatment have been reported in previous studies. These include a decrease in markers of bacterial translocation mediated by an amelioration of intestinal permeability.[39] Additionally, NSBB-related effects on markers of systemic inflammation were demonstrated in patients with acute-on-chronic liver failure.[40] Therefore, it should be investigated whether these novel biomarkers are able to reflect changes in HVPG and/or dynamic NSBB-related benefits in patients with CSPH. Ultimately, noninvasive biomarkers of CSPH should be tested for their prognostic value in patients with ACLD and if they are suited to be included in comprehensive risk scores for refined prognostication in personalized medicine.

STATE OF THE ART IN PRIMARY PROPHYLAXIS OF VARICEAL BLEEDING

Since the first reports on their beneficial effects in the 1980s, NSBBs have been the cornerstone of medical treatment in portal hypertension owing to their mitigating effects on portal pressure that are paralleled by lower risks of variceal bleeding and rebleeding. Thus, the European Association for the Study of the Liver (EASL), the American Association for the Study of the Liver (AASLD), and the Baveno VI guidelines have recommended the use of NSBBs for primary and secondary (in combination with endoscopic band ligation [EBL]) prophylaxis of variceal bleeding in cirrhotic patients with GEVs.[20,41,42] Still, concerns about the safety profile of NSBBs and potential deleterious effects in advanced cirrhosis have been raised in recent years, and the evidence for the benefits of NSBB treatment is weaker in certain patient cohorts, for example, in patients with refractory ascites.[15]

As outlined elsewhere in this article, HVPG-guided NSBB therapy is preferably used in all patients with CSPH to precisely predict and monitor the benefits of NSBB treatment and optimize the patient's clinical outcome.[43] However, we also acknowledge the limited availability of HVPG measurement, as well as its cost and invasive nature. Therefore, endoscopic screening for the presence of GEVs and, thus, evaluation for the risk of variceal bleeding, is currently used most widely. The subsequent overview on the evidence for best clinical practice for primary and secondary prophylaxis of variceal bleeding is, therefore, based on the prestratification of patients by the presence or absence of GEVs. This strategy provides a clinically relevant and widely feasible approach for a tailored NSBB treatment for the primary and secondary prophylaxis of variceal hemorrhage, which is complemented by data on the choice of NSBB type and doses in distinct clinical scenarios.

Primary Prophylaxis: Patients with No or Small Varices

The benefit of NSBB treatment in patients without varices was thoroughly investigated in a study by Groszmann and colleagues,[23] in which patients with cirrhosis and portal hypertension as defined by an HVPG of 6 mmHg or greater were randomly assigned to timolol or placebo. Patients were followed for a median of almost 5 years, and about 40% in both treatment groups reached the primary end point that comprised development of varices or variceal bleeding. Importantly, decreases in HVPG of 10% or greater were more frequent in the timolol group, as compared with placebo (53% vs 38%); however, the authors also reported a significantly higher rate of serious adverse events in the timolol group (18% vs 6%). Thus, there is no evidence for NSBB treatment for (pre-)primary prophylaxis in patients without CSPH and without varices as of today.

Recently, the PREDESCI study that was conducted by Villanueva and colleagues[44] demonstrated that patients with compensated cirrhosis with CSPH without high-risk varices show lower rates of first decompensation under ongoing NSBB therapy. In a cohort of 201 patients (propranolol: n = 67; carvedilol: n = 33; inactive treatment: n = 101), the primary end point that was defined as ascites development, bleeding, or hepatic encephalopathy occurred in 16 patients (16%) in the active treatment cohort, as compared with 27 patients (27%) in the placebo cohort (hazard ratio, 0.51 [95% confidence interval, 0.26–0.97], $P = .041$). Serious adverse events were comparable between the 2 cohorts. This study demonstrated that NSBBs not only decrease the risk for variceal bleeding, but also modify the risk of first decompensation in compensated cirrhosis in general. The ultimate conclusion of this study is, thus, to consider initiation of NSBB therapy upon diagnosis of CSPH because NSBB seem to increase decompensation-free survival, regardless of varix status. Of note, this recommendation has not yet been implemented into international guidelines.

However, there are controversial results on preprimary prophylaxis of variceal bleeding and on prevention of varix size progression from randomized controlled trials (RCTs) and a subsequent meta-analysis available.[45–47] These conflicting results were likely obtained owing to the fact that different proportions of patients without varices and, importantly, also without CSPH were enrolled. Consequently, our research group repeated the meta-analysis, including only studies on patients with small varices (CSPH) at baseline,[48] also considering the results of the RCT by Bhardwaj and colleagues[49] observing a lower risk for progression from small to large varices with carvedilol therapy. Our updated meta-analysis revealed a trend toward a lower risk of large varix development under NSBB therapy in the fixed effect model. Of note, NSBB treatment is not recommended by recent guidelines for preprimary prophylaxis or for the prevention of varix progression. However, we argue for further research on the beneficial effects of NSBB as soon as the diagnosis of CSPH has been established, regardless of the presence or absence of varices.

Primary Prophylaxis: Patients with Medium to Large or High-Risk Small Varices

The current guidelines recommend the use of NSSBs to prevent variceal bleeding in patients with medium to large varices or high-risk small varices.[20,41,42] NSBB treatment in primary prophylaxis is associated with an absolute risk reduction of −10% (25% vs 15%, as compared with inactive treatment) during 2-year follow-up, which translates into a number needed to treat (NNT) of 10 (10 patients need to be treated with NSBBs to prevent one episode of variceal hemorrhage within 2 years of follow-up).[50] When only treating patients with medium to large varices, the absolute risk reduction is −16% (NNT = 6).[50] Slightly different criteria for the definition of high-risk small varices have been proposed: Although the AASLD definition encompasses small varices in Child-Turcotte-Pugh score (Child) stage B/C or the presence of red wale marks,[42] the EASL definition is restricted to small varices in Child C patients or the presence of red wale marks.[41]

Concern about NSBB treatment owing to small varices without red wale marks in Child B/C was raised by Kalambokis and colleagues.[51,52] In their cohort study, they demonstrated an increased risk of the hepatorenal syndrome and of overall mortality related to propranolol treatment in patients with Child B/C disease. Accordingly, it may be wise to base the decision of NSBB treatment initiation both on endoscopic findings of red wale marks and the severity of liver dysfunction, that is, Child stage. Still, no adequately powered prospective study specifically addressed the effects of NSBB treatment in patients with small varices and advanced liver dysfunction as of this writing, and we encourage future studies on this field of primary prophylaxis.

In patients who have already developed medium to large varices, NSBB treatment or EBL are recommended for the primary prophylaxis of variceal bleeding.[20,41,42] The choice between NSBB treatment or EBL should consider patient preference, availability of proficient endoscopy personnel and infrastructure, and patient intolerance or adverse events under treatment. A meta-analysis including 19 studies showed no difference in overall mortality or bleeding-related mortality between primary prophylaxis with NSBB versus EBL.[53] However, a more recent meta-analysis including 32 RCTs with a total of 3362 patients with large varices and no prior history of bleeding showed that NSBB monotherapy was associated with a better safety profile and an improvement in overall mortality, as compared with EBL.[54] Importantly, although EBL is associated with a lower rate of adverse events overall, it may cause more severe and potentially life-threatening complications, such as EBL-associated ulcer bleeding. Moreover, in contrast with medical therapy with NSBBs, EBL does not impact the underlying levels of portal pressure and has no hemodynamic or disease-modifying effects. Last, EBL is associated with significantly lower time and cost efficiency as compared with NSBB treatment. However, EBL treatment is prone to achieve variceal obliteration that could lead to long anxiety-free intervals in high-risk patients and does not rely as much on treatment adherence, which is why EBL might be preferable in some scenarios.[55] In contrast, it may be hypothesized that the results of the PRE-DESCI study—although excluding patients with high-risk varices—extend to all compensated patients under NSBB treatment for primary bleeding prophylaxis. Thus, patients might benefit more from NSBB treatment because it may lead to longer decompensation-free survival, as compared with endoscopic therapy.[44] Ultimately, both treatment options are validated for use in primary prophylaxis in patients with medium to large varices, and clinicians should always consider the individual patient's opinion in the process of shared decision-making.

Carvedilol Versus Propranolol and Other Conventional Nonselective Beta-Blockers

Carvedilol, in contrast with conventional NSBBs, has additional anti-α-1-adrenergic activity, which makes the compound more potent in decreasing portal pressure.[56] It was shown in a meta-analysis that carvedilol leads to stronger decreases in portal pressure levels, as compared with propranolol (−22% vs −16%).[57] Importantly, carvedilol may lead to stronger decreases in mean arterial pressure owing to its anti-α-1-adrenergic activity in comparison with conventional NSBBs. In a meta-analysis by Sinagra and associates,[57] carvedilol showed a tendency toward a stronger decrease of mean arterial pressure levels, as compared with propranolol treatment (weighed mean difference, −10.40% vs 6.35%). Moreover, it seems that higher doses of carvedilol (>12.5 mg/d) do not lead to further reductions of HVPG, although they are associated with lower mean arterial pressure levels.[11] Therefore, carvedilol should not be used in doses higher than 12.5 mg/d, with the exception of patients who show increased levels of arterial blood pressure and would need higher doses of carvedilol for antihypertensive treatment anyway.

In the setting of primary prophylaxis, an RCT comparing carvedilol versus EBL found lower rates of bleeding in the carvedilol cohort (10% vs EBL, 23%), although no differences regarding bleeding-related and overall mortality were found.[12] A second RCT by Shah and colleagues[58] also showed a trend toward lower bleeding rates with carvedilol (6.9% vs EBL, 8.5%). Of note, serious adverse events were more common in the EBL group.

Although there is no head-to-head RCT that investigated the effects of carvedilol versus propranolol in primary prophylaxis, in a study that was conducted by our group, we found that carvedilol treatment led to HVPG response, that is, a 20% or greater decrease in the HVPG or a decrease to an absolute HVPG value of less than 12 mmHg, in a high proportion (58%) of patients who did not respond to propranolol treatment.[11] Hemodynamic nonresponders to carvedilol were treated with EBL. Lower rates of variceal bleeding (carvedilol, 5%; propranolol, 11%; EBL, 25%) and mortality (carvedilol, 11%; propranolol, 14%; EBL, 31%) were observed among hemodynamic responders to NSBB treatment, as compared with EBL treatment. In conclusion, we recommend carvedilol for the primary prophylaxis of variceal bleeding in patients with compensated cirrhosis owing to its higher potency to reduce portal pressure as compared with propranolol.

Two RCTs compared carvedilol versus nadolol with or without isosorbidmononitrate in the setting of secondary prophylaxis.[59,60] In the study conducted by Lo and colleagues,[59] comparable rebleeding rates (61% and 62%) were found, the survival was similar, and serious adverse events were more common in the nadolol with or without isosorbidmononitrate group. Stanley and colleagues,[60] who conducted the second RCT, found a rebleeding rate of 36%, irrespective of treatment. Notably, there was a trend toward an increased survival in the carvedilol group, whereas serious adverse event rates were similar between the 2 groups. Despite the promising results of these 2 RCTs, standalone carvedilol treatment has never been compared with the current state-of-the-art therapy for secondary prophylaxis, that is, combined NSBB and EBL treatment; thus, the Baveno VI faculty did not recommend its use for secondary prophylaxis.[20] In summary, carvedilol is a potent compound for the reduction of portal pressure both in primary and secondary prophylaxis. However, we do not recommend the use of carvedilol in patients with severe ascites, because carvedilol seems to impair circulatory homeostasis and this setting.[15]

STATE OF THE ART IN SECONDARY PROPHYLAXIS OF VARICEAL BLEEDING

The current guidelines recommend a combination of NSBB treatment and EBL for the secondary prophylaxis of recurrent variceal bleeding.[20,41,42] These recommendations are based on 2 meta-analyses that confirmed the protective benefits of combined medical (NSBBs with or without isosorbidmononitrate) and endoscopic therapy, that is, EBL.[61,62] Importantly, both meta-analyses showed a trend toward a lower risk of overall mortality in the combined treatment group, as compared with the EBL monotherapy group, whereas the addition of EBL to NSBB treatment was not associated with decreases in mortality. Thus, NSBBs are the cornerstone of treatment in the prophylaxis of recurrent bleeding. Interestingly, the impact of NSBB treatment on mortality seems to be restricted to secondary prophylaxis,[14] and it may be hypothesized that nonhemodynamic effects, such as a decrease in bacterial translocation,[39] but possibly also anti-inflammatory effects related to NSBBs[40] might contribute to this finding.

Patients for whom NSSBs are contraindicated or who do not tolerate medical therapy, should be evaluated for alternative treatment, for example, transjugular intrahepatic portosystemic shunt implantation.[41]

DOSE TITRATION AND NONSELECTIVE BETA-BLOCKER TREATMENT IN PATIENTS WITH ASCITES

The limited availability of HVPG measurement forces many clinicians to rely on the aforementioned noninvasive signs and biomarkers for the diagnosis of portal hypertension and, thus, the initiation and monitoring of prophylactic NSBB therapy. The absence of HVPG measurement availability often necessitates empiric treatment and titration of NSBB doses, usually to a certain target heart rate at 60 bpm[63] or even 50 to 55 bpm.[41] However, this concept is challenged by the fact that, in decompensated patients, worsening of liver function is paralleled by more pronounced sympathetic nervous system activation, leading to higher heart rates and a progressive hyperdynamic state, which implies that those patients would need higher NSBB doses to achieve those target heart rates. However, cardiac reserve is limited in end-stage cirrhotic patients, for example, in patients with refractory ascites, and SerSté and colleagues[15] were the first to report deleterious effects of NSBB treatment in patients with refractory ascites. Of note, one-half of the patients (46.7%) received high-dose propranolol treatment (160 mg/d) in their prospective cohort study. Recently, it has been demonstrated in an elegant quasi-experimental, prospective proof-of-concept study by Téllez and colleagues[64] that, in patients with refractory ascites, high-dose treatment with propranolol might indeed be detrimental to patients' circulatory homeostasis and kidney function, which could potentially worsen their prognosis. Importantly, a Danish nationwide study showed a differential impact of NSBB treatment in

81 patients with spontaneous bacterial peritonitis.[65] Although high-dose propranolol treatment, that is, 160 mg/d, was associated with increased mortality after spontaneous bacterial peritonitis (hazard ratio, 2.27, unadjusted analysis), doses of 80 mg or less per day were associated with decreased mortality after spontaneous bacterial peritonitis (hazard ratio, 0.56).

Although the potential harmful effects of (high-dose) NSBB treatment in patients with advanced disease warrant further investigation, there is evidence that carefully titrated and closely monitored NSBB treatment is not harmful to patients with ascites in general.[66–69] This finding was corroborated by the results of 2 meta-analyses. The first one concluded that NSBB treatment was not associated with an increased risk of mortality in patients with ascites or refractory ascites,[16] and the second one found that the achievement of an HVPG response was associated with a significantly lower odds of decompensation, liver transplantation, and death, regardless of the presence of ascites.[17]

The results of these studies indicate that, in patients with advanced disease, NSBB treatment seems to be a valid option for the prophylaxis of variceal bleeding, although hemodynamic treatment targets and maximum doses may have to be reconsidered. However, no RCT has thoroughly investigated the titration schemes of NSBB treatment, and the need for international recommendations remains unmet. In the absence of evidence-based guidelines on NSBB dose regimens in advanced decompensated cirrhosis, clinicians should make decisions based on individual risk/benefit considerations.[20] Signs of systemic circulatory dysfunction, severe hyponatremia,[70] a low mean arterial pressure,[71] low cardiac output,[72] and increasing levels of serum creatinine[73] allow for the identification of vulnerable patients, in which dose reduction or transient or permanent treatment discontinuation might be warranted.

Therefore, the Baveno VI consensus proposed that, in patients with refractory ascites and (i) a systolic arterial blood pressure of less than 90 mmHg, or (ii) a serum creatinine of greater than 1.5 mg/dL, or (iii) hyponatremia of less than 130 mmol/L, dose reduction or treatment discontinuation should be considered.[20]

SUMMARY: A TAILORED APPROACH TO NONSELECTIVE BETA-BLOCKER TREATMENT

NSBB treatment markedly reduces the risk of variceal bleeding in primary (absolute risk reduction, 25%–15%; NNT = 10) and secondary prophylaxis (absolute risk reduction, 63%–42%; NNT = 5), as compared with inactive treatment.[50] Accordingly, NSBBs are recommended both in primary and secondary prophylaxis by current guidelines. Although NSBBs are the first choice of medical therapy for the prevention of variceal bleeding, a considerable number of patients have to be treated to prevent a single episode of variceal hemorrhage. In addition, a large proportion of patients do not achieve the HVPG response that is associated with considerably lower bleeding rates and a lower risk of mortality.[21,50] Therefore, clinicians need to be endowed with reliable, feasible methods to accurately predict the benefit of NSBB treatment in their individual patients.

A summary of our proposed treatment algorithm is given in **Fig. 1**. Sequential HVPG measurements before and under ongoing NSBB remain the most reliable but invasive tool to assess the individual patient's response to treatment: Achieving a chronic HVPG response, that is, a reduction of 10% or more (primary prophylaxis) or 20% or more (secondary prophylaxis), or to an absolute value 12 mmHg or less is associated with a strong decrease in bleeding rates and increase in survival in secondary prophylaxis.[7,74] The evaluation of an acute response to NSBB can predict

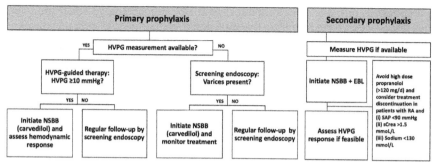

Fig. 1. A tailored approach to NSBB therapy for the prevention of first and recurrent variceal bleeding in patients with portal hypertension. The treatment algorithm for the use of NSBBs for the prevention of variceal bleeding in primary and secondary prophylaxis is shown. In primary prophylaxis, we recommend carvedilol/NSBB as the treatment of choice, whereas EBL is an alternative to NSBB therapy in case of safety or tolerability concerns or patient preference. The doses of carvedilol/NSBB should be slowly titrated and may not exceed 12.5 mg/d for carvedilol or 120 mg/d for propranolol. Close monitoring is warranted in patients with advanced liver disease considering Baveno VI recommendations for the use of NSBB therapy in patients with refractory ascites. EBL, endoscopic banding ligature; RA, refractory ascites; SAP, systolic arterial pressure; sCrea, serum creatinine.

decompensating events accurately, but still requires 1 invasive HVPG measurement.[27,75] Despite its obvious limitations in the daily clinical routine, we argue for HVPG-guided therapy in all stages of portal hypertension, because its implementation can improve clinical outcomes in patients with portal hypertension.[43] Nonetheless, the field of noninvasive surrogates for the monitoring of NSBB treatment effects remains highly relevant, and promising results were demonstrated for sequential ultrasound-based elastography assessment of the spleen.[35]

If endoscopic evaluation for GEVs is the only means of assessing portal hypertension, the initiation of NSBB treatment is recommended in all patients with medium to large varices or with high-risk varices.[20,41,42] Although patients without varices should undergo regular follow-up endoscopy for early detection of varix development, we recommend NSBB therapy also for patients with small varices even without additional risk factors such as red spot signs or advanced liver dysfunction, that is, Child stages B or C. Recent data also suggest that NSBBs prolong decompensation-free survival in compensated patients with CSPH without high-risk varices, potentially owing to nonhemodynamic effects, and thus, we recommend NSBB treatment in all of these patients.[44] In primary prophylaxis, we prefer carvedilol over propranolol owing to its greater potency to decrease portal pressure that is accompanied by a similar safety profile, as compared with propranolol.[11,12,57,58] In patients with low arterial pressure or slow heart rate, cautious dose titration under close monitoring of side effects is warranted.[20]

NSBBs combined with EBL for variceal obliteration remains the standard of care for secondary prophylaxis of variceal bleeding.[20,41,42] In patients with end-stage liver disease, for example, patients with refractory ascites, we tend to avoid carvedilol given the current lack of prospective studies that specifically addressed its use in this setting. In patient with ascites, the NSBB dose should be carefully titrated, and changing to EBL treatment in patients with refractory ascites who show a systolic arterial pressure of less than 90 mmHg, hyponatremia of less than 130 mmol/L, or a serum creatinine of more than 1.5 mg/dL should be considered.[20] We want to emphasize, however, that in contrast with EBL monotherapy, NSBB treatment does not only decrease the risk of bleeding and even mortality in secondary prophylaxis, but it is also associated with potential nonhemodynamic benefits as compared with EBL.[39,40]

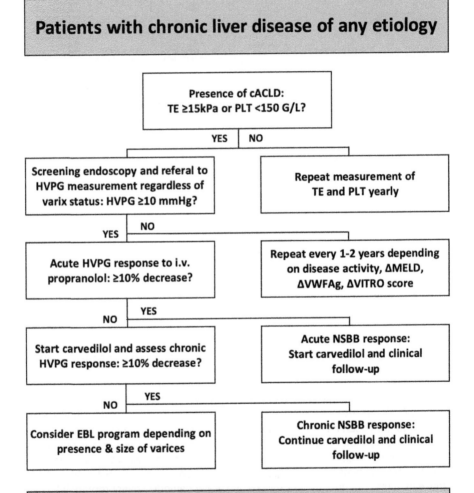

Patients with chronic liver disease of any etiology

Presence of cACLD:
TE ≥15kPa or PLT <150 G/L?

YES | NO

Screening endoscopy and referal to HVPG measurement regardless of varix status: HVPG ≥10 mmHg?

Repeat measurement of TE and PLT yearly

YES | NO

Acute HVPG response to i.v. propranolol: ≥10% decrease?

Repeat every 1-2 years depending on disease activity, ΔMELD, ΔVWFAg, ΔVITRO score

NO | YES

Start carvedilol and assess chronic HVPG response: ≥10% decrease?

Acute NSBB response: Start carvedilol and clinical follow-up

NO | YES

Consider EBL program depending on presence & size of varices

Chronic NSBB response: Continue carvedilol and clinical follow-up

Clinical follow-up for acute decompensation (AD) or ACLF:
1) Evaluate NSBB type and dose during AD/ACLF
2) Try to keep patient on NSBB if possible or reinitiate therapy after stabilazation
3) Assess ΔMELD, ΔVWFAg, ΔVITRO after stabilazation
4) Consider reassessment of HVPG
5) In case of variceal beeding: start EBL program in addition to NSBB

Fig. 2. The Viennese HVPG-based NSBB treatment algorithm in patients with cACLD. A summary of the Viennese algorithm on HVPG-guided NSBB therapy in patients with cACLD. ACLF, acute-on-chronic liver failure; AD, acute decompensation; cACLD, compensated advanced chronic liver disease; EBL, endoscopic banding ligature; MELD, Model for End-stage Liver Disease; PLT, platelet count; TE, transient elastography; VITRO, von Willebrand factor/PLT ratio; VWFAg, von Willebrand factor antigen activity.

We propose a patient-centered, tailored approach for the prevention of bleeding in patients with portal hypertension that considers the distinct stage of CSPH and preferably the individual patient's HVPG levels, or endoscopic varix stage for stratification.

OUTLOOK: THE VIENNESE APPROACH TO HEPATIC VENOUS PRESSURE GRADIENT-GUIDED NONSELECTIVE BETA-BLOCKER THERAPY IN PATIENTS WITH COMPENSATED ADVANCED CHRONIC LIVER DISEASE

Considering recent evidence[44,48,76] on top of international (Baveno VI,[20] AASLD,[42] EASL[41]) and national recommendations (Billroth III consensus),[77] we propose an individualized NSBB treatment algorithm for patients with compensated ACLD (**Fig. 2**). Our algorithm is based on 2 principles: (i) noninvasive risk stratification and (ii) HVPG-guided diagnosis and treatment of CSPH. In patients with suspected compensated ACLD as evident by significantly elevated liver stiffness ($\geq$15 kPa) or thrombocytopenia (platelet count of <150 g/L) we conduct screening endoscopy for the early detection of varices, but always also recommend HVPG measurement for the early detection of CSPH. If CSPH is present and the patient shows an acute 10% or greater HVPG response to intravenously applied propranolol, carvedilol (titrated to 12.5 mg/d) therapy is initiated. In case of nonresponse to intravenous propranolol, we initiate carvedilol nonetheless and assess chronic hemodynamic response after 4 to 5 weeks. In patients who achieve a chronic HVPG response to carvedilol, we keep the patient on carvedilol. However, in patients who do not achieve a chronic HVPG response to carvedilol, EBL is recommended for primary prophylaxis in case of large varices and/or red spot signs.

When patients progress from compensated to decompensated disease, we recommend reevaluating the type and dose of NSBB (eg, switch to propranolol or decrease the dose of NSBB in patients with refractory ascites and low arterial blood pressure). Importantly, NSBB treatment should not be discontinued in acute decompensation as long as the patient is hemodynamically stable, and therapy should be reinitiated as soon as possible in patients in whom transient treatment discontinuation cannot be avoided. In case of significant increases in Model for End-stage Liver Disease score or other noninvasive biomarkers for disease severity (such as von Willebrand factor antigen activity or the VITRO score), we aim for a reassessment of HVPG after stabilization of the patient. Last, if acute variceal bleeding occurs, we add EBL to NSBB-based therapy for secondary prophylaxis of variceal bleeding. A summary of our Viennese approach to HVPG-guided therapy in patients with compensated ACLD is given in **Fig. 2**.

CLINICS CARE POINTS

- The measurement of the hepatic venous pressure gradient (HVPG) is the gold standard for assessing the severity of portal hypertension and enables the detection of clinically significant portal hypertension (CSPH, i.e. HVPG $\geq$10 mmHg) before varices or other CSPH-related complications develop.

- NSBB treatment should be initated in all patients with CSPH, and HVPG-guided therapy should be applied whenever available. In settings where the measurement of the HVPG is not available, screening endoscopy should be performed. NSBB therapy should be initiated upon detection of varices.

- In patients with compensated liver cirrhosis, carvedilol is the treatment of choice for primary prophylaxis of variceal bleeding – dosed at 12.5 mg once daily.

322 Jachs & Reiberger

- In patients with advanced disease, i.e. refractory ascites, propranolol should be preferred over carvedilol treatment but high doses of propranolol (>120 mg daily) should be avoided due to potential deleterious effects on circulatory homestasis by blunting critical sympathetic compensatory mechanisms.
- In case of intolerance or contraindications to NSBB treatment, endoscopic band ligation (EBL) should be considered for primary prophylaxis. Combined NSBB and EBL is the treatment of choice in secondary prophylaxis.

DISCLOSURE

M. Jachs has nothing to declare. T. Reiberger received grant support from AbbVie, Boehringer-Ingelheim, Gilead, MSD, Philips Healthcare, Gore; speaking honoraria from AbbVie, Gilead, Gore, Intercept, Roche, MSD; consulting/advisory board fee from AbbVie, Bayer, Boehringer-Ingelheim, Gilead, Intercept, MSD, Siemens; and travel support from Boehringer-Ingelheim, Gilead and Roche.

REFERENCES

1. Iwakiri Y. Pathophysiology of portal hypertension. Portal Hypertens 2014;18(2): 281–91.
2. Bolognesi M, Di Pascoli M, Verardo A, et al. Splanchnic vasodilation and hyperdynamic circulatory syndrome in cirrhosis. World J Gastroenterol 2014;20(10): 2555–63.
3. Simón-Talero M, Roccarina D, Martínez J, et al. Association between portosystemic shunts and increased complications and mortality in patients with cirrhosis. Gastroenterology 2018;154(6):1694–705.e4.
4. Reiberger T, Schwabl P, Trauner M, et al. Measurement of the hepatic venous pressure gradient and transjugular liver biopsy. J Vis Exp 2020;(160).
5. Reverter E, Tandon P, Augustin S, et al. A MELD-based model to determine risk of mortality among patients with acute variceal bleeding. Gastroenterology 2014; 146(2):412–9.e3.
6. Poynard T, Calès P, Pasta L, et al. Beta-adrenergic-antagonist drugs in the prevention of gastrointestinal bleeding in patients with cirrhosis and esophageal varices. An analysis of data and prognostic factors in 589 patients from four randomized clinical trials. Franco-Italian Multicenter Study Group. N Engl J Med 1991;324(22):1532–8.
7. Groszmann RJ, Bosch J, Grace ND, et al. Hemodynamic events in a prospective randomized trial of propranolol versus placebo in the prevention of a first variceal hemorrhage. Gastroenterology 1990;99(5):1401–7.
8. Schepke M, Kleber G, Nürnberg D, et al. Ligation versus propranolol for the primary prophylaxis of variceal bleeding in cirrhosis. Hepatology 2004;40(1):65–72.
9. Lebrec D, Poynard T, Hillon P, et al. Propranolol for prevention of recurrent gastrointestinal bleeding in patients with cirrhosis: a controlled study. N Engl J Med 1981;305(23):1371–4.
10. Gonzalez R, Zamora J, Gomez-Camarero J, et al. Meta-analysis: combination endoscopic and drug therapy to prevent variceal rebleeding in cirrhosis. Ann Intern Med 2008;149(2):109.
11. Reiberger T, Ulbrich G, Ferlitsch A, et al. Carvedilol for primary prophylaxis of variceal bleeding in cirrhotic patients with haemodynamic non-response to propranolol. Gut 2013;62(11):1634–41.

12. Tripathi D, Ferguson JW, Kochar N, et al. Randomized controlled trial of carvedilol versus variceal band ligation for the prevention of the first variceal bleed. Hepatology 2009;50(3):825–33.
13. Schwarzer R, Kivaranovic D, Paternostro R, et al. Carvedilol for reducing portal pressure in primary prophylaxis of variceal bleeding: a dose-response study. Aliment Pharmacol Ther 2018;47(8):1162–9.
14. Pfisterer N, Dexheimer C, Fuchs E-M, et al. Betablockers do not increase efficacy of band ligation in primary prophylaxis but they improve survival in secondary prophylaxis of variceal bleeding. Aliment Pharmacol Ther 2018;47(7):966–79.
15. Sersté T, Melot C, Francoz C, et al. Deleterious effects of beta-blockers on survival in patients with cirrhosis and refractory ascites. Hepatology 2010;52(3): 1017–22.
16. Chirapongsathorn S, Valentin N, Alahdab F, et al. Nonselective β-blockers and survival in patients with cirrhosis and ascites: a systematic review and meta-analysis. Clin Gastroenterol Hepatol 2016;14(8):1096–104.e9.
17. Turco L, Villanueva C, La Mura V, et al. Lowering portal pressure improves outcomes of patients with cirrhosis, with or without ascites: a meta-analysis. Clin Gastroenterol Hepatol 2020;18(2):313–27.e6.
18. Bosch J, Abraldes JG, Berzigotti A, et al. The clinical use of HVPG measurements in chronic liver disease. Nat Rev Gastroenterol Hepatol 2009;6(10):573–82.
19. Ripoll C, Groszmann R, Garcia-Tsao G, et al. Hepatic venous pressure gradient predicts clinical decompensation in patients with compensated cirrhosis. Gastroenterology 2007;133(2):481–8.
20. de Franchis R, Baveno VI Faculty. Expanding consensus in portal hypertension: report of the Baveno VI Consensus Workshop: stratifying risk and individualizing care for portal hypertension. J Hepatol 2015;63(3):743–52.
21. Thalheimer U. Monitoring target reduction in hepatic venous pressure gradient during pharmacological therapy of portal hypertension: a close look at the evidence. Gut 2004;53(1):143–8.
22. Villanueva C, Albillos A, Genescà J, et al. Development of hyperdynamic circulation and response to β-blockers in compensated cirrhosis with portal hypertension. Hepatology 2016;63(1):197–206.
23. Groszmann RJ, Garcia-Tsao G, Bosch J, et al. Beta-blockers to prevent gastroesophageal varices in patients with cirrhosis. N Engl J Med 2005;353(21): 2254–61.
24. Mandorfer M, Hernández-Gea V, Reiberger T, et al. Hepatic venous pressure gradient response in non-selective beta-blocker treatment—is it worth measuring? Curr Hepatol Rep 2019;18(2):174–86.
25. Villanueva C, López-Balaguer JM, Aracil C, et al. Maintenance of hemodynamic response to treatment for portal hypertension and influence on complications of cirrhosis. J Hepatol 2004;40(5):757–65.
26. Merkel C, Bolognesi M, Berzigotti A, et al. Clinical significance of worsening portal hypertension during long-term medical treatment in patients with cirrhosis who had been classified as early good-responders on haemodynamic criteria. J Hepatol 2010;52(1):45–53.
27. Villanueva C, Aracil C, Colomo A, et al. Acute hemodynamic response to β-blockers and prediction of long-term outcome in primary prophylaxis of variceal bleeding. Gastroenterology 2009;137(1):119–28.
28. Reiberger T, Ferlitsch A, Payer BA, et al. Noninvasive screening for liver fibrosis and portal hypertension by transient elastography—a large single center experience. Wien Klin Wochenschr 2012;124(11–12):395–402.

29. Colecchia A, Montrone L, Scaioli E, et al. Measurement of spleen stiffness to evaluate portal hypertension and the presence of esophageal varices in patients with HCV-related cirrhosis. Gastroenterology 2012;143(3):646–54.
30. Abraldes JG, Bureau C, Stefanescu H, et al. Noninvasive tools and risk of clinically significant portal hypertension and varices in compensated cirrhosis: the "Anticipate" study. Hepatology 2016;64(6):2173–84.
31. Berzigotti A, Seijo S, Arena U, et al. Elastography, spleen size, and platelet count identify portal hypertension in patients with compensated cirrhosis. Gastroenterology 2013;144(1):102–11.e1.
32. Ferlitsch M, Reiberger T, Hoke M, et al. Von Willebrand factor as new noninvasive predictor of portal hypertension, decompensation and mortality in patients with liver cirrhosis. Hepatology 2012;56(4):1439–47.
33. Augustin S, Millán L, González A, et al. Detection of early portal hypertension with routine data and liver stiffness in patients with asymptomatic liver disease: a prospective study. J Hepatol 2014;60(3):561–9.
34. Choi S-Y, Jeong WK, Kim Y, et al. Shear-wave elastography: a noninvasive tool for monitoring changing hepatic venous pressure gradients in patients with cirrhosis. Radiology 2014;273(3):917–26.
35. Kim HY, So YH, Kim W, et al. Non-invasive response prediction in prophylactic carvedilol therapy for cirrhotic patients with esophageal varices. J Hepatol 2019;70(3):412–22.
36. Palaniyappan N, Cox E, Bradley C, et al. Non-invasive assessment of portal hypertension using quantitative magnetic resonance imaging. J Hepatol 2016; 65(6):1131–9.
37. Trebicka J, von Heydebrand M, Lehmann J, et al. Assessment of response to beta-blockers by expression of βArr2 and RhoA/ROCK2 in antrum mucosa in cirrhotic patients. J Hepatol 2016;64(6):1265–73.
38. Reverter E, Lozano JJ, Alonso C, et al. Metabolomics discloses potential biomarkers to predict the acute HVPG response to propranolol in patients with cirrhosis. Liver Int 2019;39(4):705–13.
39. Reiberger T, Ferlitsch A, Payer BA, et al. Non-selective betablocker therapy decreases intestinal permeability and serum levels of LBP and IL-6 in patients with cirrhosis. J Hepatol 2013;58(5):911–21. https://doi.org/10.1016/j.jhep.2012.12.011.
40. Mookerjee RP, Pavesi M, Thomsen KL, et al. Treatment with non-selective beta blockers is associated with reduced severity of systemic inflammation and improved survival of patients with acute-on-chronic liver failure. J Hepatol 2016;64(3):574–82.
41. Angeli P, Bernardi M, Villanueva C, et al. EASL Clinical Practice Guidelines for the management of patients with decompensated cirrhosis. J Hepatol 2018;69(2):406–60.
42. Garcia-Tsao G, Abraldes JG, Berzigotti A, et al. Portal hypertensive bleeding in cirrhosis: risk stratification, diagnosis, and management: 2016 practice guidance by the American Association for the study of liver diseases. Hepatology 2017; 65(1):310–35.
43. Villanueva C, Graupera I, Aracil C, et al. A randomized trial to assess whether portal pressure guided therapy to prevent variceal rebleeding improves survival in cirrhosis. Hepatology 2017;65(5):1693–707.
44. Villanueva C, Albillos A, Genescà J, et al. β blockers to prevent decompensation of cirrhosis in patients with clinically significant portal hypertension (PREDESCI):

a randomised, double-blind, placebo-controlled, multicentre trial. Lancet 2019; 393(10181):1597–608.

45. Merkel C, Marin R, Angeli P, et al. A placebo-controlled clinical trial of nadolol in the prophylaxis of growth of small esophageal varices in cirrhosis 1. Gastroenterology 2004;127(2):476–84.

46. Sarin SK, Mishra SR, Sharma P, et al. Early primary prophylaxis with beta-blockers does not prevent the growth of small esophageal varices in cirrhosis: a randomized controlled trial. Hepatol Int 2013;7(1):248–56.

47. Qi X-S. Nonselective beta-blockers in cirrhotic patients with no or small varices: a meta-analysis. World J Gastroenterol 2015;21(10):3100.

48. Mandorfer M, Peck-Radosavljevic M, Reiberger T. Prevention of progression from small to large varices: are we there yet? An updated meta-analysis. Gut 2017; 66(7):1347–9.

49. Bhardwaj A, Kedarisetty CK, Vashishtha C, et al. Carvedilol delays the progression of small oesophageal varices in patients with cirrhosis: a randomised placebo-controlled trial. Gut 2017;66(10):1838–43.

50. D'Amico G, Pagliaro L, Bosch J. Pharmacological treatment of portal hypertension: an evidence-based approach. Semin Liver Dis 1999;19(04):475–505.

51. Kalambokis GN, Christodoulou D, Baltayiannis G, et al. Propranolol use beyond 6 months increases mortality in patients with Child-Pugh C cirrhosis and ascites: correspondence. Hepatology 2016;64(5):1806–8.

52. Kalambokis GN, Baltayiannis G, Christou L, et al. Red signs and not severity of cirrhosis should determine non-selective β-blocker treatment in Child-Pugh C cirrhosis with small varices: increased risk of hepatorenal syndrome and death beyond 6 months of propranolol use. Gut 2016;65(7):1228–30.

53. Gluud LL, Krag A. Banding ligation versus beta-blockers for primary prevention in oesophageal varices in adults. Cochrane Hepato-Biliary Group, ed. Cochrane Database Syst Rev 2012;(8):CD004544.

54. Sharma M, Singh S, Desai V, et al. Comparison of therapies for primary prevention of esophageal variceal bleeding: a systematic review and network meta-analysis. Hepatology 2019;69(4):1657–75.

55. Lo G-H. Letter to the editor: beta-blockers are preferable to banding ligation for primary prophylaxis of variceal bleeding? Hepatology 2019;70(5):1876.

56. Bosch J. Carvedilol: the β-blocker of choice for portal hypertension? Gut 2013; 62(11):1529–30.

57. Sinagra E, Perricone G, D'Amico M, et al. Systematic review with meta-analysis: the haemodynamic effects of carvedilol compared with propranolol for portal hypertension in cirrhosis. Aliment Pharmacol Ther 2014;39(6):557–68.

58. Shah HA, Azam Z, Rauf J, et al. Carvedilol vs. esophageal variceal band ligation in the primary prophylaxis of variceal hemorrhage: a multicentre randomized controlled trial. J Hepatol 2014;60(4):757–64.

59. Lo G-H, Chen W-C, Wang H-M, et al. Randomized, controlled trial of carvedilol versus nadolol plus isosorbide mononitrate for the prevention of variceal rebleeding: prevention of variceal rebleeding. J Gastroenterol Hepatol 2012;27(11): 1681–7.

60. Stanley AJ, Dickson S, Hayes PC, et al. Multicentre randomised controlled study comparing carvedilol with variceal band ligation in the prevention of variceal rebleeding. J Hepatol 2014;61(5):1014–9.

61. Thiele M, Krag A, Rohde U, et al. Meta-analysis: banding ligation and medical interventions for the prevention of rebleeding from oesophageal varices. Aliment Pharmacol Ther 2012;35(10):1155–65.

62. Puente A, Hernández-Gea V, Graupera I, et al. Drugs plus ligation to prevent rebleeding in cirrhosis: an updated systematic review. Liver Int 2014;34(6):823–33.
63. Patch D, Sabin CA, Goulis J, et al. A randomized, controlled trial of medical therapy versus endoscopic ligation for the prevention of variceal rebleeding in patients with cirrhosis. Gastroenterology 2002;123(4):1013–9.
64. Téllez L, Ibáñez-Samaniego L, Pérez del Villar C, et al. Non-selective beta-blockers impair global circulatory homeostasis and renal function in cirrhotic patients with refractory ascites. J Hepatol 2020;73:1404–14.
65. Madsen BS, Nielsen KF, Fialla AD, et al. Keep the sick from harm in spontaneous bacterial peritonitis: dose of beta blockers matters. J Hepatol 2016;64(6):1455–6.
66. D'Amico G, Malizia G, Bosch J. Beta-blockers in 2016: still the safest and most useful drugs for portal hypertension? D'Amico et al. Hepatology 2016;63(6): 1771–3.
67. Garcia-Tsao G. Beta blockers in cirrhosis: the window re-opens. J Hepatol 2016; 64(3):532–4.
68. Bossen L, Krag A, Vilstrup H, et al. Nonselective β-blockers do not affect mortality in cirrhosis patients with ascites: post hoc analysis of three randomized controlled trials with 1198 patients: liver Failure/Cirrhosis/Portal Hypertension. Hepatology 2016;63(6):1968–76.
69. Leithead JA, Rajoriya N, Tehami N, et al. Non-selective β-blockers are associated with improved survival in patients with ascites listed for liver transplantation. Gut 2015;64(7):1111–9.
70. Sersté T, Gustot T, Rautou P-E, et al. Severe hyponatremia is a better predictor of mortality than MELDNa in patients with cirrhosis and refractory ascites. J Hepatol 2012;57(2):274–80.
71. Llach J, Ginès P, Arroyo V, et al. Prognostic value of arterial pressure, endogenous vasoactive systems, and renal function in cirrhotic patients admitted to the hospital for the treatment of ascites. Gastroenterology 1988;94(2):482–7.
72. Krag A, Bendtsen F, Henriksen JH, et al. Low cardiac output predicts development of hepatorenal syndrome and survival in patients with cirrhosis and ascites. Gut 2010;59(01):105–10.
73. Ruiz-del-Arbol L. Systemic, renal, and hepatic hemodynamic derangement in cirrhotic patients with spontaneous bacterial peritonitis. Hepatology 2003;38(5): 1210–8.
74. Feu F, García-Pagán JC, Bosch J, et al. Relation between portal pressure response to pharmacotherapy and risk of recurrent variceal haemorrhage in patients with cirrhosis. Lancet 1995;346(8982):1056–9.
75. La Mura V, Abraldes JG, Raffa S, et al. Prognostic value of acute hemodynamic response to i.v. propranolol in patients with cirrhosis and portal hypertension. J Hepatol 2009;51(2):279–87.
76. Reiberger T, Bucsics T, Paternostro R, et al. Small esophageal varices in patients with cirrhosis-should we treat them? Curr Hepatol Rep 2018;17(4):301–15.
77. Reiberger T, Püspök A, Schoder M, et al. Austrian consensus guidelines on the management and treatment of portal hypertension (Billroth III). Wien Klin Wochenschr 2017;129(Suppl 3):135–58.

The Role of Hepatic Venous Pressure Gradient in the Management of Cirrhosis

Daniel Veldhuijzen van Zanten, MD, MBA[a],
Elizabeth Buganza, MD[b], Juan G. Abraldes, MD, MMSc[c],*

KEYWORDS

• Portal hypertension • Varices • β-blockers

KEY POINTS

- Liver catheterization with hepatic venous pressure gradient (HVPG) is the standard test for estimating the degree of portal hypertension in patients with cirrhosis.
- Patients with cirrhosis with an HVPG $\geq$ 10 mm Hg have clinically significant portal hypertension and are at risk of complications.
- The assessment of changes in HVPG is the standard for investigating new drugs for the treatment of portal hypertension.

INTRODUCTION

Cirrhosis causes an increased resistance to portal blood flow. This increased resistance results in an increase in portal pressure that subsequently activates several pathophysiologic mechanisms that lead to an increased splanchnic blood inflow, which perpetuates and aggravates portal hypertension despite the development of portal systemic collaterals.[1] Portal hypertension plays a causal mediation role in most complications of cirrhosis, including variceal bleeding, ascites, kidney dysfunction, hepatic encephalopathy, and infections. It is well established that the degree of portal hypertension is closely associated with the risk of these complications.[2] In addition, a decrease in portal pressure, either in response to specific treatments to improve portal hemodynamics or related to an improvement in the cause of cirrhosis, is associated with an improvement in prognosis. Therefore, quantifying the degree of portal hypertension provides useful information to estimate prognosis and to evaluate new therapies for portal hypertension. This article addresses the applications of measuring portal pressure in cirrhosis.

[a] Department of Medicine, University of Alberta, 13-103 Clinical Sciences Building, 11350-83 Avenue, Edmonton, Alberta T6G 2G3, Canada; [b] Division of Gastroenterology, Zeidler Ledcor Centre, University of Alberta, 8540 112 St NW, Edmonton, Alberta T6G 2X8, Canada; [c] Division of Gastroenterology, University of Alberta, 8540 112 St NW, 1-38 Zeidler Ledcor Centre, Edmonton, Alberta T6G 2X8, Canada
* Corresponding author.
E-mail address: juan.g.abraldes@ualberta.ca

Clin Liver Dis 25 (2021) 327–343
https://doi.org/10.1016/j.cld.2021.01.002
liver.theclinics.com
1089-3261/21/© 2021 Elsevier Inc. All rights reserved.

MEASURING PORTAL PRESSURE GRADIENT IN CLINICAL PRACTICE: THE HEPATIC VENOUS PRESSURE GRADIENT
Technique

The wedge hepatic venous pressure as a readout of portal venous pressure

The portal vein is located between two capillary territories and, therefore direct measurements of the portal vein pressure require the puncture of the portal vein through the liver parenchyma, using percutaneous,[3] transjugular,[4] or, more recently, a transgastric/transduodenal approach (under endoscopic ultrasonography guidance).[5] Direct measurements are seldom used in clinical practice because of their invasiveness. In 1951, Myers and Taylor,[6] first introduced the indirect measurement of portal venous pressure by measuring the wedge hepatic venous pressure (WHVP). The principle of the technique is that if a catheter is introduced, usually through the right femoral or jugular vein into a hepatic venous radicle until it can go no further (**Fig. 1**A), occluding the vein and stopping the blood flow, the static column of blood transmits the pressure that is present in the preceding vascular territory; that is, the hepatic sinusoids. Although this is a measurement of liver sinusoidal pressure, it reflects portal pressure in the absence of pre-sinusoidal obstruction.[3] Note that because WHVP reflects the pressure in the portal vein, it does not solely measure the changes occurring in the section of the liver occluded by the catheter (ie, it does not sample a small portion of the liver). Portal pressure is determined by the structural and functional changes in the whole liver (because the entire liver contributes to hepatic resistance) and by the upstream changes in the splanchnic circulation, and these are all further modulated by the development of collaterals (**Fig. 2**). Therefore, WHVP measurement

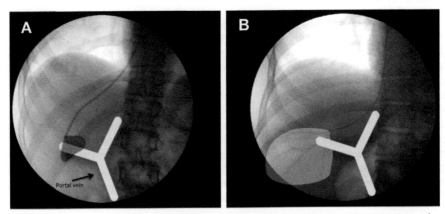

Fig. 1. End-hole catheter (*A*) and balloon catheter (*B*) techniques to measure WHVP. After occluding the hepatic vein, the static column of blood transmits the pressure of the preceding vascular territory: the hepatic sinusoids. In the absence of a presinusoidal obstruction, this equates to the pressure in the portal vein. The volume of liver transmitting pressure, painted in purple in (*A*) and in yellow in (*B*), is much larger (and thus less prone to artifacts) with the balloon catheter than with the end-hole catheter. Note that the WHVP measurement is not sampling the specific area of liver that is coloured in the figure because WHVP is a measure of portal pressure that depends on whole-liver hepatic resistance, portal blood flow, and the degree of collateralization. Once WHVP is measured, the free hepatic venous pressure (FHVP) is measured with the catheter freely floating in the hepatic vein. This FHVP permits the determination of HVPG, which can be calculated with the equation HVPG = WHVP − FHVP.

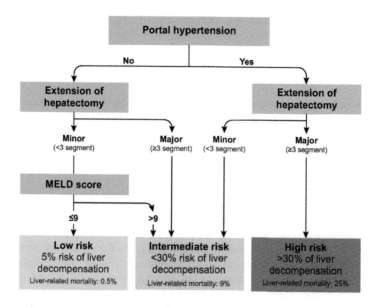

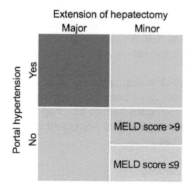

Fig. 2. Role of portal hypertension as a decision tool to select patients with early hepatocellular carcinoma for liver resection. This algorithm from the EASL guidelines for the management of liver cancer[53] is based on the hierarchical model proposed by Citterio and colleagues.[54] European Association for the Study of the Liver (EASL) guidelines define clinically relevant portal hypertension as HVPG > 10 mm Hg, which is equivalent to the concept of clinically significant portal hypertension. In the original publication of this algorithm,[54] portal hypertension was defined by the presence of esophageal varices or the coexistence of low platelet count (<100 × 10^3/mm^3) and splenomegaly (>120 mm in diameter). MELD, Model for End-stage Liver Disease. (Figure reproduced from European Association for the Study of the Liver. Electronic address eee, European Association for the Study of the L. EASL Clinical Practice Guidelines: Management of hepatocellular carcinoma. *J Hepatol.* 2018;69(1):182-236, with permission. (Figure 4 in original).)

integrates the contribution of all hemodynamic pathophysiologic events occurring in cirrhosis.

WHVP has been shown to accurately reflect portal pressure in alcoholic and viral cirrhosis.[3] However, recent data suggest that, in patients with advanced nonalcoholic fatty liver disease (NAFLD) cirrhosis undergoing transjugular intrahepatic portosystemic shunt (TIPS), there is lower agreement between WHVP and direct portal pressure than in patients with alcohol/hepatitis C.[7] In addition, WHVP was a mean 1.3 mm Hg lower than portal pressure, suggesting that WHVP tends to underestimate portal pressure in patients with NAFLD.[7] Whether this is the case at earlier stages of NAFLD cirrhosis is still uncertain.

The free hepatic venous pressure and the hepatic venous pressure gradient

Once WHVP is measured, the catheter is withdrawn to measure the free hepatic venous pressure (FHVP), which provides an internal zeroing for portal pressure and allows calculating the portal pressure gradient across the liver. Using this internal zero provides several additional advantages. Because the measurements are expressed as a gradient, the potential variations introduced by the height of the external zero (normally a water column at the level of the midaxillary line of the patient) are neutralized. In addition, it discounts the variation induced by the intra-abdominal pressure, which might be significant in patients with ascites or obesity.[4]

In 1979, Groszmann and colleagues[8] described a variation of the technique in which the FHVP and the WHVP were obtained by deflating and inflating a balloon at the tip of the catheter (**Fig. 1**B). This variation offers several advantages. Firstly, inflation and deflation of a balloon is much simpler than moving the catheter in and out of the wedged position. Secondly, it permits repeated pressure measurements of hepatic venous pressure gradient (HVPG) without moving the catheter, thus decreasing artifacts. Thirdly, the volume of the liver circulation transmitting the portal pressure is much larger than that attained by wedging the catheter, which reduces the variability of the measurements[9] (see **Fig. 1**B). A specifically designed balloon catheter that improves the rate of direct cannulation of the hepatic vein has recently been developed.[10]

Guidelines for reliable HVPG measurements have been published by different research groups,[11–15] and there have been new, recent attempts of standardization with the use of HVPG as a surrogate marker for drug development in NAFLD.[16–19] These studies have shown the feasibility of homogenizing the quality of HVPG measurements in multicenter studies.

The Controversy of Internal Zeroing

In recent years, and especially since the introduction of TIPS, many reports have used the right atrial pressure (RAP) as the internal zero reference to calculate portal pressure gradient (hepatic-atrial pressure gradient [HAPG]),[20] the rationale being that in a small number of patients, the anatomy of the hepatic vein does not allow a free-floating position of the catheter. In addition, because the esophageal varices drain mainly through the azygos vein near the right atrium, it could be hypothesized that the gradient between WHVP and RAP better reflects the hemodynamics of these varices. However, in a large cross-sectional study, La Mura and colleagues[21] showed that the HAPG had a poor agreement with HVPG. More importantly, although HVPG response to pharmacologic therapy showed an excellent predictive value for bleeding risk and survival, the response measured with HAPG did not.[21] This issue is still a source of controversy. A subsequent more recent study showed high variability in FHVP measurement depending on the position of the tip of the catheter and hepatic vein morphology, thereby recommending the use of HAPG.[20] However, until data showing a prognostic value of HAPG become available, HVPG measured with the FHVP should be the standard for diagnosis and prognosis prediction.

Another source of controversy has been the use of inferior vena cava (IVC) pressure rather than FHVP as the internal reference, especially when the difference between the

FHVP and IVC pressure is >2 mm Hg, because this suggests that the catheter is not in a fully free-floating position, or it is causing a partial obstruction of the hepatic vein. This question was addressed in a recent study showing that, even in these cases, HVPG calculated with the FHVP offers a better prognostic estimate than HVPG calculated with IVC.[22]

Complications and Tolerance

Only 1% of patients show major complications at the puncture site, including local bleeding, hematoma, and more rarely arteriovenous fistulae or Horner syndrome in the case of jugular puncture. Because of these risks, ultrasonographic guidance should always be used when available. Supraventricular arrhythmias may also occur because of the passage of the catheter through the right atrium,[13] but they are self-limiting in more than 90% of cases.

Catheterization of the hepatic vein can be performed under light sedation (midazolam, up to 0.02 mg/Kg),[23] and overall is well tolerated, although this can decrease with longer procedures (such as those assessing hemodynamic response to drugs) and is associated with worse tolerance.[24] Higher doses of midazolam or deep sedation significantly alter pressure measurements.[4,23]

APPLICATIONS OF HEPATIC VENOUS PRESSURE GRADIENT IN CIRRHOSIS
Differential Diagnosis of Portal Hypertension

Cirrhosis is the most common cause of portal hypertension in the Western world and is often easily diagnosed with specific clinical history, laboratory data, and imaging findings. However, in certain clinical contexts, alternative differential diagnosis exists.[25] Examples of these are the presence of varices without obvious morphologic changes of cirrhosis, where the main differential is noncirrhotic portal hypertension,[25,26] or ascites of unclear origin. In the latter, HVPG measurement might help differentiate between a cardiac origin (increase in both FHVP and WHVP, with normal HVPG, but, with progression to cardiac cirrhosis, HVPG might increase), tumoural ascites (normal FHVP, WHVP, and HVPG) or ascites caused by portal hypertension in the setting of cirrhosis (increased HVPG).

Table 1 shows how HVPG measurements can aid in classifying portal hypertension according to the cause and the location of the increased resistance to portal flow.

Risk Stratification in Cirrhosis

Compensated cirrhosis
The natural history of liver cirrhosis can be divided into two main phases: a long, compensated phase (median survival of 12 years) and a much shorter decompensated phase (median survival of 2 years).[27] Although there are excellent prognostic models to predict outcomes in patients with decompensated cirrhosis,[28,29] tools for risk stratification in compensated cirrhosis are limited. A major driver for decompensation in patients with cirrhosis is the development of clinically significant portal hypertension (CSPH), defined as an HVPG $\geq$ 10 mm Hg. This definition is based on cross-sectional studies that found that patients with an HVPG < 10 mm Hg did not develop esophageal varices or complications related to portal hypertension.[30] More importantly, longitudinal studies have also shown that the 5-year risk of progression to decompensation is minimal (<10%) in patients without CSPH, whereas, in patients with CSPH, the risk increases to 30-40%.[2] This concept was initially described in series in which the main causes were untreated hepatitis C and alcohol,[2] and has recently been confirmed in patients with nonalcoholic steatohepatitis (NASH)–related cirrhosis.[19] The impact of the degree of portal hypertension showed a remarkable

Table 1
Hepatic vein pressure measurements in the different types of portal hypertension

Type of PH[a]	Wedged (WHVP)	Free (FHVP)	Gradient[b] (HVPG)
	Hepatic Vein Pressure Measurement		
Prehepatic (portal vein thrombosis)	Normal	Normal	Normal
Presinusoidal (cirrhosis attributed to cholestatic liver disease, schistosomiasis, and idiopathic portal hypertension)[c]	Normal	Normal	Normal
Sinusoidal (cirrhosis attributed to alcohol/HCV/NASH)	↑	Normal	↑
Postsinusoidal Sinusoidal obstruction syndrome (hepatic veno-occlusive disease)	↑	Normal	↑
Budd-Chiari syndrome	Unable to catheterize hepatic vein		
Posthepatic Right heart failure	↑	↑	Normal

Abbreviations: FHVP, free hepatic venous pressure; HCV, hepatitis C virus; NASH, nonalcoholic steatohepatitis; PH, portal hypertension.
[a] PH is classified by the site of increased resistance to blood flow.
[b] Gradient or HVPG is calculated by subtracting the FHVP from the WHVP: HVPG = WHVP - FHVP.
[c] In advanced stages of presinusoidal causes of PH, the WHVP and HVPG may increase.

consistency across these studies: for every 1 mm Hg that the baseline HVPG was higher, the risk of decompensation increased by 11%.[2,31]

The development of CSPH also has major therapeutic consequences. Firstly, in patients without CSPH, treatments specifically designed to decrease portal pressure are unlikely to have a role in the management of cirrhosis, thus the main goal is to target its cause. Secondly, and as detailed later in this article, in those patients that have already reached the threshold of CSPH, elimination of the cause of cirrhosis does not always result in a regression of portal hypertension to levels less than 10 mm Hg.[32–35] Therefore, these patients require, in addition to etiologic treatments, specific treatments to decrease portal pressure to prevent decompensation. Thirdly, reaching the threshold of CSPH has an impact on the pathophysiology of portal hypertension. Only after reaching the threshold of CSPH does the increased portal blood inflow become a relevant contributor to increasing portal pressure.[36] Consequently, only patients with CSPH are likely to benefit from treatments to reduce splanchnic blood flow, such as nonselective β-blockers (NSBBs).[36,37] A recent randomized controlled trial (RCT), focused on patients with compensated cirrhosis with CSPH, showed a major decrease in the risk of decompensation with the use of NSBBs.[38] The results of this trial have markedly increased the relevance of identifying patients with CSPH. However, performing HVPG in every patient with compensated cirrhosis is unfeasible, thus highlighting the relevance of non-invasive methods to identify patients with CSPH, who would then benefit from treatment with β-blockers. This topic is covered elsewhere.[39]

Decompensated cirrhosis
HVPG measurements have also been shown to predict prognosis in patients with decompensated cirrhosis.[40–42] An HVPG ≥ 16 mm Hg is independently associated

with increased mortality in series of patients with overall decompensated cirrhosis,[40,43–45] and in patients with acute variceal bleeding, an HVPG of ≥ 20 mm Hg is an independent predictor of rebleeding and of mortality.[46–48] These findings are relevant to understanding the role of portal pressure causing further decompensation. However, alternative risk prediction models such as Model for End-stage Liver Disease (MELD)[28] or Child-Pugh[29,48] are more commonly used to predict prognosis in different clinical scenarios of decompensated cirrhosis.

Risk of decompensation after liver surgery

Patients with hepatocellular carcinoma (HCC) in the context of compensated cirrhosis and normal liver function are frequently considered for curative surgery if this is technically feasible. However, many of these patients have asymptomatic CSPH. An initial small series identified an HVPG ≥ 10 mm Hg as an independent predictor of overt cirrhosis decompensation after liver surgery.[49] Subsequent studies and a recent meta-analysis[50,51] confirmed that the presence of CSPH was a negative prognostic marker in patients undergoing surgery for HCC. The odds of 3-year and 5-year mortality were roughly double in patients with CSPH compared with patients without CSPH, and the odds of clinical decompensation after surgery were increased by approximately three times in patients with CSPH.

However, recent guidelines[52,53] modulate the message of avoiding liver resection in early HCC with CSPH, acknowledging that advances in surgical techniques have allowed for good outcomes in patients with CSPH that have preserved liver function requiring a minor extension hepatectomy (<3 segments).[54] Latest European Association for the Study of the Liver (EASL) recommendations are based on the model proposed by Citterio and colleagues[54] and are summarized in **Fig. 2**.

Surgical risk in extrahepatic surgery

Cirrhosis is associated with increased morbidity and mortality in extrahepatic surgery. These patients have an increased risk of complications, including infections, renal failure, decompensation, blood transfusion, reintervention, and mortality.[55] Because portal hypertension in cirrhosis is associated with marked systemic and splanchnic hemodynamic changes that can contribute to postsurgical complications, it is plausible that measuring portal pressure could help in estimating the surgical risk in cirrhosis. This possibility was tested in a multicenter study including 140 patients with cirrhosis undergoing extrahepatic surgery.[56] HVPG was independently associated with transplant-free survival. An algorithm to predict 30-day, 90-day, and 1-year transplant-free survival was provided (**Fig. 3**), which could help in decision making. This study also sets a conceptual rationale for assessing the role of preemptive TIPS before surgery in patients with severe portal hypertension.

Assessment of the Hemodynamic Response to Drug Therapy for Portal Hypertension

Several cohort studies have shown that, if the HVPG decreases to less than 12 mm Hg, either by pharmacologic therapy[57,58] or spontaneously (because of an improvement in liver disease),[41] esophageal variceal bleeding is markedly reduced. This pressure threshold of 12 mm Hg is less precise for predicting bleeding from fundal gastric varices, and occasionally bleeding may occur below this threshold.[59] In addition, even if this target is not achieved, a decrease in HVPG of at least 20%[58,60,61] from baseline levels offers substantial protection from variceal bleeding in the long-term. In patients surviving a bleeding episode, achievement of these targets (reduction <12 mm Hg or >20% from baseline) constitutes a strong independent predictor of protection from subsequent variceal bleeding, reduces the risk of other portal hypertension–

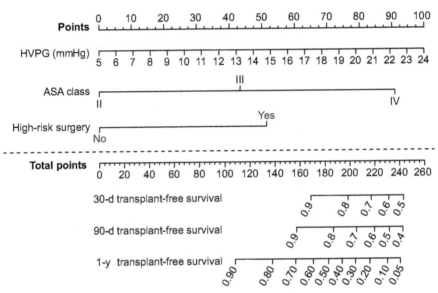

Fig. 3. Nomogram for 30-day, 90-day, and 1-year transplant-free survival predictions in patients with cirrhosis undergoing extrahepatic surgery, according to HVPG, American Society of Anesthesiologists (ASA) class, and low-risk versus high-risk surgery. To calculate the risk score, first estimate the points contributed by each variable using the points scale at the top. Then add all points and bring the total number of points to the second scale, which estimates the transplant-free survival. The high-risk group of surgeries included cardiovascular, thoracic, and open abdominal surgeries, whereas the low-risk group included laparoscopic and abdominal wall surgeries, orthopedic surgeries, and others. (Reproduced from Reverter E, Cirera I, Albillos A, et al. The prognostic role of hepatic venous pressure gradient in cirrhotic patients undergoing elective extrahepatic surgery. *J Hepatol.* 2019;71(5):942-950, with permission. (Figure 2 in original).)

related complications (eg, ascites, spontaneous bacterial peritonitis), and is associated with an improved survival.[60–63] Interestingly, this survival benefit could not be attributed to an improvement in liver function.[64] In compensated patients, a decrease by 10% in HVPG might be enough to achieve protection from complications of cirrhosis.[38,65,66]

The clinical application of the prognostic value of changes in HVPG is hampered by the need for repeated measurements of HVPG, and by the fact that a significant number of patients might bleed before a second HVPG measurement is taken.[67] Two studies have shown that evaluation of the acute HVPG response to intravenous propranolol therapy is a useful tool in predicting the prognosis in patients treated with nonselective β-blockers for the prevention of first bleeding or rebleeding.[65,68] The acute HVPG response to propranolol was independently associated with survival in these patients.[68] The threshold reduction in HVPG that defines a good response (associated with decreased bleeding and mortality) in these studies was a decline of 10-12% from baseline (instead of the 20% decrease that applies when using the chronic response).

Issues in defining what constitutes a clinically relevant decrease in portal pressure
Although the studies mentioned earlier are of capital conceptual relevance because they show that decreasing portal pressure improves prognosis in cirrhosis, there is no biological rationale or clinical evidence to suggest that there is a minimal threshold

of portal pressure decrease that yields a clinical benefit. If the association between the HVPG and prognosis is a continuum,[2,31] then likely the association between a reduction in portal pressure and improved prognosis is also a continuum, and recent data (Ref.[69], published in abstract form) suggest that even reductions in portal pressure of 1 mm Hg could have therapeutic benefit. It has been questioned whether HVPG has enough resolution to detect differences as low as 1 mm Hg (which would be <7% in a patient, for example, with a baseline HVPG of 15 mm Hg). When considering the variation in before and after HVPG measurements in the placebo groups of several recent trials,[17,70,71] such differences, or even substantially greater differences, cannot be detected at the individual level. However, in the context of a randomized clinical trial, in which only the mean group responses (but not individual responses) have an interpretation,[72] differences as small as 1 mm Hg between placebo and treated patients can be detected with only 40-50 patients per treatment arm.

Hepatic venous pressure gradient measurements to guide pharmacologic therapy for portal hypertension

A relevant question is whether there is any benefit in monitoring pharmacologic therapy for portal hypertension with HVPG in day-to-day practice. One of the limitations of this approach is that the relative invasiveness and the cost of HVPG limit the possibility of obtaining several measurements at different time points to assess the response to a drug (such as is done with arterial hypertension, a physiologic variable with wide physiologic variability, where repeated measurements or 24-hour monitoring are used to assess response and escalate therapy).[73]

In the context of trials, it precludes conducting several crossover studies, which would be required to reliably detect individual treatment responses.[72] These considerations require caution over approaches to tailoring pharmacologic therapy according to individual HVPG response or to indicate an escalation of therapy in nonresponders, and emphasizes the notion that these strategies should be extensively validated in RCTs before being implemented in practice. In addition, although the patients achieving a target reduction in portal pressure with β-blockers have much better prognosis than hemodynamic nonresponders, the labeling of these patients as nonresponders led to the (wrong) concept that these patients do not benefit from β-blockers.[74] Randomized trials showing the benefits of β-blockers compared with placebo were conducted without guiding treatment according to HVPG response.[75] Because these were parallel randomized trials, conclusions regarding the benefits of NSBBs apply to the whole group of patients treated in those trials, and it cannot be inferred that the efficacy of NSBBs was limited to hemodynamic responders.

To our knowledge, three RCTs have compared HVPG-guided therapy with alternative treatments, one in patients with compensated cirrhosis and two for the secondary prevention of variceal bleeding.

The 2019 PREDESCI trial compared β-blockers with placebo for the prevention of decompensation in patients with CSPH.[38] During baseline HVPG study, the acute hemodynamic response to propranolol was tested, and those patients that were responders received propranolol (or placebo), and nonresponders received carvedilol (or placebo). This optimization of the use of β-blockers, which would be unfeasible in practice, was likely unnecessary. With current knowledge about the hemodynamic effects of propranolol and carvedilol,[76] hemodynamic response to β-blockers in compensated patients can be optimized by treating all patients with carvedilol.

In a multicenter randomized trial in Germany, TIPS was compared with a medical/ endoscopic treatment arm guided by HVPG as first-line therapy for the prevention of variceal rebleeding.[77] In this treatment arm, patients achieving a good hemody-namic response to β-blockers plus nitrates were treated with drug therapy only, whereas nonresponders were switched to endoscopic variceal ligation only. Rebleed-ing in the HVPG-guided treatment arm was higher than in the TIPS arm and not relevantly different from the rebleeding risk reported in previous RCTs in the same setting.

Finally, in an open single-center randomized trial,[78] 172 patients were randomized to pharmacologic HVPG-guided therapy (using nadolol alone, nadolol plus nitrates, or nadolol plus prazosin to optimize the response, adding ligation in those nonre-sponders after the third HVPG measurement) or to empiric treatment with β-blockers plus nitrates plus ligation. Rebleeding and survival were better in the HVPG-guided group. Therefore, the evidence to use HVPG-guided therapy, is very limited and of questionable applicability because of the need for repeated (up to 3) HVPG measurements.

Assessment of New Therapeutic Agents for the Treatment of Portal Hypertension

The rationale for the development of new drugs for the treatment of portal hyperten-sion has been that the patients' disease phenotypes can be modified by decreasing portal pressure. Therefore, the effect of a candidate drug on HVPG has been used to triage new drugs to be subsequently assessed in randomized trials with clinical end points.[79,80] The considerations made earlier to quantify what is a relevant decrease in portal pressure also apply for trial design. Furthermore, additional read-outs of potential hemodynamic effects (either beneficial or harmful) such as liver blood flow (with clearance techniques) or azygos blood flow, might contribute in clarifying the potential of the drug for the management of patients with cirrhosis and portal hy-pertension.[79,80] In addition, although HVPG measurements are still needed for proof-of-concept studies (phase II clinical trials), HVPG reduction is not yet an accepted surrogate for drug approval in phase III trials. For this, more evidence relating changes in HVPG with outcomes at each of the stages and substages of compensated and decompensated cirrhosis would be needed.

Achieving such validation would be relevant in patients with compensated cirrhosis, because the rate of clinical events is low. Having a surrogate end point such as HVPG would facilitate the early completion of trials and faster approval of drugs that can pre-vent cirrhosis decompensation. This validation is close to being available. In the trial by Groszmann and colleagues[37] comparing timolol versus placebo for the prevention of the development of varices, timolol did not achieve a decrease in portal pressure compared with placebo, and timolol did not provide clinical benefit. However, a spon-taneous decrease in portal pressure was associated with improvement in the risk of decompensation.[2] In the trial by Villanueva and colleagues,[38] comparing β-blockers with placebo to prevent decompensation, β-blockers did achieve a moderate decrease in portal pressure (−1.9 mm Hg compared with placebo), and β-blocker treatment was associated with a hazard ratio of 0.6 for decompensation-free survival (~40% relative reduction), which was within the range of expected benefit observed with a spontaneous decrease in portal pressure in the timolol trial.[69] A reasonable pro-visional proposal could combine the efficacy of the new drug decreasing portal pres-sure with the overall profile of the drug (favourable or unfavourable depending on convenience of administration, potential additional benefits, side effects, and costs) to define an area of potential drug approval, as depicted in **Fig. 4**.

In settings such as secondary prophylaxis of bleeding, in which relevant clinical end points are frequent, the relevance of HVPG as a surrogate would be much lower.[79] Therefore, trials in secondary prophylaxis can be efficiently designed and conducted

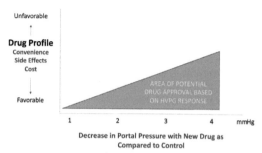

Fig. 4. A proposal for potential drug approval to treat portal hypertension in compensated cirrhosis combining the capacity of the drug to decrease portal pressure with the overall profile in terms of safety, easiness of administration, and costs. Drugs inducing mild decreases in portal pressure but associated with an overall favourable profile could be considered for approval. Drugs with less favourable profile require stronger portal pressure–reducing effects to be considered for approval based on HVPG response.

based on relevant clinical outcomes, without the need for surrogate end points such as HVPG response.[81] However, HVPG studies would obviously be required in trials assessing a therapeutic arm of HVPG-guided therapy and could provide useful additional explanatory information to understand the effects (or lack thereof) of novel drugs on relevant clinical endpoints.

In addition, HVPG has also been proposed as a potential endpoint to assess the effects of etiologic treatments.[82] Because disease progression is reflected as an increase in portal pressure, the assumption for using HVPG as a readout in these trials would be that an improvement in the underlying disease that causes cirrhosis would be associated with a decrease in portal pressure. Although this is a reasonable assumption (as discussed next) changes in HVPG might be slow after removing the causative agent and might not capture in full the potential benefit of suppressing the activity of the underlying liver disease. Therefore, HVPG is probably much better suited to assess hemodynamic drugs, which act through a vasoactive mechanism, rather than to assess the effects of etiologic treatments for cirrhosis.

Assessment of the Regression of Portal Hypertension After Treating the Underlying Liver Disease

Several studies have assessed the effects on portal pressure of treating the underlying liver disease, and how these relate to prognosis. By assessing the liver as a whole, including the potential functional changes in the hepatic microvasculature, the assessment of HVPG changes after therapy might provide a more comprehensive understanding of the effects of therapy rather than histology.[18]

A landmark prospective study by Vorobioff and colleagues[41] conducted in patients with cirrhosis related to alcohol, with esophageal varices but no previous bleeding, showed that alcohol abstinence is followed by a sustained decrease in portal pressure, which was associated with improved outcomes (bleeding and survival). Because none of these patients had received any form of prophylaxis for their first variceal bleeds, the study suggests that this improvement was the result of a reversible component of the disease.

In patients with cirrhosis from viral causes (mainly hepatitis C), several studies have assessed in recent years the impact of curing the viral disease on portal hypertension, initially with interferon-based therapies, in which only a small proportion of patients achieved sustained viral response (SVR)[34] and more recently with direct antivirals, which achieve SVR in most patients with cirrhosis.[32,33,35,83,84]

Collectively, these studies show consistent results that can be summarized as follows. Patients without CSPH at the time of viral eradication do not progress to CSPH and remain compensated. In patients in whom SVR is achieved when CSPH is already present, even if most patients show some degree of decrease in HVPG, only a fraction (~30%) regress to an HVPG < 10 mm Hg in the short term. The higher the baseline HVPG, the lower the probability of regressing to non-CSPH. Patients remain at risk of decompensation if CSPH persists after SVR, although a decrease in HVPG > 10% after SVR is associated with decreased risk of decompensation. The decrease in portal pressure probably continues over the years, and the proportion of patients regressing to non-CSPH increases with time. This last result is still difficult to interpret, because in these studies only a small subset of patients were assessed for long-term HVPG response, likely representing a selected group of patients not experiencing events in the interim. Altogether, these results suggest that most patients with CSPH at baseline, even if they achieve SVR, require treatment of portal hypertension (nowadays with β-blockers) to prevent decompensation. Again, this suggests the need for noninvasive markers to identify post-SVR patients with persistent CSPH. This topic is covered elsewhere.

SUMMARY

HVPG reflects disease severity and has strong prognostic value with regard to survival and decompensation in patients with cirrhosis. Furthermore, repeated measurements of HVPG provide information on the response to the medical treatment to decrease portal pressure and represent an essential tool for drug development for portal hypertension. Moreover, because changes in HVPG also correlate with the extent of structural changes in the liver, assessing the trajectory of HVPG after etiologic therapies (mainly hepatitis C) has provided new insights into the patterns and clinical consequences of portal hypertension regression after removing the causative agent of cirrhosis. Because of the wide range of applications of this measurement, hepatologists should be familiar with the procedure for assessing HVPG and interpretation of the results.

CLINICS CARE POINTS

- Various methods for measuring or estimating the portal hepatic pressure gradient exist but catheterization remains the gold standard.
- Clinically significant portal hypertension (CSPH) defined as hepatic venous pressure gradient (HVPG) ≥ 10mmHg is the threshold above which many of the complications from cirrhosis occur.
- Assessing the trajectory of CSPH after the underlying etiology of cirrhosis has been treated can help predict ongoing occurrences of such complications.

DISCLOSURE

Dr J.G. Abraldes reports grants and personal fees from Gilead, and personal fees from Intercept, Lupin, Ferring, Boehringer-Ingelheim, and Genfit outside the submitted work. Drs D. Veldhuijzen van Zanten and E. Buganza declare no conflicts.

REFERENCES

1. Groszmann RJ, Abraldes JG. Portal hypertension: from bedside to bench. J Clin Gastroenterol 2005;39(4 Suppl):S215.
2. Ripoll C, Groszmann R, Garcia-Tsao G, et al. Hepatic venous pressure gradient predicts clinical decompensation in patients with compensated cirrhosis. Gastroenterology 2007;133(2):481–8.
3. Perello A, Escorsell A, Bru C, et al. Wedged hepatic venous pressure adequately reflects portal pressure in hepatitis C virus-related cirrhosis. Hepatology 1999; 30(6):1393–7.
4. Reverter E, Blasi A, Abraldes JG, et al. Impact of deep sedation on the accuracy of hepatic and portal venous pressure measurements in patients with cirrhosis. Liver Int 2014;34(1):16–25.
5. Samarasena JB, Huang JY, Tsujino T, et al. EUS-guided portal pressure gradient measurement with a simple novel device: a human pilot study. VideoGIE 2018; 3(11):361–3.
6. Myers JD, Taylor WJ. An estimation of portal venous pressure by occlusive catheterization of an hepatic venule. J Clin Invest 1951;30:662.
7. Ferrusquia-Acosta J, Bassegoda O, Turco L, et al. Agreement between wedged hepatic venous pressure and portal pressure in non-alcoholic steatohepatitis-related cirrhosis. J Hepatol 2020. https://doi.org/10.1016/j.jhep.2020.10.003.
8. Groszmann RJ, Glickman M, Blei AT, et al. Wedged and free hepatic venous pressure measured with a balloon catheter. Gastroenterology 1979;76(2):253–8.
9. Zipprich A, Winkler M, Seufferlein T, et al. Comparison of balloon vs. straight catheter for the measurement of portal hypertension. Aliment Pharmacol Ther 2010; 32(11–12):1351–6.
10. Ferlitsch A, Bota S, Paternostro R, et al. Evaluation of a new balloon occlusion catheter specifically designed for measurement of hepatic venous pressure gradient. Liver Int 2015;35(9):2115–20.
11. Groszmann RJ, Wongcharatrawee S. The hepatic venous pressure gradient: anything worth doing should be done right. Hepatology 2004;39(2):280–2.
12. Bosch J, Abraldes JG, Berzigotti A, et al. The clinical use of HVPG measurements in chronic liver disease. Nat Rev Gastroenterol Hepatol 2009;6:576–82.
13. Abraldes JG, Sarlieve P, Tandon P. Measurement of portal pressure. Clin Liver Dis 2014;18(4):779–92.
14. Tandon P, Ripoll C, Assis D, et al. The interpretation of hepatic venous pressure gradient tracings - excellent interobserver agreement unrelated to experience. Liver Int 2016;36(8):1160–6.
15. Reiberger T, Schwabl P, Trauner M, et al. Measurement of the hepatic venous pressure gradient and transjugular liver biopsy. J Vis Exp 2020;(160). https://doi.org/10.3791/58819.
16. Chalasani N, Abdelmalek MF, Garcia-Tsao G, et al. Effects of belapectin, an inhibitor of Galectin-3, in patients with nonalcoholic steatohepatitis with cirrhosis and portal hypertension. Gastroenterology 2020;158(5):1334–45.e5.
17. Garcia-Tsao G, Bosch J, Kayali Z, et al. Randomized placebo-controlled trial of emricasan for non-alcoholic steatohepatitis-related cirrhosis with severe portal hypertension. J Hepatol 2020;72(5):885–95.
18. Garcia-Tsao G, Fuchs M, Shiffman M, et al. Emricasan (IDN-6556) lowers portal pressure in patients with compensated cirrhosis and severe portal hypertension. Hepatology 2019;69(2):717–28.

19. Harrison SA, Abdelmalek MF, Caldwell S, et al. Simtuzumab is ineffective for patients with bridging fibrosis or compensated cirrhosis caused by nonalcoholic steatohepatitis. Gastroenterology 2018;155(4):1140–53.
20. Rossle M, Blanke P, Fritz B, et al. Free hepatic vein pressure is not useful to calculate the portal pressure gradient in cirrhosis: a morphologic and hemodynamic study. J Vasc Interv Radiol 2016;27(8):1130–7.
21. La Mura V, Abraldes JG, Berzigotti A, et al. Right atrial pressure is not adequate to calculate portal pressure gradient in cirrhosis: a clinical-hemodynamic correlation study. Hepatology 2010;51(6):2108–16.
22. Silva-Junior G, Baiges A, Turon F, et al. The prognostic value of hepatic venous pressure gradient in patients with cirrhosis is highly dependent on the accuracy of the technique. Hepatology 2015;62(5):1584–92.
23. Steinlauf AF, Garcia-Tsao G, Zakko MF, et al. Low-dose midazolam sedation: an option for patients undergoing serial hepatic venous pressure measurements. Hepatology 1999;29(4):1070–3.
24. Casu S, Berzigotti A, Abraldes JG, et al. A prospective observational study on tolerance and satisfaction to hepatic haemodynamic procedures. Liver Int 2015;35(3):695–703.
25. Berzigotti A, Abraldes JG, Tandon P, et al. Ultrasonographic evaluation of liver surface and transient elastography in clinically doubtful cirrhosis. J Hepatol 2010;52(6):846–53.
26. Seijo S, Reverter E, Miquel R, et al. Role of hepatic vein catheterisation and transient elastography in the diagnosis of idiopathic portal hypertension. Dig Liver Dis 2012;44(10):855–60.
27. D'Amico G, Garcia-Tsao G, Pagliaro L. Natural history and prognostic indicators of survival in cirrhosis: a systematic review of 118 studies. J Hepatol 2006;44(1): 217–31.
28. Jepsen P, Watson H, Macdonald S, et al. MELD remains the best predictor of mortality in outpatients with cirrhosis and severe ascites. Aliment Pharmacol Ther 2020;52(3):492–9.
29. Kok B, Abraldes JG. Child-Pugh classification: time to abandon? Semin Liver Dis 2019;39(1):96–103.
30. Garcia-Tsao G, Groszmann RJ, Fisher RL, et al. Portal pressure, presence of gastroesophageal varices and variceal bleeding. Hepatology 1985;5(3):419–24.
31. Sanyal AJ, Harrison SA, Ratziu V, et al. The natural history of advanced fibrosis due to nonalcoholic steatohepatitis: data from the simtuzumab trials. Hepatology 2019;70(6):1913–27.
32. Lens S, Alvarado-Tapias E, Marino Z, et al. Effects of all-oral anti-viral therapy on HVPG and systemic hemodynamics in patients with hepatitis C virus-associated cirrhosis. Gastroenterology 2017;153(5):1273–83.e1.
33. Lens S, Baiges A, Alvarado E, et al. Clinical outcome and hemodynamic changes following HCV eradication with oral antiviral therapy in patients with clinically significant portal hypertension. J Hepatol 2020;73(6):1415–24.
34. Lens S, Rincon D, Garcia-Retortillo M, et al. Association between severe portal hypertension and risk of liver decompensation in patients with hepatitis c, regardless of response to antiviral therapy. Clin Gastroenterol Hepatol 2015;13(10): 1846–53.e1.
35. Mandorfer M, Kozbial K, Schwabl P, et al. Changes in hepatic venous pressure gradient predict hepatic decompensation in patients who achieved sustained virologic response to interferon-free therapy. Hepatology 2020;71(3):1023–36.

36. Villanueva C, Albillos A, Genesca J, et al. Development of hyperdynamic circulation and response to beta-blockers in compensated cirrhosis with portal hypertension. Hepatology 2016;63(1):197–206.
37. Groszmann RJ, Garcia-Tsao G, Bosch J, et al. Beta-blockers to prevent gastroesophageal varices in patients with cirrhosis. N Engl J Med 2005;353(21): 2254–61.
38. Villanueva C, Albillos A, Genesca J, et al. Beta blockers to prevent decompensation of cirrhosis in patients with clinically significant portal hypertension (PREDESCI): a randomised, double-blind, placebo-controlled, multicentre trial. Lancet 2019;393(10181):1597–608.
39. Mandorfer M, Hernandez-Gea V, Garcia-Pagan JC, et al. Noninvasive diagnostics for portal hypertension: a comprehensive review. Semin Liver Dis 2020; 40(3):240–55.
40. Merkel C, Bolognesi M, Bellon S, et al. Prognostic usefulness of hepatic vein catheterization in patients with cirrhosis and esophageal varices. Gastroenterology 1992;102(3):973–9.
41. Vorobioff J, Groszmann RJ, Picabea E, et al. Prognostic value of hepatic venous pressure gradient measurements in alcoholic cirrhosis: a 10-year prospective study. Gastroenterology 1996;111(3):701–9.
42. Ripoll C, Banares R, Rincon D, et al. Influence of hepatic venous pressure gradient on the prediction of survival of patients with cirrhosis in the MELD Era. Hepatology 2005;42(4):793–801.
43. Patch D, Armonis A, Sabin C, et al. Single portal pressure measurement predicts survival in cirrhotic patients with recent bleeding. Gut 1999;44(2):264–9.
44. Berzigotti A, Rossi V, Tiani C, et al. Prognostic value of a single HVPG measurement and Doppler-ultrasound evaluation in patients with cirrhosis and portal hypertension. J Gastroenterol 2011;46(5):687–95.
45. La Mura V, Garcia-Guix M, Berzigotti A, et al. A new prognostic algorithm based on stage of cirrhosis and HVPG to improve risk-stratification after variceal bleeding. Hepatology 2020;72(4):1353–65.
46. Monescillo A, Martinez-Lagares F, Ruiz-del-Arbol L, et al. Influence of portal hypertension and its early decompression by TIPS placement on the outcome of variceal bleeding. Hepatology 2004;40(4):793–801.
47. Moitinho E, Escorsell A, Bandi JC, et al. Prognostic value of early measurements of portal pressure in acute variceal bleeding. Gastroenterology 1999;117(3): 626–31.
48. Abraldes JG, Villanueva C, Banares R, et al. Hepatic venous pressure gradient and prognosis in patients with acute variceal bleeding treated with pharmacologic and endoscopic therapy. J Hepatol 2008;48(2):229–36.
49. Bruix J, Castells A, Bosch J, et al. Surgical resection of hepatocellular carcinoma in cirrhotic patients: prognostic value of preoperative portal pressure. Gastroenterology 1996;111(4):1018–22.
50. Llovet JM, Fuster J, Bruix J. Intention-to-treat analysis of surgical treatment for early hepatocellular carcinoma: resection versus transplantation. Hepatology 1999;30(6):1434–40.
51. Berzigotti A, Reig M, Abraldes JG, et al. Portal hypertension and the outcome of surgery for hepatocellular carcinoma in compensated cirrhosis: a systematic review and meta-analysis. Hepatology 2015;61(2):526–36.
52. Heimbach JK, Kulik LM, Finn RS, et al. AASLD guidelines for the treatment of hepatocellular carcinoma. Hepatology 2018;67(1):358–80.

53. European Association for the Study of the Liver. EASL clinical practice guidelines: management of hepatocellular carcinoma. J Hepatol 2018;69(1):182–236.

54. Citterio D, Facciorusso A, Sposito C, et al. Hierarchic interaction of factors associated with liver decompensation after resection for hepatocellular carcinoma. JAMA Surg 2016;151(9):846–53.

55. Simonetto DA, Shah VH, Kamath PS. Surgery in patients with cirrhosis: as much an art as science. Hepatology 2020. https://doi.org/10.1002/hep.31643.

56. Reverter E, Cirera I, Albillos A, et al. The prognostic role of hepatic venous pressure gradient in cirrhotic patients undergoing elective extrahepatic surgery. J Hepatol 2019;71(5):942–50.

57. Groszmann RJ, Bosch J, Grace ND, et al. Hemodynamic events in a prospective randomized trial of propranolol versus placebo in the prevention of a first variceal hemorrhage [see comments]. Gastroenterology 1990;99(5):1401–7.

58. Feu F, Garcia-Pagan JC, Bosch J, et al. Relation between portal pressure response to pharmacotherapy and risk of recurrent variceal haemorrhage in patients with cirrhosis. Lancet 1995;346(8982):1056–9.

59. Stanley AJ, Jalan R, Ireland HM, et al. A comparison between gastric and oesophageal variceal haemorrhage treated with transjugular intrahepatic portosystemic stent shunt (TIPSS). Aliment Pharmacol Ther 1997;11(1):171–6.

60. Abraldes JG, Tarantino I, Turnes J, et al. Hemodynamic response to pharmacological treatment of portal hypertension and long-term prognosis of cirrhosis. Hepatology 2003;37(4):902–8.

61. Turco L, Villanueva C, La Mura V, et al. Lowering portal pressure improves outcomes of patients with cirrhosis, with or without ascites: a meta-analysis. Clin Gastroenterol Hepatol 2020;18(2):313–27.e6.

62. Albillos A, Banares R, Gonzalez M, et al. Value of the hepatic venous pressure gradient to monitor drug therapy for portal hypertension: a meta-analysis. Am J Gastroenterol 2007;102(5):1116–26.

63. D'Amico G, Garcia-Pagan JC, Luca A, et al. Hepatic vein pressure gradient reduction and prevention of variceal bleeding in cirrhosis: a systematic review. Gastroenterology 2006;131(5):1611–24.

64. Villanueva C, Lopez-Balaguer JM, Aracil C, et al. Maintenance of hemodynamic response to treatment for portal hypertension and influence on complications of cirrhosis. J Hepatol 2004;40(5):757–65.

65. Villanueva C, Aracil C, Colomo A, et al. Acute hemodynamic response to beta-blockers and prediction of long-term outcome in primary prophylaxis of variceal bleeding. Gastroenterology 2009;137(1):119–28.

66. Hernandez-Gea V, Aracil C, Colomo A, et al. Development of ascites in compensated cirrhosis with severe portal hypertension treated with beta-blockers. Am J Gastroenterol 2012;107(3):418–27.

67. Garcia-Pagan JC, Villanueva C, Albillos A, et al. Nadolol plus isosorbide mononitrate alone or associated with band ligation in the prevention of recurrent bleeding: a multicenter randomized controlled trial. Gut 2009;58(8):1144–50.

68. La Mura V, Abraldes JG, Raffa S, et al. Prognostic value of acute hemodynamic response to i.v. propranolol in patients with cirrhosis and portal hypertension. J Hepatol 2009;51(2):279–87.

69. Abraldes JG, Garcia-Tsao G, Ripoll C, et al. Dynamic prediction of the risk of decompensation/death in patients with compensated cirrhosis based on serial hepatic venous pressure gradient (HVPG) measurements. Hepatology 2018; 68(Suppl 1). Abstract.

70. Abraldes JG, Albillos A, Banares R, et al. Simvastatin lowers portal pressure in patients with cirrhosis and portal hypertension: a randomized controlled trial. Gastroenterology 2009;136(5):1651–8.
71. Lebrec D, Bosch J, Jalan R, et al. Hemodynamics and pharmacokinetics of tezosentan, a dual endothelin receptor antagonist, in patients with cirrhosis. Eur J Clin Pharmacol 2012;68(5):533–41.
72. Senn S. Mastering variation: variance components and personalised medicine. Stat Med 2016;35(7):966–77.
73. Available at: https://guidelines.hypertension.ca/diagnosis-assessment/ diagnosis/. Accessed July 4, 2020.
74. Moctezuma-Velazquez C, Kalainy S, Abraldes JG. Reply. Liver Transplant 2017; 23(10):1353.
75. Moctezuma-Velazquez C, Kalainy S, Abraldes JG. Beta-blockers in patients with advanced liver disease: has the dust settled? Liver Transplant 2017;23(8): 1058–69.
76. Sinagra E, Perricone G, D'Amico M, et al. Systematic review with meta-analysis: the haemodynamic effects of carvedilol compared with propranolol for portal hypertension in cirrhosis. Aliment Pharmacol Ther 2014;39(6):557–68.
77. Sauerbruch T, Mengel M, Dollinger M, et al. Prevention of rebleeding from esophageal varices in patients with cirrhosis receiving small-diameter stents vs hemodynamically controlled medical therapy. Gastroenterology 2015;149(3):660–8.e1.
78. Villanueva C, Graupera I, Aracil C, et al. A randomized trial to assess whether portal pressure guided therapy to prevent variceal rebleeding improves survival in cirrhosis. Hepatology 2017;65(5):1693–707.
79. Abraldes JG, Garcia-Tsao G. The design of clinical trials in portal hypertension. Semin Liver Dis 2017;37(1):73–84.
80. Abraldes JG, Trebicka J, Chalasani N, et al. Prioritization of therapeutic targets and trial design in cirrhotic portal hypertension. Hepatology 2019;69(3):1287–99.
81. de Franchis R, Baveno VIF. Expanding consensus in portal hypertension: Report of the Baveno VI Consensus Workshop: Stratifying risk and individualizing care for portal hypertension. J Hepatol 2015;63(3):743–52.
82. Sanyal AJ, Friedman SL, McCullough AJ, et al. Challenges and opportunities in drug and biomarker development for nonalcoholic steatohepatitis: findings and recommendations from an American association for the study of liver diseases-U.S. Food and drug administration Joint Workshop. Hepatology 2015;61(4): 1392–405.
83. Diez C, Berenguer J, Ibanez-Samaniego L, et al. Persistence of clinically significant portal hypertension after eradication of HCV in patients with advanced cirrhosis. Clin Infect Dis 2020. https://doi.org/10.1093/cid/ciaa502.
84. Mandorfer M, Kozbial K, Schwabl P, et al. Sustained virologic response to interferon-free therapies ameliorates HCV-induced portal hypertension. J Hepatol 2016;65(4):692–9.

Treatment of Acute Variceal Bleeding in 2021—When to Use Transjugular Intrahepatic Portosystemic Shunts?

Anna Baiges, MD, PhD[a,b], Marta Magaz, MD[a,b], Fanny Turon, MD[a,b],
Virginia Hernández-Gea, MD, PhD[a,b],
Juan Carlos García-Pagán, MD, PhD[a,b,*]

KEYWORDS

- TIPS • Preemptive TIPS • Portal hypertension • Acute variceal bleeding

KEY POINTS

- Preemptive transjugular intrahepatic portosystemic shunt (TIPS) should be the standard of care in patients with high-risk acute variceal bleeding (Child-Turcotte-Pugh stage B plus active bleeding on endoscopy or stage C with 10–13 points).
- The implementation of preemptive TIPS in clinical practice still requires further efforts.
- Lack of control of bleeding or early rebleeding within 5 days should be managed by rescue/salvage TIPS. Esophageal stents should be considered as the treatment of choice as a bridge until TIPS placement.

Continued

A. Baiges and M. Magaz share first coauthorship.

Conflict of Interest Statement: V. Hernández-Gea and F. Turon receive speaker fees from Gore. J.C. García-Pagán advisory for GORE, Cook, and Shionogi. The remaining authors declare no conflicts of interests.

Financial Support Statement: This study was supported by the Ministry of Education and Science (SAF-2016-75767-R); Instituto de Salud Carlos III (ISCIII) and Fondo Europeo de Desarrollo Regional (FEDER) (PIE15/00027); and Centro de Investigación Biomédica en Red de Enfermedades Hepáticas y Digestivas (CIBERehd), funded by the Instituto de Salud Carlos III. J.C. García-Pagán also received a grant from Secretariat for Universities and Research of the Department of Economy and Knowledge (SGR17_00517). A. Baiges is a recipient of a Juan Rodés grant from Instituto de Salud Carlos III, Spain. M. Magaz is a recipient of a Río Hortega grant from Instituto de Salud Carlos III, Spain.

[a] Barcelona Hepatic Hemodynamic Laboratory, Liver Unit, Hospital Clínic, Institut de Investigacions Biomèdiques August Pi i Sunyer (IDIBAPS), University of Barcelona, Villarroel 170, Barcelona 08036, Spain; [b] CIBEREHD (Centro de Investigación Biomédica en Red Enfermedades Hepáticas y Digestivas), HealthCare Provider of the European Reference Network on Rare Liver Disorders (ERN-Liver)

* Corresponding author. Barcelona Hepatic Hemodynamic Laboratory, Liver Unit, Hospital Clinic, Villarroel 170, Barcelona 08036, Spain.

E-mail address: jcgarcia@clinic.cat

Clin Liver Dis 25 (2021) 345–356
https://doi.org/10.1016/j.cld.2021.01.001
1089-3261/21/© 2021 Elsevier Inc. All rights reserved.

Continued

- Currently, there is not enough evidence to use TIPS as a first-line treatment to prevent rebleeding.
- TIPS also may play a role in gastric varices, gastropathy of portal hypertension, and ectopic varices bleeding.

INTRODUCTION

Cirrhosis is a progressive disease that impairs liver function and decreases life expectancy.[1] The prognosis of patients with cirrhosis is highly dependent on the presence or not of portal hypertension (PH) and also on the presence or not of hepatic decompensation (mainly ascites, variceal bleeding, or hepatic encephalopathy [HE]). PH is defined by a pathologic increase in portal pressure gradient between the portal vein and inferior vena cava (portal pressure gradient), which is increased above the normal limit of 5 mm Hg in the setting of PH due to cirrhosis.[1] PH becomes clinically significant when the portal pressure gradient increases above the threshold of 10 mm Hg (formation of varices and ascites) or 12 mm Hg (variceal bleeding).[2–4] Clinically, the development of gastroesophageal varices (GEVs) is a hallmark in the natural history of cirrhosis, given that they represent the clinical confirmation of PH and increase the risk of decompensation. Acute variceal bleeding (AVB) is due to the rupture of GEVs and represents one of the most severe medical emergencies in cirrhosis. The prognosis of AVB has improved significantly over the past decades due to better management of the hemorrhage and its associated complications. Mortality, however, still is approximately 15% to 20%.[5,6] Moreover, variceal bleeding can trigger other complications of cirrhosis, such as bacterial infections, HE, and hepatorenal syndrome, that deteriorate prognosis further. Therefore, therapy to prevent bleeding (primary prophylaxis), to adequately control the acute bleeding episode, and to prevent rebleeding (secondary prophylaxis) is mandatory in order to improve survival. Currently, prevention and treatment of PH-related complications are based on medical treatment (nonselective β-blockers [NSBBs] administration; nitrates; diuretics; vasoactive drugs, such as somatostatin/terlipressin/octreotide; and so forth), endoscopic procedures and transjugular intrahepatic portosystemic shunt (TIPS) placement. Since the introduction of TIPS, the management of PH has been radically improved. TIPS placement is a percutaneous imaging-guided procedure that, by connecting usually the right intrahepatic portal branch and the right hepatic vein with a self-expandable metal stent, drastically reduces the portocaval pressure gradient. Although TIPS also can be used to treat other complications of PH, this review focuses on the use of TIPS in the different scenarios of cirrhotic PH bleeding, which are summarized in **Fig. 1**.

TRANSJUGULAR INTRAHEPATIC PORTOSYSTEMIC SHUNTS FOR PRIMARY PROPHYLAXIS

Different disease states encompass different risks of decompensation and, specifically, of variceal bleeding. It is considered that in patients with GEVs who never have bled that the risk of TIPS implantation outweights its potential benefits and, therefore, currently TIPS is not indicated for primary prophylaxis. When TIPS is performed for another indication (ie, refractory ascites), however, variceal prophylaxis

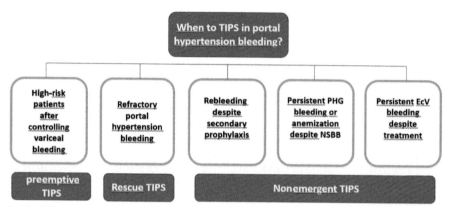

Fig. 1. When to use TIPS in the management of portal hypertension - related bleeding..

can be discontinued as long as TIPS is properly decreasing the portal pressure gradient below 12 mm Hg.

ACUTE EPISODE OF VARICEAL BLEEDING
Medical and Endoscopic Management

Vasoactive drugs, prophylactic antibiotics, and a restrictive blood transfusion constitute the cornerstone of the initial medical treatment of AVB.[7] Vasoactive drugs should be initiated as soon as AVB is suspected, because they facilitate the subsequent endoscopy and improve bleeding control.[8] Somatostatin, terlipressin, and octreotide currently are accepted vasoactive drugs; they require intravenous (IV) administration[9] and should be maintained for up to 5 days, with the aim of avoiding early rebleeding.[1] A shorter administration (48–72 h) has been suggested as effective as maintaining treatment for 5 days. More data are required, however, to strongly support this short-term administration.

Active infections that are quite frequent at admission in cirrhotic patients with acute gastrointestinal bleeding must be ruled out and treated adequately. Even if these are ruled out, prophylactic antibiotics must be given to reduce the probability of infection, improve bleeding control, and survival rates.[10] Also, it is important to apply antiencephalopathy measures and preserve renal function with adequate replacement of fluids and electrolytes. Red blood cell restitution must be restrictive, aiming at maintaining hemoglobin levels to a target level of 7 g/dL in order to avoid overexpansion.[11] Once hemodynamic stability is achieved, a gastroscopy should be performed and, if variceal bleeding is confirmed, endoscopic therapy done.[1,12] Several studies have evaluated the best timing for endoscopy after admission with divergent results.[12–15] The most accepted time interval to perform the gastroscopy, however, is within 12 hours after admission, especially in patients with hematemesis or hemodynamic instability. In patients with severe active bleeding or HE or in comatose patients, there is a high risk of aspiration. Thus, it is advisable to consider prophylactic orotracheal intubation prior to endoscopy to ensure airway protection.[7]

In the absence of contraindications (QT prolongation), administration of prokinetic agents. such as erythromycin, before the endoscopy (250 mg IV, 30–120 min before) has been shown to improve endoscopy performance and esophagogastric mucosa visibility.[16,17] Endoscopic band ligation (EBL) is more effective than sclerotherapy and presents fewer adverse effects and, therefore, must be the endoscopic treatment of choice. Sclerotherapy can be used when band ligation is not feasible.

Rescue Transjugular Intrahepatic Portosystemic Shunt

In 10% to 20% of patients, variceal bleeding is not controlled or reappears in a short period of time despite the application of the strategy, discussed previously. In mild rebleedings, a second endoscopic attempt finally may achieve hemostasis. In most cases, however, especially in those with more severe bleeding, a rescue/salvage TIPS is needed.[12] Balloon tamponade (BT) might be used as a bridge to rescue TIPS in unstable patients. BT is highly effective in controlling variceal bleeding. It can be used only for a short period of time (<24 h), however, due to its damage to the esophagus mucosa, and physicians always should be aware that bleeding recurs after deflation in more than half of the cases. In addition, BT frequently causes severe complications, such as bronchoaspiration, asphyxia, or esophageal perforation.[18,19] Esophageal stents have proved to be at least as effective as BT but, importantly, they are safer than BT in the management of AVB. Moreover, stents can be left in place for longer periods of time (usually up to 7 days), thus giving more time to achieve stabilization of the patient (ie, controlling possible sepsis or aspiration pneumonias) before placing a rescue TIPS.[20]

The studies establishing the value of TIPS as a rescue therapy were uncontrolled (due to lack of an adequate comparator) and used uncovered stents. These studies showed that rescue TIPS is associated with considerable mortality rates (30%–50%)[21–23] despite achieving high rates of bleeding control.[24,25] Therefore, additional studies in the era of covered stents are needed. Considering the lack of effective therapeutic alternatives, the main factor limiting the use of rescue TIPS is therapeutic futility, which should be evaluated in the light of a patient's eligibility for liver transplantation and in prognostic scores developed to predict survival after rescue TIPS: a consistent finding in the literature is that patients with a Child-Turcotte-Pugh score over 13 points requiring rescue TIPS rarely survive a TIPS.[26] Nevertheless, individual decisions should be taken in a case-by-case basis.

ROLE OF PREEMPTIVE TRANSJUGULAR INTRAHEPATIC PORTOSYSTEMIC SHUNT IN PATIENTS WITH VARICEAL BLEEDING AT HIGH RISK OF TREATMENT FAILURE AND OF MORTALITY

The high mortality associated with the use of TIPS as a rescue treatment raised the question on whether patients with poor prognostic indicators at admission might benefit from a more aggressive initial therapeutic approach. The concept of preemptive (p)-TIPS refers to the preventive insertion of a TIPS in patients who are at high risk both of failure to control bleeding (considering a period of 5 days) and of bleeding-related mortality. The rationale for placing a p-TIPS is that by preventing treatment failure (and, therefore, maneuvers associated with it, such as multiple blood transfusions, repeated endoscopies, used of BT, and high risk of aspiration pneumonia) and by promoting a marked reduction in PH, mortality would be reduced. Accordingly, the use of p-TIPS requires identifying which patients are at risk of having a poor prognosis during AVB. It has been reported that patients with hepatic venous pressure gradient (HVPG) greater than or equal to 20 mm Hg are 5 times more likely to experience failure to control AVB or to present early rebleeding, require more blood transfusions, and have higher mortality rates than patients with HVPG less than 20 mm Hg.[2,27,28] Likewise, the Child-Turcotte-Pugh score also has been used widely to estimate prognosis in the setting of AVB: survival in Child-Turcotte-Pugh stage A patients ranges from 96% to 100% whereas mortality is very high in patients with a Child-Turcotte-Pugh score greater than 13 points. More recently, a Model for End-Stage Liver Disease score greater than or equal to 19 also has proved an accurate marker of poor prognosis.[29] An important randomized clinical trial (RCT) confirmed the concept of better bleeding control and better survival in patients receiving p-TIPS in high-risk patients, defined as an HVPG greater than or equal to 20 mm Hg, as opposed to those receiving endoscopic treatment.[30] Nevertheless, this study was criticized because the high-risk criteria used (HVPG measurement) were not widely available and difficult to apply in many centers. More importantly, in this RCT, both arms were undertreated, according to current standards (TIPSs were placed using uncovered stents and patients in the control arm received sclerotherapy instead of band ligation). This study was followed by 2 other RCTs[29,31] and 4 observational studies,[32–35] however, that were performed using easy clinical criteria to define high-risk patients, such as (1) Child-Turcotte-Pugh stage B patients with active bleeding at diagnostic endoscopy despite receiving vasoactive drugs and (2) Child-Turcotte-Pugh stage C patients up to 13 points (regardless of endoscopy findings). All these studies used covered stents and proved that p-TIPS increases bleeding control, decreases rebleeding, improves ascites control without worsening HE, and, more importantly, reduces mortality. Mortality is reduced from 30% to 41% in patients receiving NSBBs plus EBL to 14% to 22% in the p-TIPS arm.[33–36] In the control arm (NSBBs plus EBL group), mortality is lower in Child-Turcotte-Pugh stage B plus active bleeding than in Child-Turcotte-Pugh stage C patients. Accordingly, the effects of p-TIPS on survival are more marked in Child-Turcotte-Pugh stage C patients than on the Child-Turcotte-Pugh stage B plus active bleeding group, which present more variable and heterogeneous survival results among the different studies.[33] Most of these studies, however, have limited sample size and more data are needed. In any case, also in Child-Turcotte-Pugh stage B patients, p-TIPS clearly has been shown to improve bleeding and ascites control without worsening HE, therefore making its use advisable in this setting.

Despite this evidence and despite clinical guidelines currently recommending the implementation of p-TIPS,[1] prospective surveys demonstrate that only 7% to 13%[33,34] of eligible patients currently are treated with p-TIPS, which highlights that physicians still need to incorporate p-TIPS in real-world practice. Supporting its implementation, it has been estimated that 4 high-risk patients need to be treated with p-TIPS to save 1 life, a number that is comparable to other very well-accepted invasive therapeutic strategies applied in other severe diseases, such as myocardial infarction. Also, Child-Turcotte-Pugh stage C patients have been shown to benefit from early intervention due to their higher risk of treatment failure and early death; patients with Child-Turcotte-Pugh stage B disease, even with active bleeding at the time of endoscopy, do not seem to universally benefit from preemptive intervention with TIPS; however a recent meta-analysis of individual patient data reveals improving survival and control of bleeding in both subgroups.[37]

TRANSJUGULAR INTRAHEPATIC PORTOSYSTEMIC SHUNT IN SECONDARY PROPHYLAXIS AFTER ACUTE VARICEAL BLEEDING

A combination of NSBBs plus EBL is highly effective in the secondary prevention of rebleeding and currently is the treatment of choice.[1] Several studies have compared this strategy with the initial use of TIPS in secondary prophylaxis.[23,38–40] Overall, in these studies, TIPS has been proved more effective than combination therapy in terms of preventing rebleeding but at expenses of a higher incidence of HE and no improvement in survival.[23,38–40] Although in most of these studies TIPS was performed using uncovered stents, 2 of them used covered stents[38,39] and showed similar results. Therefore, based on available data, TIPS currently cannot be recommended as a first-line treatment in secondary prophylaxis,[23] although it must be used to prevent further rebleeding when combination therapy fails.

Following the same rationale than that applied for AVB and p-TIPS, if the subpopulation of patients in whom combination therapy (NSBBs plus EBL) would fail to prevent rebleeding could be identified accurately and promptly, it might be worthy to test whether TIPS may be a better secondary prophylaxis strategy than NSBBs plus EBL in this selected group. In that regard, it already is known that patients undergoing secondary prophylaxis with EBL alone presents a higher rate of rebleeding and higher mortality than patients receiving combination therapy with NSBBs plus EBL.[41] Therefore, patients who cannot tolerate NSBBs or who present other conditions contraindicating NSBBs would be a potential high-risk population in whom other therapeutic strategies, such as TIPS, should be explored. Consequently, studies aiming at identifying patients with poor prognosis despite the use of the current standard of care for secondary prophylaxis are needed.

Probably the characteristics of the population requiring secondary prophylaxis will drastically change in the coming years if most centers adopt the use of the p-TIPS strategy for treating high-risk patients with AVB, because only the less severe patients will undergo secondary prophylaxis with NSBBs plus EBL. Future research needs to focus on exploring whether certain subgroups of patients initially considered not high-risk patients or patients who did not undergo p-TIPS for logistical reasons still may benefit from elective TIPS implantation for secondary prophylaxis.

MANAGEMENT OF GASTRIC VARICES

The prevalence of gastric varices (GVs) is lower (15%–20%) than esophageal varices (EVs) and they seem to bleed less frequently. When they do bleed, however, the bleeding usually is more severe and with a higher mortality than in EV.[42] According to Sarin and colleagues'[43] classification, there are 4 subtypes of GVs that have been shown to have different prognosis: GEVs associated with EVs along the lesser curve (gastroesophageal varices type 1 [GOV1]), GEVs associated with EVs along the along the fundus (gastroesophageal varices type 2 [GOV2]), isolated GVs (IGVs) located in the fundus (isolated gastroesophageal varices type 1 [IGV1]), and IGVs located at ectopic sites in the stomach/duodenum (isolated gastroesophageal varices type 2 [IGV2]).[43] Unfortunately, the management strategy for this subtype of varices is not as well established as in EV bleeding, given their lower prevalence and the scarce number of RCTs.[44] Additionally, in most studies, the different types of GVs are mixed and, therefore, the results are of difficult interpretation.

The initial treatment of GV bleeding is like that of EV bleeding (vasoactive drugs, volume resuscitation, and antibiotics prior to endoscopy). In a massive GV bleeding, a careful tamponade with a Linton-Nachlas balloon plays an important role as a bridge to further definitive therapy. It may achieve hemostasis in up to 80% of patients, although rebleeding may occur frequently when deflating the balloon.[45]

Studies evaluating the best endoscopic therapy for GVs are scarce and, as discussed previously, mix different GV types. Tissue adhesives, such as cyanoacrylate injection, are the more frequently endoscopic technique used,[46,47] although other possible endoscopic treatments are thrombin injection, sclerotherapy, band ligation, and their combinations. A recent RCT comparing cyanoacrylate injection versus thrombin injection for the acute management of GV hemorrhage found that, although both techniques present a similar rate of successful hemostasis, thrombin injection had a lower incidence of complications.[48] A significant percentage of patients included in this study presented GOV1 varices, which, according with current guidelines, should be treated as EV (including the use of p-TIPS in high-risk patients).[7,12,49] Remarkably, there is no consensus on the management of GOV2 and IGV1: although the American guidelines recommend TIPS as first-line therapy without prior use of endoscopic therapy,[12] Baveno VI criteria counsels cyanoacrylate injection plus NSBBs as first-line secondary prophylaxis,[1] reserving TIPS for treatment failure. Although admittedly no IGV1 or IGV2 patients were included in the p-TIPS studies, it seems reasonable to also apply the p-TIPS strategy in high-risk patients with AVB from GOV2, IGV1, and IGV2.

In experienced centers, patients with cardio-fundal varices (GOV-2 and IGV-1) and presence of an anatomic gastrorenal shunt can be treated with balloon-occluded retrograde transvenous obliteration (BRTO).[50] BRTO is a radiological procedure that aims at sclerosing the shunt feeding the varix: a balloon catheter is inserted, usually via the right femoral vein, and wedged into the left adrenal vein, achieving variceal obliteration. This technique is effective for treating bleeding fundic GVs. Patients may be at risk, however, of developing EVs after occlusion of the gastrorenal shunt[51] as well as thrombosis of the splanchnic axis. Despite the possibility of this side effects, among the BRTO advantages are lower rates of failure to control bleeding and rebleeding[52] and diminished incidence of HE. Thus, BRTO may be a good option for patients who have bled from fundic varices and are at high risk of HE or cardiac failure after TIPS.[53]

In recent studies, a modified BRTO strategy (balloon-assisted antegrade transvenous obliteration), combined with TIPS placement, has proved useful for the treatment of cardio-fundal varices (GOV2 or IGV1). This combined technique seems effective and may diminish the complications of PH, such as ascites and portal vein thrombosis.[54] These results must be interpreted with caution, however, due to the low number of patients reported and the need of more standardized studies addressing this approach.

MANAGEMENT OF ECTOPIC VARICES

Ectopic varices (EcVs) are composed of dilated portosystemic collaterals placed along the gastrointestinal tract instead of the common gastroesophageal region and account for 1% to 5% of all varices.[55] Their most frequent locations are around the insertion of stomas (40%), duodenum (23%), and rectum (17%), whereas the remaining 20% are located at other sites (20%). EcVs have a 4-fold increased risk, however, of bleeding when compared with EVs and, remarkably, can have a mortality rate as high as 40%.[56] Besides, difficulty in localizing the bleeding makes the management of these patients challenging, which can be solved by performing a computed tomographic angiography.[55]

TIPS employment in the management of EcV bleeding is based on case series.[57–59] The largest cohort published is a multicentric retrospective study that included 53 patients. The investigators concluded that TIPS may provide long-term control of bleeding in most cirrhotic patients with EcV and is effective particularly in stomal EcV, although might not be as effective in duodenal EcV (50% of rebleeding risk). A British study, including 21 patients with cirrhosis and EcV bleeding, who underwent TIPS, showed that embolization stopped the bleeding in most subjects. Therefore, combining TIPS and embolization may be a good approach in this setting.[57] In any case, therapeutic approach in EcV should be individualized based on the bleeding site and the vascular anatomy, taking into account the different points of view of a multidisciplinary team.[12]

PORTAL HYPERTENSION GASTROPATHY

PH gastropathy (PHG) is a cause of morbidity in patients with PH. Its diagnosis relies in the typical endoscopic findings of polygonal areas of variable erythema and, although not necessary for diagnosis, histologic findings may include venule and capillary dilatation, congestion, and tortuosity.[60] PHG may manifest both as chronic and overt bleeding,[61] sometimes even requiring repeated blood transfusions.[62]

The initial treatment of acute PHG bleeding should be based on vasoactive drugs, followed by NSBBs for secondary prophylaxis.[62] TIPS should be considered in patients who rebleed or continue to bleed despite adequate β-blocker therapy and in those who present persistent anemia despite iron supplementation. Unfortunately, the evidence for TIPS in the management of PHG is limited to reduced case reports and small series.[63–65] TIPS placement, however, may improve PHG and reduce the need of transfusions in most of the patients.[66]

It is important to differentiate PHG from gastric antral vascular ectasia (GAVE), which may be present in patients without PH. GAVE is characterized by red spots without a mosaic pattern, characteristically located in the antrum with a linear distribution, hence the name, *watermelon stomach*. GAVE's gold standard treatment is argon plasma coagulation and TIPS does not play a role in its management, although it could be considered in cases where PHG and GAVE coexist.[67]

CLINICS CARE POINTS

- Primary prophylaxis for AVB should be based on non-selective betablockers or endoscopic band ligation.
- The first approach to AVB is a prompt administration of vasoactive drugs, endoscopic treatment and prevention of other complications (use of antibiotics and anti-encephalopathy measures).
- In Child-Turcotte-Pugh stage B patients with active bleeding at endoscopy, and in all Child-Turcotte-Pugh stage C patients, preemptive TIPS should be considered.
- In patients presenting a rebleeding episode despite adequate secondary prophylaxis TIPS should be considered.
- TIPS ± embolization would be recommended in the setting of gastric variceal bleeding if patients rebleed despite medical and endoscopic therapy.
- In ectopic varices refractory to local therapy, TIPS could be an effective tool.
- In patients with persistent anemization and bleeding from portal hypertensive gastropathy refractory to iron and beta-blockers treatment, TIPS could also be considered.

ACKNOWLEDGMENTS

Administrative support by Oliva Ros Fargas.

REFERENCES

1. De Franchis R, Baveno V. Faculty. Expanding consensus in portal hypertension. Report of the Baveno VI Consensus Workshop: stratifying risk and individualizing care for portal hypertension. J Hepatol 2015;63:743–52.
2. Merli M, Nicolini G, Angeloni S, et al. Incidence and natural history of small esophageal varices in cirrhotic patients. J Hepatol 2003;38:266–72.
3. O'Brien J, Triantos C, Burroughs AK. Management of varices in patients with cirrhosis. Nat Rev Gastroenterol Hepatol 2013;10:402–12.
4. Ripoll C, Groszmann R, Garcia-Tsao G, et al. Hepatic venous pressure gradient predicts clinical decompensation in patients with compensated cirrhosis. Gastroenterology 2007;133:481–8.

5. Augustin S, Muntaner L, Altamirano JT, et al. Predicting early mortality after acute variceal hemorrhage based on classification and regression tree analysis. Clin Gastroenterol Hepatol 2009;7:1347–54.

6. Amitrano L, Guardascione MA, Manguso F, et al. The effectiveness of current acute variceal bleed treatments in unselected cirrhotic patients: refining short-term prognosis and risk factors. Am J Gastroenterol 2012;107:1872–8.

7. Angeli P, Bernardi M, Villanueva C, et al. EASL Clinical Practice Guidelines for the management of patients with decompensated cirrhosis. J Hepatol 2018;69:406–60.

8. Levacher S, Blaise M, Pourriat J-L, et al. Early administration of terlipressin plus glyceryl trinitrate to control active upper gastrointestinal bleeding in cirrhotic patients. Lancet 1995;346:865–8.

9. Seo YS, Park SY, Kim MY, et al. Lack of difference among terlipressin, somatostatin, and octreotide in the control of acute gastroesophageal variceal hemorrhage. Hepatology 2014;60:954–63.

10. Bernard B, Grangé J-D, Khac EN, et al. Antibiotic prophylaxis for the prevention of bacterial infections in cirrhotic patients with gastrointestinal bleeding: a meta-analysis. Hepatology 1999;29:1655–61.

11. Villanueva C, Colomo ABA. Transfusion for acute upper gastrointestinal bleeding. N Engl J Med 2013;368:1361–3.

12. Garcia-Tsao G, Abraldes JG, Berzigotti A, et al. Portal hypertensive bleeding in cirrhosis: risk stratification, diagnosis, and management: 2016 practice guidance by the American Association for the study of liver diseases. Hepatology 2017;65:310–35.

13. Lau JYW, Yu Y, Tang RSY, et al. Timing of endoscopy for acute upper gastrointestinal bleeding. N Engl J Med 2020;382:1299–308.

14. Chen P-H, Chen W-C, Hou M-C, et al. Delayed endoscopy increases re-bleeding and mortality in patients with hematemesis and active esophageal variceal bleeding: a cohort study. J Hepatol 2012;57:1207–13.

15. Huh CW, Kim JS, Jung DH, et al. Optimal endoscopy timing according to the severity of underlying liver disease in patients with acute variceal bleeding. Dig Liver Dis 2019;51:993–8.

16. Altraif I, Handoo FA, Aljumah A, et al. Effect of erythromycin before endoscopy in patients presenting with variceal bleeding: a prospective, randomized, double-blind, placebo-controlled trial. Gastrointest Endosc 2011;73:245–50.

17. Stanley AJ, Laine L. Management of acute upper gastrointestinal bleeding. BMJ 2019;364:I536.

18. Panés J, Terés J, Bosch J, et al. Efficacy of balloon tamponade in treatment of bleeding gastric and esophageal varices. Results in 151 consecutive episodes. Dig Dis Sci 1988;33:454–9.

19. Avgerinos A, Armonis A. Balloon tamponade technique and efficacy in variceal haemorrhage. Scand J Gastroenterol Suppl 1994;207:11–6.

20. Escorsell À, Pavel O, Cárdenas A, et al. Esophageal balloon tamponade versus esophageal stent in controlling acute refractory variceal bleeding: a multicenter randomized, controlled trial. Hepatology 2016;63:1957–67.

21. D'Amico G, Pagliaro L, Bosch J. The treatment of portal hypertension: a meta-analytic review. Hepatology 1995;22:332–54.

22. Bosch J. Salvage transjugular intrahepatic portosystemic shunt: is it really life-saving? J Hepatol 2001;35:658–60.

23. Escorsell A, Bañares R, García-Pagán JC, et al. TIPS versus drug therapy in preventing variceal rebleeding in advanced cirrhosis: a randomized controlled trial. Hepatology 2002;35:385–92.

24. Azoulay D, Castaing D, Majno P, et al. Salvage transjugular intrahepatic portosystemic shunt for uncontrolled variceal bleeding in patients with decompensated cirrhosis. J Hepatol 2001;35:590–7.

25. Bañares R, Casado M, Rodríguez-Láiz JM, et al. Urgent transjugular intrahepatic portosystemic shunt for control of acute variceal bleeding. Am J Gastroenterol 1998;93:75–9.

26. Patch D, Nikolopoulou V, McCormick A, et al. Factors related to early mortality after transjugular intrahepatic portosystemic shunt for failed endoscopic therapy in acute variceal bleeding. J Hepatol 1998;28:454–60.

27. D'Amico G, Morabito A, D'Amico M, et al. Clinical states of cirrhosis and competing risks. J Hepatol 2018;68:563–76.

28. D'Amico G, Luca A. Natural history. Clinical-haemodynamic correlations. Prediction of the risk of bleeding. Baillieres Clin Gastroenterol 1997;11:243–56.

29. García-Pagán JC, Caca K, Bureau C, et al. Early use of TIPS in patients with cirrhosis and variceal bleeding. N Engl J Med 2010;362:2370–9.

30. Monescillo A, Martínez-Lagares F, Ruiz-del-Arbol L, et al. Influence of portal hypertension and its early decompression by TIPS placement on the outcome of variceal bleeding. Hepatology 2004;40:793–801.

31. Lv Y, Yang Z, Liu L, et al. Early TIPS with covered stents versus standard treatment for acute variceal bleeding in patients with advanced cirrhosis: a randomised controlled trial. lancet. Gastroenterol Hepatol 2019;4:587–98.

32. Garcia-Pagán JC, Di Pascoli M, Caca K, et al. Use of early-TIPS for high-risk variceal bleeding: results of a post-RCT surveillance study. J Hepatol 2013;58:45–50.

33. Hernández-Gea V, Procopet B, Giráldez Á, et al. Preemptive-TIPS improves outcome in high-risk variceal bleeding: an observational study. Hepatology 2019;69:282–93.

34. Thabut D, Pauwels A, Carbonell N, et al. Cirrhotic patients with portal hypertension-related bleeding and an indication for early-TIPS: a large multicentre audit with real-life results. J Hepatol 2017;68:73–81.

35. Lv Y, Zuo L, Zhu X, et al. Identifying optimal candidates for early TIPS among patients with cirrhosis and acute variceal bleeding: a multicentre observational study. Gut 2018;68(7):1297–310.

36. Conejo I, Guardascione MA, Tandon P, et al. Multicenter external validation of risk stratification criteria for patients with variceal bleeding. Clin Gastroenterol Hepatol 2018;16:132–9.e8.

37. Nicoară-Farcău O, Han G, Rudler M, et al. Effects of early placement of transjugular portosystemic shunts in patients with high-risk acute variceal bleeding: a meta-analysis of individual patient data. Gastroenterology 2021;160:193–205.e10.

38. Holster IL, Tjwa ETTL, Moelker A, et al. Covered transjugular intrahepatic portosystemic shunt versus endoscopic therapy + beta-blocker for prevention of variceal rebleeding. Hepatology 2016;63:581–9.

39. Sauerbruch T, Mengel M, Dollinger M, et al. Prevention of rebleeding from esophageal varices in patients with cirrhosis receiving small-diameter stents versus hemodynamically controlled medical therapy. Gastroenterology 2015;149:660–8.e1.

40. Lin L-L, Du S-M, Fu Y, et al. Combination therapy versus pharmacotherapy, endoscopic variceal ligation, or the transjugular intrahepatic portosystemic shunt

alone in the secondary prevention of esophageal variceal bleeding: a meta-analysis of randomized controlled trials. Oncotarget 2017;8:57399–408.

41. Albillos A, Zamora J, Martínez J, et al. Stratifying risk in the prevention of recurrent variceal hemorrhage: results of an individual patient meta-analysis. Hepatology 2017;66:1219–31.

42. Kim T. Risk factors for hemorrhage from gastric fundal varices. Hepatology 1997; 25:307–12.

43. Sarin SK, Lahoti D, Saxena SP, et al. Prevalence, classification and natural history of gastric varices: a long-term follow-up study in 568 portal hypertension patients. Hepatology 1992;16:1343–9.

44. Tripathi D, Ferguson JW, Therapondos G, et al. Review article: recent advances in the management of bleeding gastric varices. Aliment Pharmacol Ther 2006; 24:1–17.

45. Terés J, Cecilia A, Bordas JM, et al. Esophageal tamponade for bleeding varices. Controlled trial between the Sengstaken-Blakemore tube and the Linton-Nachlas tube. Gastroenterology 1978;75:566–9.

46. Dhiman RK, Chawla Y, Taneja S, et al. Endoscopic sclerotherapy of gastric variceal bleeding with N-Butyl-2-Cyanoacrylate. J Clin Gastroenterol 2002;35:222–7.

47. Elsebaey MA, Tawfik MA, Ezzat S, et al. Endoscopic injection sclerotherapy versus N-Butyl-2 Cyanoacrylate injection in the management of actively bleeding esophageal varices: a randomized controlled trial. BMC Gastroenterol 2019; 19:23.

48. Lo G-H, Lin C-W, Tai C-M, et al. A prospective, randomized trial of thrombin versus cyanoacrylate injection in the control of acute gastric variceal hemorrhage. Endoscopy 2020;52(7):548–55.

49. Lo G-H, Liang H-L, Chen W-C, et al. A prospective, randomized controlled trial of transjugular intrahepatic portosystemic shunt versus cyanoacrylate injection in the prevention of gastric variceal rebleeding. Endoscopy 2007;39:679–85.

50. Luo X, Ma H, Yu J, et al. Efficacy and safety of balloon-occluded retrograde transvenous obliteration of gastric varices with lauromacrogol foam sclerotherapy: initial experience. Abdom Radiol 2018;43:1820–4.

51. Matsumoto A, Hamamoto N, Nomura T, et al. Balloon-occluded retrograde transvenous obliteration of high risk gastric fundal varices. Am J Gastroenterol 1999; 94:643–9.

52. Lipnik A, Pandhi M, Khabbaz R, et al. Endovascular treatment for variceal hemorrhage: TIPS, BRTO, and combined approaches. Semin Intervent Radiol 2018; 35:169–84.

53. Wang Y-B, Zhang J-Y, Gong J-P, et al. Balloon-occluded retrograde transvenous obliteration versus transjugular intrahepatic portosystemic shunt for treatment of gastric varices due to portal hypertension: a meta-analysis. J Gastroenterol Hepatol 2016;31:727–33.

54. Liu J, Yang C, Huang S, et al. The combination of balloon-assisted antegrade transvenous obliteration and transjugular intrahepatic portosystemic shunt for the management of cardiofundal varices hemorrhage. Eur J Gastroenterol Hepatol 2020;32:656–62.

55. Etik D, Oztas E, Okten S, et al. Ectopic varices in portal hypertension. Eur J Gastroenterol Hepatol 2011;23:620–2.

56. Saad WEA, Lippert A, Saad NE, et al. Ectopic varices: anatomical classification, hemodynamic classification, and hemodynamic-based management. Tech Vasc Interv Radiol 2013;16:108–25.

57. Vangeli M, Patch D, Terreni N, et al. Bleeding ectopic varices—treatment with transjugular intrahepatic porto-systemic shunt (TIPS) and embolisation. J Hepatol 2004;41:560–6.
58. Vidal V, Joly L, Perreault P, et al. Usefulness of transjugular intrahepatic portosystemic shunt in the management of bleeding ectopic varices in cirrhotic patients. Cardiovasc Intervent Radiol 2006;29:216–9.
59. Kochar N, Tripathi D, Mcavoy NC, et al. Bleeding ectopic varices in cirrhosis: the role of transjugular intrahepatic portosystemic stent shunts. Aliment Pharmacol Ther 2008;28:294–303.
60. Gjeorgjievski M, Cappell MS. Portal hypertensive gastropathy: a systematic review of the pathophysiology, clinical presentation, natural history and therapy. World J Hepatol 2016;8:231–62.
61. D'Amico G, Montalbano L, Traina M, et al. Natural history of congestive gastropathy in cirrhosis. Gastroenterology 1990;99:1558–64.
62. Ripoll C, Garcia-Tsao G. Treatment of gastropathy and gastric antral vascular ectasia in patients with portal hypertension. Curr Treat Options Gastroenterol 2007; 10:483–94.
63. Mezawa S, Homma H, Ohta H, et al. Effect of transjugular intrahepatic portosystemic shunt formation on portal hypertensive gastropathy and gastric circulation. Am J Gastroenterol 2001;96:1155–9.
64. Ashraf P, Shah GM, Shaikh H, et al. Transjugular intrahepatic portosystemic stenting in portal hypertensive gastropathy. J Coll Physicians Surg Pak 2009;19: 584–5.
65. Urata J, Yamashita Y, Tsuchigame T, et al. The effects of transjugular intrahepatic portosystemic shunt on portal hypertensive gastropathy. J Gastroenterol Hepatol 1998;13:1061–7.
66. Kamath PS, Lacerda M, Ahlquist DA, et al. Gastric mucosal responses to intrahepatic portosystemic shunting in patients with cirrhosis. Gastroenterology 2000; 118:905–11.
67. Tripathi D, Stanley AJ, Hayes PC, et al. Transjugular intrahepatic portosystemic stent-shunt in the management of portal hypertension. Gut 2020;15. gutjnl-2019-320221.

Bacterial Infections in Cirrhosis as a Cause or Consequence of Decompensation?

Salvatore Piano, MD, PhD*, Paolo Angeli, MD, PhD

KEYWORDS

- Sepsis • Cirrhosis • Decompensation • Ascites • Hepatic encephalopathy
- Variceal bleeding • Acute-on-chronic liver failure

KEY POINTS

- Patients with cirrhosis are at high risk of developing bacterial infections because of cirrhosis-associated immune dysfunction, increased intestinal permeability and gut dysbiosis.
- Bacterial infections induce systemic inflammation, oxidative stress and worsen portal hypertension and circulatory dysfunction, triggering decompensation and organ failures.
- In patients at high risk for developing infections, antibiotic prophylaxis reduces the incidence of infections and improve prognosis.
- Infections should be rapidly ruled out in all patients hospitalized with decompensated cirrhosis; antibiotic treatment should not be delayed.
- Patients with spontaneous bacterial peritonitis should receive volume expansion with human albumin to decrease the incidence of renal failure and improve survival.

INTRODUCTION

Liver cirrhosis is one of the leading causes of death worldwide. According to data from the Global Burden of Disease study 2017, cirrhosis is the 13th cause of death worldwide and was responsible for almost 200,000 deaths on 2017.[1] Most of death occurs after decompensation of the disease. In fact, liver cirrhosis is characterized by a compensated phase, in which the liver disease is asymptomatic or paucisymptomatic and the prognosis is quite good (median survival, 12 years).[2] However, the occurrence of complications of cirrhosis (ascites, variceal bleeding, hepatic encephalopathy, or jaundice) marks the transition to the decompensated phase, which is associated to a poor prognosis (median survival, 2 years).[2] Portal hypertension is the main driver of decompensation and has been a relevant target for

Unit of Internal Medicine and Hepatology (UIMH), Department of Medicine – DIMED, University and Hospital of Padova, Via Giustiniani 2, Padova 35100, Italy
* Corresponding author. Unit of Internal Medicine and Hepatology, Department of Medicine – DIMED, University of Padova, Via Giustiniani 2, Padova 35100, Italy.
E-mail address: salvatore.piano@unipd.it

Clin Liver Dis 25 (2021) 357–372
https://doi.org/10.1016/j.cld.2021.01.006
1089-3261/21/© 2021 Elsevier Inc. All rights reserved.

preventing decompensation in patients with cirrhosis.[3,4] However, other factors can facilitate the occurrence of decompensation. Among them, bacterial infections (BIs) are increasingly recognized as the most common precipitating event of acute decompensation of cirrhosis.[5] Indeed, patients with cirrhosis have a high risk of developing BIs, which can trigger decompensation. In turns, after decompensation, the risk of developing BIs further increases, being associated with further episodes of decompensation. The net results of this vicious circle is a 4-fold increase in mortality rate in patients with cirrhosis and infections,[6] which has led some authors to consider BIs as a distinct stage of liver disease.[6,7] Beyond cirrhosis staging definitions, there is no doubt that strategies to prevent and/or early recognize and treat infections are key to improve prognosis of patients with cirrhosis.[8] Herein we review the role of BIs as a cause and consequence of decompensation in patients with cirrhosis.

CIRRHOSIS PREDISPOSES TO BACTERIAL INFECTIONS

Patients with cirrhosis have more than twice the risk of developing an infection than general population.[9] The most common infections in these patients are spontaneous bacterial peritonitis (SBP), urinary tract infections, pneumonia, skin and soft tissues infections, and spontaneous bacteremia.[7,10–13] Several mechanisms are responsible for predisposing patients with cirrhosis to BIs, which involves changes in adaptive and acquired immunity, alteration of intestinal barrier with an increase in intestinal permeability and changes in quantity and quality of gut microbiome.[14]

Cirrhosis is associated with several abnormalities in the innate and adaptive components of the immune system's response to bacteria, leading to a state of immunodeficiency.[15] Circulating immune cells, such as neutrophils and lymphocytes, decrease in frequency and exhibit an alteration in bacterial phagocytosis and killing abilities. The defective production of complement and soluble pattern recognition receptors impairs the capability of bacterial recognition and opsonization. Finally, the disruption of liver architecture and portosystemic shunts compromise the immune surveillance function of the liver.[15]

The increase in intestinal permeability is caused by ultrastructural changes in the intestinal mucosa (tight junctions disruption, widening of intracellular spaces, vascular congestion, wall thickening, etc), oxidative stress, local inflammation, and hyperactivity of the autonomic nervous system.[16] More recently, bile acids showed to exerts a relevant role on promoting intestinal barrier integrity toward the activation of farnesoid X receptors (FXR), which are nuclear receptors expressed in the gut and the liver.[17] In cirrhosis, the decrease in gut bile acids availability is associated with an increased intestinal permeability and bacterial translocation, which can be reverted with the administration of FXR agonists.[17]

The gut microbiome in patients with cirrhosis is profoundly altered. The decrease in small bowel motility and the decrease in antimicrobial peptides such as α-defensins facilitates bacterial overgrowth. However, also the quality of bacteria is changed, with the depletion of the beneficial phyla *Lachnospiraceae* and enrichment of the phyla *Proteobacteria* (mainly *Enterobacteriaceae*) and *Enterococcaceae*.[18,19] *Enterobacteriaceae* and *Enterococcaceae* are more adapted to translocate from the gut to systemic circulation and are also the most common pathogens responsible for spontaneous infections in patients with cirrhosis.[10] More recently, metagenomics studies showed a decrease in gut microbial diversity in patients with cirrhosis, which was further reduced in decompensated cirrhosis and ACLF and associated with risk of being hospitalized.[20,21] Finally, experimental models of cirrhosis suggest that gut dysbiosis impairs the intestinal immune response and leads to disrupted barrier function, promoting bacterial translocation.[22]

Putting all these data together, the balance of the host–pathogen interaction is altered in patients with cirrhosis with a reduction in barrier function, altered immune response and increase in pathogens abundance (**Box 1**).

BACTERIAL INFECTIONS AS A CAUSE OF DECOMPENSATION

Overall, almost 40% of patients hospitalized for an acute decompensation of cirrhosis experience a BI during the hospitalization.[11,23] About two-thirds of these infections are present at hospital admission, and 25% to 30% are nosocomial.[10,11] Several studies found an association between BIs and decompensating events such as hepatic encephalopathy,[24] gastrointestinal bleeding,[25,26] and ascites.[23] However, there is a paucity of studies clearly demonstrating whether BIs occurred before decompensation, thus triggering decompensation, or were a consequence of decompensation. In a large series of patients with compensated viral cirrhosis, Nahon and colleagues[27] showed that BIs occurred before decompensation in more than 80% of cases. Patients with BIs had a higher risk of developing decompensation (5-year incidence of decompensation of 45% vs 15% in patients with or without infections, respectively; $P<.001$).[27] In a post hoc analysis of the PREDESCI trial,[28] a trial investigating the ability of beta-blockers in preventing decompensation in patients with clinically significant portal hypertension, Villanueva and colleagues[29] showed that the occurrence of BIs significantly increases the risk of developing ascites and worsens survival.

When BIs occurs they frequently cause dysfunction and failure of organs other than the liver.[30] In fact BIs are recognized as the most common precipitating event of acute kidney injury (AKI)[23,31–33] and of ACLF, a syndrome characterized by acute decompensation of cirrhosis, organ failures, systemic inflammation, and high short-term mortality.[5] Furthermore, when ACLF is triggered by BIs, short-term mortality further increases.[34] After the first decompensation of cirrhosis, BIs facilitates further

---

Box 1
Summary of the host–pathogen changes occurring in patients with liver cirrhosis and predisposing to the development of infections

Host alterations
   Hypersplenism decreases circulating neutrophils and lymphocytes
   A decrease in complement and acute phase protein production with decreased opsonization of bacteria by immune cells
   Monocytes and neutrophils show an impaired bacterial phagocytosis and bacterial killing ability
   Portal hypertension induces ultrastructural changes in the intestinal mucosa (tight junctions disruption, widening of intracellular spaces, vascular congestion, wall thickening), increasing intestinal permeability
   A decreased availability of bile acids in the gut impairs the FXR signaling, disrupting the intestinal barrier function and increasing intestinal permeability
   Reticuloendothelial removal capacity is reduced because of alteration of liver structure and portosystemic shunts

Pathogen alterations
   Intestinal bacterial overgrowth
   Changes in microbiome composition with enrichment in pathogenic *Enterobacteriaceae* and *Enterococcaceae* and a decrease in beneficial *Lachnospiraceae*
   Decrease in gut microbial diversity

decompensation, such as variceal rebleeding,[35] recurrent hepatic encephalopathy,[36] and hepatorenal syndrome.[37] Finally, after BIs patients with cirrhosis have a high risk of early hospital readmissions.[38,39]

Pathophysiology of Decompensation Induced by Bacterial Infections

For several years, the hemodynamics consequences of portal hypertension have been considered the main drivers of decompensation of cirrhosis.[4] Portal hypertension is responsible for splanchnic arterial vasodilation, which causes a reduction of effective circulating volume and activation of endogenous vasoconstrictor systems (renin–angiotensin–aldosterone system, sympathetic nervous system, and nonosmotic release of vasopressin), which are responsible for sodium and water retention and thus the appearance of ascites and edema.[40] Portal hypertension induces the appearance of varices, which are responsible for bleeding. Finally, portal hypertension causes the appearance of portosystemic shunts, which are involved in the pathogenesis of hepatic encephalopathy.

More recently, systemic inflammation was shown to play a relevant role in promoting decompensation.[41] In fact, it has been shown that the levels of inflammatory cytokines increase in patients with ascites,[42] hepatic encephalopathy,[43] and organ failures.[44] Systemic inflammation in cirrhosis is caused by the interaction of immune system with pathogens-associated molecular pattern (PAMPs), which are molecule expressed by pathogens (eg, lipopolysaccharide for gram-negative bacteria) and danger-associated molecular patterns, which are molecules released by cell death. The recognition of PAMPs and danger-associated molecular patterns on pattern recognition receptors (such as Toll-like receptors) induces the production of inflammatory cytokines, nitric oxide (NO), the recruitment of leukocytes, and the release of reactive oxygen species.[41]

Sterile inflammation in cirrhosis is determined by translocation of PAMPs from the gut to the mesenteric lymph nodes and/or owing to the release of danger-associated molecular patterns after an acute hepatic inflammatory process. However, when overt BIs occur, the inflammatory response is quite higher.[44] The inflammatory response is crucial for providing defense against pathogens; however, it comes with relevant undesired drawbacks (**Fig. 1**). In cirrhotic rats, PAMPs aggravates portal hypertension by increasing the severity of intrahepatic microvascular dysfunction, exacerbating hepatic inflammation, increasing oxidative stress, and recruiting hepatic stellate cells.[45] Inflammation induces the production of NO in splanchnic circulation, further worsening arterial vasodilation.[41] Furthermore, experimental data suggests that inflammatory cytokines such as tumor necrosis factor-α cause an increase in the expression of inducible NO synthase and production of NO in the heart of cirrhotic rats, impairing cardiac contractility.[46,47] The consequent reduction in cardiac output causes a further drop in effective circulating volume. These hemodynamic changes favor the chain of events responsible for the development of ascites, dilutional hyponatremia and hepatorenal syndrome.

As for the brain, in vitro studies showed that inflammatory cytokines (tumor necrosis factor-α, IL-1, IL-6 and IFN-γ) induce astrocyte swelling to a similar extent of ammonia. Furthermore, stimulation of astrocytes previously exposed to ammonia, further increased astrocyte swelling.[48] Finally, in vivo studies showed an increase in brain water content and protein nitration in bile duct ligated rats after stimulation with lipopolysaccharide.[49]

Severe inflammation is also responsible for the release of reactive oxygen species, which can cause mitochondrial dysfunction, decreasing the oxidative phosphorylation with a consequent shift of metabolism to glycolysis.[50] Glycolysis is more rapid, but

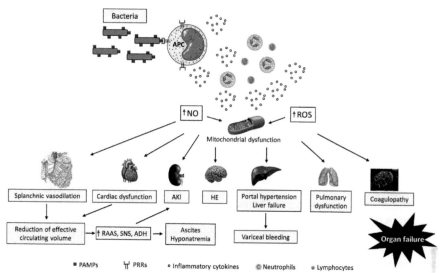

Fig. 1. The pathophysiology of decompensation induced by bacterial infections. Bacterial PAMPs are recognized by pattern recognition receptors on APCs, which promotes the production of inflammatory cytokines, and recruitment of inflammatory cells, which further enhances the inflammatory response. Inflammation induces the production of NO, which worsens splanchnic vasodilation and induces cardiac dysfunction. The result is a reduction in effective circulating volume which promotes the activation of vasoconstrictor systems and promotes water and sodium retention and renal hypoperfusion. Inflammation worsens intrahepatic microvascular dysfunction and oxidative stress increasing portal hypertension. Inflammation worsens brain edema and favors the occurrence of hepatic encephalopathy. NO and oxidative stress induces mitochondrial dysfunction which can cause organ failures. ADH, antidiuretic hormone; APC, antigen presenting cells; HE, hepatic encephalopathy; pattern recognition receptors, pattern recognition receptors; RAAS, renin-angiotensin-aldosterone system; ROS, reactive oxygen species; SNS, sympathetic nervous system.

less efficient than oxidative phosphorylation and in case of severe inflammation, cells can be unable to meet their metabolic needs. Mitochondrial dysfunction is well known to occur in sepsis, but more recently, a metabolomic study in patients with decompensated cirrhosis and ACLF found features suggesting inhibition of mitochondrial energy production, which may contribute to the development of organ failures.[51]

BACTERIAL INFECTIONS AS A CONSEQUENCE OF DECOMPENSATION

After decompensation, patients with cirrhosis have a relevant risk for developing BIs. Variceal bleeding is a relevant risk factor for the development of infections in patients with cirrhosis. In fact, although about 20% of patients with variceal bleeding is already infected at the time of bleeding, infections can complicate the clinical course in almost 50% of patients.[52] When infections occur, they are associated with an increased rate of failure to control bleeding, rebleeding, and hospital mortality.[35,53] Patients with ascites are at risk of developing infections, in particular SBP.[52] Specific risk factors in this group are a low protein content in ascitic fluid and high levels of bilirubin.[54,55] Patients with hepatic encephalopathy are fragile and at risk of developing aspiration pneumonia. In patients with decompensated cirrhosis, BIs are associated with the risk of developing AKI, hepatorenal syndrome, organ failures and ACLF.[5,23,31] Remarkably, patients with ACLF have an increased risk of developing BIs, which increases mortality rate.[34] Among organ dysfunction or failures, relative adrenal insufficiency has been associated with an increased risk of infections and sepsis.[56,57] In summary, a vicious circle links BIs and decompensation of cirrhosis, where decompensation can cause infections, which can cause further decompensation, further infections, organ failures and mortality (**Fig. 2**).

Pathophysiology of Bacterial Infections as a Consequence of Decompensation

After decompensation of cirrhosis, characteristics predisposing to BIs (immune dysfunction, gut dysbiosis, increased intestinal permeability) are further enhanced.[16] After variceal bleeding, the high amount of blood reaches the gut, altering intestinal flora and promoting bacterial translocation. Furthermore, hematemesis per se is a risk factor for aspiration pneumonia. In patients with ascites, the decrease in reticulo-endothelial removal capacity is associated with the risk of developing infections.[58] Furthermore, the decrease in complement in ascites affects the ability of immune cells to opsonize of bacteria predisposing patients to the development of infections.[59] Hepatic encephalopathy is associated with portosystemic shunts, which lower the liver's ability to clear intestinal bacteria and are associated with the occurrence of SBP.[60] Furthermore, patients with severe hepatic encephalopathy are at risk for aspiration pneumonia.

As for patients with ACLF, it has been demonstrated that, despite a severe inflammatory response, ACLF is frequently associated with immune dysfunction, which impairs pathogen killing ability by macrophages and neutrophils.[61,62] This condition of immune paralysis is associated with the risk of developing infections.[34]

PREVENTION OF INFECTIONS AS A STRATEGY TO PREVENT DECOMPENSATION AND/OR FURTHER DECOMPENSATION IN CIRRHOSIS

Infections have such an important role in inducing decompensation and/or further decompensation that several strategies have been developed to prevent BIs in cirrhosis (**Table 1**).

Antibiotic Prophylaxis

Antibiotic prophylaxis has been used to prevent infections in patients with decompensated cirrhosis at high risk of developing BIs. In patients with gastrointestinal bleeding, antibiotic prophylaxis decrease the incidence of BIs, rebleeding and mortality.[63] Norfloxacin (400 mg 2 times per day) was shown to be effective for this purpose; however, it is less effective than ceftriaxone (1 g/d) in patients with advanced

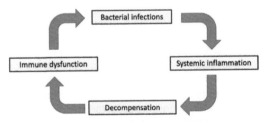

Fig. 2. Bacterial infections and decompensation: the ominous vicious circle. Bacterial infections can trigger hepatic decompensation by increasing systemic inflammation, oxidative stress and portal pressure. After decompensation, cirrhosis-associated immune dysfunction and dysbyosis worsens, favoring the appearance of infections, which triggers further decompensation.

Table 1
Evidence-based strategies to prevent bacterial infections and decompensation in cirrhosis

Treatment	Target Population	Effects
Norfloxacin 400 mg qd	Patients with previous episodes of SBP	Decreased incidence of SBP
Norfloxacin 400 mg qd	Patients with ascites, ascites protein of <15 g/L and advanced cirrhosis[a]	Decreased incidence of SBP, HRS and trends toward better survival
Ceftriaxone 2g[b] Norfloxacin 400 mg bid	Patients with variceal bleeding	Decreased incidence of infections, failure to control bleeding, rebleeding and mortality

Abbreviations: bid, 2 times per day; HRS, hepatorenal syndrome; qd, daily.
  [a] Child-Turcotte-Pugh score of ≥9 points with a serum bilirubin of ≥3 mg/dL or a serum creatinine of ≥1.2 mg/dL/urea of ≥25 mg/dL, or serum sodium of ≤130 mmol/L.
  [b] Ceftriaxone is more effective than norfloxacin in patients with advanced cirrhosis (≥2 of the following: ascites, severe malnutrition, encephalopathy, or bilirubin of >3 mg/dL).

cirrhosis (ie, ≥2 of the following: ascites, severe malnutrition, encephalopathy, or bilirubin >3 mg/dL).[64] However, norfloxacin is no more available in many countries (including the United States) and it should be avoided in countries with a high rate of quinolone resistant bacteria.[4]

In patients with ascites and a high risk of developing SBP (ie, ascitic fluid protein of <1.5 g/dL plus ≥1 among [i] a Child-Turcotte-Pugh score of ≥9 points with serum bilirubin ≥3 mg/dL; [ii] a serum creatinine of ≥1.2 mg/dL or a urea of ≥25 mg/dL; or [iii] a serum sodium of ≤130 mmol/L) norfloxacin prophylaxis (400 mg/d) decrease the incidence of SBP and hepatorenal syndrome, with a trend toward an improved survival.[65] More recently, a post hoc analysis of a randomized placebo-controlled trial showed improved survival in patients with cirrhosis, ascites, and Child-Turcotte-Pugh class C.[66] However, the survival benefit was observed only in patients with an ascitic fluid protein of less than 1.5 g/dL and quinolone prophylaxis should be reserved to these high-risk patients.

After the first episode of SBP, the recurrence of infection is almost 70% at 1 year. Prophylaxis with norfloxacin (400 mg/d) decreases the recurrence of SBP.[67]

Antibiotic prophylaxis can induce the development of multidrug-resistant bacteria,[68] which are a relevant emerging problem worldwide[10]; therefore, it should be reserved to high-risk patients.

Rifaximin, a nonabsorbable antibiotic, has been shown to prevent the recurrence of hepatic encephalopathy[69] and to decrease endotoxemia[70] in patients with cirrhosis. Whether rifaximin could replace quinolone in the prevention of SBP remain to be proven in well-designed randomized controlled trial. Anyway, it could represent an interesting strategy for preventing infections and decompensation.

Nonantibiotic Strategies to Prevent Infections

Antibiotics can lead to the development of multidrug-resistant bacteria and nonantibiotic strategies should be implemented to prevent infections in cirrhosis (**Table 2**). Among nonantibiotic strategies, the first relevant point is to avoid unnecessary and potentially hazardous drugs. Proton pump inhibitors use is frequently inappropriate in patients with cirrhosis and has been associated with the risk of SBP and non-SBP infections[71]; therefore, their use should be avoided unless clearly indicated.

Table 2
Promising strategies to prevent bacterial infections and decompensation in cirrhosis

Treatment	Mechanism	Preliminary and Established Evidence
Rifaximin	Nonabsorbable antibiotic	Decrease the recurrence of hepatic encephalopathy Decreases endotoxemia
Nonselective beta-blockers	Inhibition of β1 and β2 adrenergic receptors, Decrease in portal pressure	Decreased incidence of SBP Decreased incidence of decompensation Decrease intestinal permeability, bacterial translocation and ameliorates immune dysfunction
Long-term use of albumin	Scavenging of PAMPs Counteracting reduction of effective circulating volume	Decreased incidence of infections, HRS, and refractory ascites Improved survival[b] Attenuates immune dysfunction, systemic inflammation and circulatory dysfunction
Statins	Pleiotropic effects with anti-inflammatory and antifibrotic effects Decrease in the portal pressure	Improved survival[a] Preclinical evidence of reduced inflammation and liver damage after the administration of PAMPs
FXR agonists	Activation of FXR signaling	Preclinical evidence of improved intestinal barrier integrity and decrease in bacterial translocation
Fecal microbiome transplantation	Counteracts dysbiosis	Decreased recurrence of *Clostridium difficile* infection Preliminary data suggesting decreased the hospitalization rate

Abbreviations: HRS, hepatorenal syndrome; PAMPs, pathogens associated molecular patterns.
[a] In patients with ascites and requiring ≥200 mg of antialdosteronic drugs and 25 mg of furosemide.
[b] In patients with variceal bleeding.

Among drugs to be used, it is remarkable that beta-blockers were associated with a reduced risk of SBP in patients with cirrhosis.[72] Beta-blockers were shown to decrease intestinal permeability, bacterial translocation, and levels of inflammatory cytokines.[73] These findings, which were partially independent of hemodynamic changes, could involve the effects of beta-adrenergic blockade on immune function. In fact, the administration of beta-blockers in cirrhotic rats ameliorates systemic and splenic immune dysfunction.[74]

Albumin administration is widely used to prevent or treat the complications of cirrhosis such as postparacentesis circulatory dysfunction and hepatorenal syndrome.[52] More recently, the long-term use of albumin (40 g twice a week for 2 weeks followed by 40 g per week) has been shown to improve survival in patients with cirrhosis and ascites requiring at least 200 mg of an antialdosteronic drug and 25 mg of furosemide.[75,76] Interestingly, in addition to improving the control of ascites, albumin also decreased the incidence of SBP and non-SBP infections, hepatorenal syndrome, and hepatic encephalopathy.[75,76] These effects could be related to the nononcotic properties of albumin, which attenuated the immune dysfunction in experimental models of cirrhosis,[77] and decreased systemic inflammation and cardiocirculatory dysfunction in patients with decompensated cirrhosis.[78] However, the beneficial effects of the long-term use of albumin were not confirmed in a randomized placebo-controlled trial (with a different design, a smaller sample size, and a lower dose of albumin).[79]

Other interesting strategies to be explored in future studies involves the use of statins, FXR agonists, and fecal microbiota transplantation. Statins had anti-inflammatory and antifibrotic effects, and were shown to decrease the portal pressure in patients with cirrhosis, as well as improving survival in those with variceal bleeding.[80] In experimental models of cirrhosis simvastatin decreased lipopolysaccharide-induced inflammation and liver damage. Therefore, statins represent an interesting drug. However, owing to the potential hepatotoxicity and muscular toxicity of simvastatin,[81] further studies are needed before its implementation in clinical practice. In experimental cirrhosis, FXR agonists showed to promote intestinal barrier integrity and to reduce bacterial translocation[82] and may represent a promising nonantibiotic strategy to prevent SBP. Finally, fecal microbial transplantation showed to be effective in preventing recurrence of *Clostridium difficile* infection and it is currently under investigation to prevent complications of cirrhosis.[83]

TREATMENT OF INFECTIONS AS A STRATEGY TO PREVENT DECOMPENSATION AND/ OR FURTHER DECOMPENSATION IN CIRRHOSIS

The early identification and management of BIs is crucial to prevent and treat decompensation of cirrhosis (**Table 3**). In fact, without an effective treatment of infections, the occurrence of AKI, hepatorenal syndrome, and ACLF dramatically increases.[10] Infections should be rapidly ruled out in all patients hospitalized for an acute decompensation of cirrhosis (chest radiographs; blood, urine, and ascites cultures; and diagnostic paracentesis).

Antibiotic Management of Bacterial Infections

Antibiotic treatment should be started as soon as possible in patients with cirrhosis and BIs, because the early initiation of an effective empirical antibiotic treatment is the most important measure to improve survival these patients.[10,11] Ideally, the antibiotic treatment should cover all bacteria potentially responsible for infections, which depends on the site of infection, local epidemiology and contact with health care.[14,52] The spread of multidrug resistant bacteria made more challenging the management of infections in patients with cirrhosis.[10,11] On clinical ground, the selection of antibiotic is based on the following principles: (a) site of infection, (b) risk factors for multidrug resistant bacteria (nosocomial infections, previous use of antibiotics, recent hospitalization), (c) the severity of the infection, and (d) the local epidemiology.[8] In patients with SBP, third-generation cephalosporins are the first choice for community acquired SBP, although they are poorly effective in nosocomial infections and a broader spectrum treatment should be considered.[68] In centers with a high rate of multidrug resistant species, meropenem plus daptomycin was more effective than a third-generation cephalosporins in treating nosocomial SBP.[84] Similarly, in centers with a high rate of multidrug resistant in health care–associated infections (eg, those occurring in patients hospitalized in the previous 3 months, resident in nursing home facilities, etc), a broader spectrum antibiotic treatment is associated with higher efficacy and improved survival.[85] In patients with sepsis, septic shock, and ACLF clinicians should

Table 3
Strategies for the management of bacterial infections in cirrhosis

Strategy	Intervention	Clinical Significance
Early diagnosis of infections in patients with acute decompensation of cirrhosis	Rule out infections (chest radiographs, diagnostic paracentesis, urinalysis, cultures of blood, ascites and urine)	Delay in diagnosis and treatment of infections is associated with worse outcomes
Early initiation of empirical antibiotic treatment	Administer antibiotic treatment as soon as possible in patients with infections	Delay in administering antibiotic treatment is associated with worse outcomes
Optimal selection of antibiotic treatment	Antibiotic treatment should be selected according to the following: a. Type of infections b. Severity of infection c. Contact with health care system d. Recent use of antibiotics e. Local epidemiology	Patients with nosocomial infections/previous contact with health care system, or recent use of antibiotics are at risk of multidrug resistant bacteria. Broader spectrum antibiotics should be considered in these cases. Local epidemiology is heterogeneous
De-escalation of antibiotic	In case of positive cultures narrow the antibiotic treatment whenever possible	Broad spectrum antibiotics can select multidrug resistant bacteria. De-escalation is safe
Prevention of AKI	Albumin administration[a] is recommended in patients with cirrhosis and SBP	Albumin is associated with reduced incidence of AKI and improved survival
Avoid nephrotoxic drugs	Aminoglycosides and NSAIDs should be avoided in patients with cirrhosis and bacterial infections	Aminoglycosides and NSAIDs are associated with a high risk of AKI

Abbreviation: NSAIDs, nonsteroidal anti-inflammatory drugs.
[a] Give 1.5 g/kg of body weight at diagnosis followed by 1 g/kg of body weight on day 3.

consider to start early a broad spectrum antibiotic treatment, because any delay in starting an effective therapy increases the mortality rate.[52] In any case, biological samples for cultures should be collected and antibiotic treatment should be de-escalated whenever possible.

Nonantibiotic Management of Bacterial Infections

Nonantibiotic management of infections involve both the general management (treatment of organ dysfunction and failures) and strategies to prevent AKI. Nephrotoxic drugs such as aminoglycosides and nonsteroidal anti-inflammatory agents should be avoided. In patients with SBP, the use of albumin solution (1.5 g/kg of body weight on day 1 followed by 1 g/kg of body weight on day 3) decreased the incidence of AKI and improve survival.[86] As for other infections, results were controversial. Guevara and colleagues[87] found an improvement in renal function in patients treated with albumin, which was found an independent predictive factor of survival. Thévenot and colleagues[88] showed a delay in the incidence of renal failure in patients treated with albumin, however, no benefit in survival was found with the use of albumin. More recently, in the INFECIR-2 trial, in-hospital mortality was similar between those who received albumin versus controls. However, patients receiving albumin were sicker at baseline and, during the follow-up period, had a higher rate of ACLF resolution and a lower rate second infections.[89]

SUMMARY

Patients with cirrhosis have a high risk of developing BIs, which are a relevant trigger of decompensation, organ failure, and ACLF. After decompensation the risk of developing infections further increases in an ominous vicious circle. Antibiotic prophylaxis is indicated in patients with variceal bleeding, previous episodes of SBP and in patients with ascites and high risk of developing SBP. Nonantibiotic strategies targeting microbiome, intestinal permeability and immune response are needed to prevent both infections and decompensation. BIs should be diagnosed and treated as soon as possible in all patients with decompensated cirrhosis and antibiotic treatment should not be delayed.

CLINICS CARE POINTS

- Bacterial infections can be sublte in cirrhosis. All in patients with cirrhosis should be investigated for infections at admission and in case of clinical deterioration.
- Broad spectrum antibiotic treatment (high doses, short time) should not be delayed in patients with cirrhosis and sepsis.
- Broad spectrum antibiotic treatment improve survival in patients with cirrhosis and BIs at high risk of MDR bacteria.
- De-escalation of antibiotics (whenever possible) is a good clinical practice and may help to reduce the spread of MDR bacteria.
- Albumin administration prevents AKI and improve survival in SBP.
- Antibiotic prophylaxis should be limited to evidence based indications.
- Non antibiotic strategies are urgently needed to prevent infections in cirrhosis and limit the further spread of MDR bacteria.

DISCLOSURE

The authors states that they have no conflicts of interest regarding the content of this article. The authors did not receive any grants and/or financial support for this manuscript.

REFERENCES

1. Roth GA, Abate D, Abate KH, et al. Global, regional, and national age-sex-specific mortality for 282 causes of death in 195 countries and territories, 1980-2017: a systematic analysis for the Global Burden of Disease Study 2017. Lancet 2018;392:1736–88.

2. D'Amico G, Garcia-Tsao G, Pagliaro L. Natural history and prognostic indicators of survival in cirrhosis: a systematic review of 118 studies. J Hepatol 2006;44: 217–31.

3. Ripoll C, Groszmann R, Garcia-Tsao G, et al. Hepatic venous pressure gradient predicts clinical decompensation in patients with compensated cirrhosis. Gastroenterology 2007;133:481–8.

4. de Franchis R. Expanding consensus in portal hypertension. J Hepatol 2015; 63(3):743–52.

5. Moreau R, Jalan R, Gines P, et al. Acute-on-chronic liver failure is a distinct syndrome that develops in patients with acute decompensation of cirrhosis. Gastroenterology 2013;144:1426–37.e9.

6. Arvaniti V, D'Amico G, Fede G, et al. Infections in patients with cirrhosis increase mortality four-fold and should be used in determining prognosis. Gastroenterology 2010;139:1246–56.e5.

7. Dionigi E, Garcovich M, Borzio M, et al. Bacterial infections change natural history of cirrhosis irrespective of liver disease severity. Am J Gastroenterol 2017;112: 588–96.

8. Piano S, Brocca A, Mareso S, et al. Infections complicating cirrhosis. Liver Int 2018;38:126–33.

9. Foreman MG, Mannino DM, Moss M. Cirrhosis as a risk factor for sepsis and death: analysis of the national hospital discharge survey. Chest 2003;124: 1016–20.

10. Piano S, Singh V, Caraceni P, et al. Epidemiology and effects of bacterial infections in patients with cirrhosis worldwide. Gastroenterology 2019;156: 1368–80.e10.

11. Fernández J, Prado V, Trebicka J, et al. Multidrug-resistant bacterial infections in patients with decompensated cirrhosis and with acute-on-chronic liver failure in Europe. J Hepatol 2019;70:398–411.

12. Borzio M, Salerno F, Piantoni L, et al. Bacterial infection in patients with advanced cirrhosis: a multicentre prospective study. Dig Liver Dis 2001;33:41–8.

13. Bajaj JS, O'Leary JG, Reddy KR, et al. Second infections independently increase mortality in hospitalized patients with cirrhosis: the north American Consortium for the study of end-stage liver disease (NACSELD) experience. Hepatology 2012; 56:2328–35.

14. Jalan R, Fernandez J, Wiest R, et al. Bacterial infections in cirrhosis: a position statement based on the EASL Special Conference 2013. J Hepatol 2014;60: 1310–24.

15. Albillos A, Lario M, Álvarez-Mon M. Cirrhosis-associated immune dysfunction: distinctive features and clinical relevance. J Hepatol 2014;61:1385–96.

16. Wiest R, Lawson M, Geuking M. Pathological bacterial translocation in liver cirrhosis. J Hepatol 2014;60:197–209.

17. Albillos A, de Gottardi A, Rescigno M. The gut-liver axis in liver disease: pathophysiological basis for therapy. J Hepatol 2020;72(3):558–77. https://doi.org/10.1016/j.jhep.2019.10.003.

18. Bajaj JS, Heuman DM, Hylemon PB, et al. Altered profile of human gut microbiome is associated with cirrhosis and its complications. J Hepatol 2014;60: 940–7.

19. Qin N, Yang F, Li A, et al. Alterations of the human gut microbiome in liver cirrhosis. Nature 2014;513:59–64.

20. Bajaj JS, Idilman R, Mabudian L, et al. Diet affects gut microbiota and modulates hospitalization risk differentially in an international cirrhosis cohort. Hepatology 2018;68:234–47.
21. Sole C, Llopis M, Solà E, et al. Gut microbiome is profoundly altered in acute-on-chronic liver failure as evaluated by quantitative metagenomics. Relationship with liver cirrhosis severity. J Hepatol 2018;68:S11–2.
22. Muñoz L, Borrero M-J, Úbeda M, et al. Intestinal immune dysregulation driven by dysbiosis promotes barrier disruption and bacterial translocation in rats with cirrhosis. Hepatology 2019;70:925–38.
23. Fasolato S, Angeli P, Dallagnese L, et al. Renal failure and bacterial infections in patients with cirrhosis: epidemiology and clinical features. Hepatology 2007;45: 223–9.
24. Merli M, Lucidi C, Pentassuglio I, et al. Increased risk of cognitive impairment in cirrhotic patients with bacterial infections. J Hepatol 2013;59:243–50.
25. Bleichner G, Boulanger R, Squara P, et al. Frequency of infections in cirrhotic patients presenting with acute gastrointestinal haemorrhage. Br J Surg 1986;73: 724–6.
26. Soriano G, Guarner C, Tomas A, et al. Norfloxacin prevents bacterial infection in cirrhotics with gastrointestinal hemorrhage. Gastroenterology 1992;103:1267–72.
27. Nahon P, Lescat M, Layese R, et al. Bacterial infection in compensated viral cirrhosis impairs 5-year survival (ANRS CO12 CirVir prospective cohort). Gut 2017;66:330–41.
28. Villanueva C, Albillos A, Genescà J, et al. β blockers to prevent decompensation of cirrhosis in patients with clinically significant portal hypertension (PREDESCI): a randomised, double-blind, placebo-controlled, multicentre trial. Lancet 2019; 393:1597–608.
29. Villanueva C, Albillos A, Genescà J, et al. Bacterial infections in patients with compensated cirrhosis and clinically significant portal hypertension: implications on the risk of developing decompensation and on survival. Hepatology 2019; 70(Suppl):36–37A.
30. Piano S, Bartoletti M, Tonon M, et al. Assessment of sepsis-3 criteria and quick SOFA in patients with cirrhosis and bacterial infections. Gut 2018;67:1892–9.
31. Terra C, Guevara M, Torre A, et al. Renal failure in patients with cirrhosis and sepsis unrelated to spontaneous bacterial peritonitis: value of MELD score. Gastroenterology 2005;129:1944–53.
32. Huelin P, Piano S, Solà E, et al. Validation of a staging system for acute kidney injury in patients with cirrhosis and association with acute on chronic liver failure. Clin Gastroenterol Hepatol 2017;15:438–45.
33. Angeli P, Gines P, Wong F, et al. Diagnosis and management of acute kidney injury in patients with cirrhosis: revised consensus recommendations of the International Club of Ascites. Gut 2015;64:531–7.
34. Fernández J, Acevedo J, Wiest R, et al. Bacterial and fungal infections in acute-on-chronic liver failure: prevalence, characteristics and impact on prognosis. Gut 2018;67:1870–80.
35. Bernard B, Cadranel JF, Valla D, et al. Prognostic significance of bacterial infection in bleeding cirrhotic patients: a prospective study. Gastroenterology 1995; 108:1828–34.
36. Vilstrup H, Amodio P, Bajaj J, et al. Hepatic encephalopathy in chronic liver disease: 2014 practice guideline by the American Association for the Study of Liver Diseases and the European Association for the Study of the Liver. Hepatology 2014;60:715–35.

37. Angeli P, Tonon M, Pilutti C, et al. Sepsis-induced acute kidney injury in patients with cirrhosis. Hepatol Int 2016;10:115–23.
38. Bajaj JS, Reddy KR, Tandon P, et al. The 3-month readmission rate remains unacceptably high in a large North American cohort of patients with cirrhosis. Hepatology 2016;64:200–8.
39. Piano S, Morando F, Carretta G, et al. Predictors of early readmission in patients with cirrhosis after the resolution of bacterial infections. Am J Gastroenterol 2017; 112:1575–83.
40. Schrier RW, Arroyo V, Bernardi M, et al. Peripheral arterial vasodilation hypothesis: a proposal for the initiation of renal sodium and water retention in cirrhosis. Hepatology 1988;8:1151–7.
41. Bernardi M, Moreau R, Angeli P, et al. Mechanisms of decompensation and organ failure in cirrhosis: from peripheral arterial vasodilation to systemic inflammation hypothesis. J Hepatol 2015;63:1272–84.
42. Turco L, Garcia-Tsao G, Magnani I, et al. Cardiopulmonary hemodynamics and C-reactive protein as prognostic indicators in compensated and decompensated cirrhosis. J Hepatol 2018;68:949–58.
43. Romero-Gómez M, Montagnese S, Jalan R. Hepatic encephalopathy in patients with acute decompensation of cirrhosis and acute-on-chronic liver failure. J Hepatol 2015;62:437–47.
44. Clària J, Stauber RE, Coenraad MJ, et al. Systemic inflammation in decompensated cirrhosis: characterization and role in acute-on-chronic liver failure. Hepatology 2016;64:1249–64.
45. Tripathi DM, Vilaseca M, Lafoz E, et al. Simvastatin prevents progression of acute on chronic liver failure in rats with cirrhosis and portal hypertension. Gastroenterology 2018;155:1564–77.
46. Yang Y-Y, Liu H, Nam SW, et al. Mechanisms of TNFα-induced cardiac dysfunction in cholestatic bile duct-ligated mice: interaction between TNFα and endocannabinoids. J Hepatol 2010;53:298–306.
47. Bortoluzzi A, Ceolotto G, Gola E, et al. Positive cardiac inotropic effect of albumin infusion in rodents with cirrhosis and ascites: molecular mechanisms. Hepatology 2013;57(1):266–76.
48. Rama Rao KV, Jayakumar AR, Tong X, et al. Marked potentiation of cell swelling by cytokines in ammonia-sensitized cultured astrocytes. J Neuroinflammation 2010;7:66.
49. Wright G, Davies NA, Shawcross DL, et al. Endotoxemia produces coma and brain swelling in bile duct ligated rats. Hepatology 2007;45:1517–26.
50. Wang A, Luan HH, Medzhitov R. An evolutionary perspective on immunometabolism. Science 2019;363:eaar3932.
51. Moreau R, Clària J, Aguilar F, et al. Blood metabolomics uncovers inflammation-associated mitochondrial dysfunction as a potential mechanism underlying ACLF. J Hepatol 2020;72:688–701.
52. Angeli P, Bernardi M, Villanueva C, et al. EASL clinical practice guidelines for the management of patients with decompensated cirrhosis. J Hepatol 2018;69: 406–60.
53. Goulis J, Armonis A, Patch D, et al. Bacterial infection is independently associated with failure to control bleeding in cirrhotic patients with gastrointestinal hemorrhage. Hepatology 1998;27:1207–12.
54. Llach J, Rimola A, Navasa M, et al. Incidence and predictive factors of first episode of spontaneous bacterial peritonitis in cirrhosis with ascites: relevance of ascitic fluid protein concentration. Hepatology 1992;16:724–7.

55. Andreu M, Sola R, Sitges-Serra A, et al. Risk factors for spontaneous bacterial peritonitis in cirrhotic patients with ascites. Gastroenterology 1993;104:1133–8.
56. Acevedo J, Fernández J, Prado V, et al. Relative adrenal insufficiency in decompensated cirrhosis: relationship to short-term risk of severe sepsis, hepatorenal syndrome, and death. Hepatology 2013;58(5):1757–65.
57. Piano S, Favaretto E, Tonon M, et al. Including relative adrenal insufficiency in definition and classification of acute-on-chronic liver failure. Clin Gastroenterol Hepatol 2020;18:1188–96.e3.
58. Bolognesi M, Merkel C, Bianco S, et al. Clinical significance of the evaluation of hepatic reticuloendothelial removal capacity in patients with cirrhosis. Hepatology 1994;19:628–34.
59. Runyon BA, Morrissey RL, Hoefs JC, et al. Opsonic activity of human ascitic fluid: a potentially important protective mechanism against spontaneous bacterial peritonitis. Hepatology 1985;5:634–7.
60. Simón-Talero M, Roccarina D, Martínez J, et al. Association between portosystemic shunts and increased complications and mortality in patients with cirrhosis. Gastroenterology 2018;154:1694–705.e4.
61. Bernsmeier C, Pop OT, Singanayagam A, et al. Patients with acute-on-chronic liver failure have increased numbers of regulatory immune cells expressing the receptor tyrosine kinase MERTK. Gastroenterology 2015;148(3):603–15.e14.
62. Bernsmeier C, Triantafyllou E, Brenig R, et al. CD14(+) CD15(-) HLA-DR(-) myeloid-derived suppressor cells impair antimicrobial responses in patients with acute-on-chronic liver failure. Gut 2018;67:1155–67.
63. Chavez-Tapia NC, Barrientos-Gutierrez T, Tellez-Avila F, et al. Meta-analysis: antibiotic prophylaxis for cirrhotic patients with upper gastrointestinal bleeding – an updated Cochrane review. Aliment Pharmacol Ther 2011;34:509–18.
64. Fernández J, del Arbol LR, Gómez C, et al. Norfloxacin vs ceftriaxone in the prophylaxis of infections in patients with advanced cirrhosis and hemorrhage. Gastroenterology 2006;131:1049–56.
65. Fernández J, Navasa M, Planas R, et al. Primary prophylaxis of spontaneous bacterial peritonitis delays hepatorenal syndrome and improves survival in cirrhosis. Gastroenterology 2007;133:818–24.
66. Moreau R, Elkrief L, Bureau C, et al. Effects of long-term norfloxacin therapy in patients with advanced cirrhosis. Gastroenterology 2018;155:1816–27.e9.
67. Ginès P, Rimola A, Planas R, et al. Norfloxacin prevents spontaneous bacterial peritonitis recurrence in cirrhosis: results of a double-blind, placebo-controlled trial. Hepatology 1990;12:716–24.
68. Fernández J, Acevedo J, Castro M, et al. Prevalence and risk factors of infections by multiresistant bacteria in cirrhosis: a prospective study. Hepatology 2012;55:1551–61.
69. Bass NM, Mullen KD, Sanyal A, et al. Rifaximin treatment in hepatic encephalopathy. N Engl J Med 2010;362:1071–81.
70. Kimer N, Pedersen JS, Busk TM, et al. Rifaximin has no effect on hemodynamics in decompensated cirrhosis: a randomized, double-blind, placebo-controlled trial. Hepatology 2017;65:592–603.
71. Wang J, Wu Y, Bi Q, et al. Adverse outcomes of proton pump inhibitors in chronic liver disease: a systematic review and meta-analysis. Hepatol Int 2020;14:385–98.
72. Senzolo M, Cholongitas E, Burra P, et al. β-Blockers protect against spontaneous bacterial peritonitis in cirrhotic patients: a meta-analysis. Liver Int 2009;29:1189–93.

73. Reiberger T, Ferlitsch A, Payer BA, et al. Non-selective betablocker therapy decreases intestinal permeability and serum levels of LBP and IL-6 in patients with cirrhosis. J Hepatol 2013;58:911–21.
74. Tsai H-C, Hsu C-F, Huang C-C, et al. Propranolol suppresses the T-Helper cell depletion-related immune dysfunction in cirrhotic mice. Cells 2020;9(3):604.
75. Caraceni P, Riggio O, Angeli P, et al. Long-term albumin administration in decompensated cirrhosis (ANSWER): an open-label randomised trial. Lancet 2018;391: 2417–29.
76. Di Pascoli M, Fasolato S, Piano S, et al. Long-term administration of human albumin improves survival in patients with cirrhosis and refractory ascites. Liver Int 2019;39:98–105.
77. O'Brien AJ, Fullerton JN, Massey KA, et al. Immunosuppression in acutely decompensated cirrhosis is mediated by prostaglandin E2. Nat Med 2014;20: 518–23.
78. Fernández J, Clària J, Amorós A, et al. Effects of albumin treatment on systemic and portal hemodynamics and systemic inflammation in patients with decompensated cirrhosis. Gastroenterology 2019;157:149–62.
79. Solà E, Solé C, Simón-Talero M, et al. Midodrine and albumin for prevention of complications in patients with cirrhosis awaiting liver transplantation. A randomized placebo-controlled trial. J Hepatol 2018;69:1250–9.
80. Abraldes JG, Villanueva C, Aracil C, et al. Addition of simvastatin to standard therapy for the prevention of variceal rebleeding does not reduce rebleeding but increases survival in patients with cirrhosis. Gastroenterology 2016;150: 1160–70.e3.
81. Pose E, Napoleone L, Amin A, et al. Safety of two different doses of simvastatin plus rifaximin in decompensated cirrhosis (LIVERHOPE-SAFETY): a randomised, double-blind, placebo-controlled, phase 2 trial. Lancet Gastroenterol Hepatol 2020;5:31–41.
82. Sorribas M, Jakob MO, Yilmaz B, et al. FXR modulates the gut-vascular barrier by regulating the entry sites for bacterial translocation in experimental cirrhosis. J Hepatol 2019;71:1126–40.
83. Bajaj JS, Khoruts A. Microbiota changes and intestinal microbiota transplantation in liver diseases and cirrhosis. J Hepatol 2020;72:1003–27.
84. Piano S, Fasolato S, Salinas F, et al. The empirical antibiotic treatment of nosocomial spontaneous bacterial peritonitis: results of a randomized, controlled clinical trial. Hepatology 2016;63:1299–309.
85. Merli M, Lucidi C, Di Gregorio V, et al. An empirical broad spectrum antibiotic therapy in health-care–associated infections improves survival in patients with cirrhosis: a randomized trial. Hepatology 2016;63(5):1632–9.
86. Sort P, Navasa M, Arroyo V, et al. Effect of intravenous albumin on renal impairment and mortality in patients with cirrhosis and spontaneous bacterial peritonitis. N Engl J Med 1999;341:403–9.
87. Guevara M, Terra C, Nazar A, et al. Albumin for bacterial infections other than spontaneous bacterial peritonitis in cirrhosis. A randomized, controlled study. J Hepatol 2012;57:759–65.
88. Thévenot T, Bureau C, Oberti F, et al. Effect of albumin in cirrhotic patients with infection other than spontaneous bacterial peritonitis. A randomized trial. J Hepatol 2015;62:822–30.
89. Fernández J, Angeli P, Trebicka J, et al. Efficacy of albumin treatment for patients with cirrhosis and infections unrelated to spontaneous bacterial peritonitis. Clin Gastroenterol Hepatol 2020;18:963–73.e14.

Nutritional Evaluation and Treatment of the Cirrhotic Patient

Shira Zelber-Sagi, RD, PhD[a,b,*], Dana Ivancovsky-Wajcman, RD[a], Liane Rabinowich, MD[b,c], Itay Bentov, MD, PhD[d], Liat Deutsch, MD[b,c]

KEYWORDS

- Malnutrition • Cirrhosis • Sarcopenia • Nutritional support • Late-evening snack

KEY POINTS

- Sarcopenia is one of the most common complications of cirrhosis, leading to functional deterioration and frailty.
- Sarcopenia also may occur in obese patients, but, due to the coexistence of obesity, it might be overlooked.
- Sarcopenia and frailty predict lower survival in patients with cirrhosis and patients undergoing liver transplantation, independent of the Model for End-Stage Liver Disease score.
- Dietary and moderate exercise interventions in patients with cirrhosis are consistently beneficial and safe, but large long-term studies are needed.
- Lifestyle intervention with a goal of moderate weight reduction can be offered to compensate obese cirrhotic patients, with diet consisting of reduced caloric intake, achieved by reduction of carbohydrate and fat intake, while maintaining high protein intake.

NUTRITIONAL STATUS OF THE CIRRHOTIC PATIENT

Malnutrition in liver cirrhosis is common, occurring in 20% of patients with compensated cirrhosis and more than 50% of patients with decompensated liver disease.[1] Among cirrhotic patients awaiting liver transplantation (LT), there is a high prevalence of malnutrition and sarcopenia, affecting more than 50% to 60% of patients,[2–4] associated with higher rates of waiting list morbidity and mortality.[5] The preoperative nutritional status is predictive of a longer post-LT intensive care unit and hospital stay, need for mechanical ventilation, and higher risk of infections. Sarcopenia also is suggested to have an impact on post-LT mortality, emphasizing the importance of

[a] School of Public Health, University of Haifa, 199 Aba Khoushy Ave, Haifa 3498838, Israel; [b] Liver Unit, Department of Gastroenterology, Tel-Aviv Medical Center, 6 Weizmann Street, Tel Aviv 6423906, Israel; [c] Sackler Faculty of Medicine, Tel Aviv University, P.O. Box 39040, Tel Aviv 6997801, Israel; [d] Department of Anesthesiology and Pain Medicine, University of Washington, Harborview Medical Center, 325 Ninth Avenue, Seattle, WA 98104, USA
* Corresponding author. School of Public Health, University of Haifa, Haifa, Israel.
E-mail address: zelbersagi@bezeqint.net

Clin Liver Dis 25 (2021) 373–392
https://doi.org/10.1016/j.cld.2021.01.007
1089-3261/21/© 2021 Elsevier Inc. All rights reserved.

considering the nutritional status while planning patients' perioperative management and placement.[6,7]

Sarcopenia, defined by a progressive decline in skeletal muscle mass and function, is a major component of malnutrition and is associated with a higher rate of complications, such as susceptibility to infections, hepatic encephalopathy (HE), and ascites. Furthermore, sarcopenia independently predicts lower survival in patients with cirrhosis and patients undergoing LT.[1] Sarcopenic obesity, in which low skeletal muscle mass is associated with high adipose tissue mass, may be overlooked due to the coexistence of obesity. It occurs mostly in nonalcoholic steatohepatitis (NASH) cirrhosis and is found in a significant number of patients with cirrhosis pre-LT and post-LT.[8–10] Post-transplant obesity and metabolic syndrome are common, and weight gain after transplantation has been considered primarily due to an increase in the adipose tissue, with a concomitant loss in skeletal muscle mass and function.[9,11] Obesity and sarcopenic obesity worsen the prognosis of patients with liver cirrhosis.[10,12,13] Importantly, decreased muscle mass and function are more prevalent among cirrhotic patients with either minimal HE (MHE) or overt HE (OHE) compared with no HE, and protein malnutrition is an independent risk factor for both OHE (odds ratio [OR] 3.4; 95% CI, 1.4–6.9) and MHE (OR 2.15; 95% CI, 1.1–4.1).[14]

SCREENING AND ASSESSMENT OF MALNUTRITION SARCOPENIA AND FRAILTY

Given the worse prognosis associated with malnutrition, all patients with advanced chronic liver disease are advised to undergo a rapid nutritional screen; those identified at risk of malnutrition should complete a more detailed nutritional assessment to confirm its presence and severity,[15] as summarized in European Association for the Study of the Liver (EASL) clinical practice guidelines[1] (**Fig. 1**). Briefly, most screening tools for malnutrition were not validated in cirrhotic patients and are prone to bias in cases of fluid retention. The Royal Free Hospital (RFH)–Nutritional Prioritizing Tool score was designed for liver disease patients and reported to correlate with the severity of disease, clinical complications, and survival.[16] The components of a detailed nutritional assessment include evaluation of muscle mass, muscle contractile function, frailty and an option to utilize global assessment tools.

Sarcopenia is defined as loss of skeletal muscle mass and function. Quantification of muscle can be accomplished by computed tomographic (CT) image analysis. Cross-sectional imaging of abdominal skeletal muscle area at the level of the L3 vertebra provides an accurate assessment of muscle mass and is normalized to stature as skeletal muscle index (cm^2/m^2). Although the use of CT specifically for this purpose is limited by cost and concerns regarding radiation exposure, it still can be utilized in clinical practice because it frequently is performed in cirrhotic patients for other reasons (screening for hepatocellular carcinoma or evaluation of vascular shunts and portal vein thrombosis). Suggested cutoff values to define sarcopenia by CT (<50 cm^2/m^2 for men and <39 cm^2/m^2 for women) are based on clinical outcomes of cirrhotic patients on the LT waiting list.[17]

In a meta-analysis of 19 studies (3803 patients) with CT-assessed skeletal muscle mass, the prevalence of sarcopenia ranged from 22% to 70% across studies. The pooled hazard ratios (HRs) of sarcopenia independent of Model for End-Stage Liver Disease (MELD) score were 1.84 (95% CI, 1.11–3.05) and 1.72 (95% CI, 0.99–3.00) for post-transplantation and waiting list mortality, respectively.[18] Additionally, in 452 patients with cirrhosis (42% with sarcopenia) during a median follow-up period of 21.2 months, after adjusting for MELD and Child–Pugh scores (CPSs), sarcopenia was associated with higher mortality (HR 2.253; 95% CI, 1.442–3.519). The impact

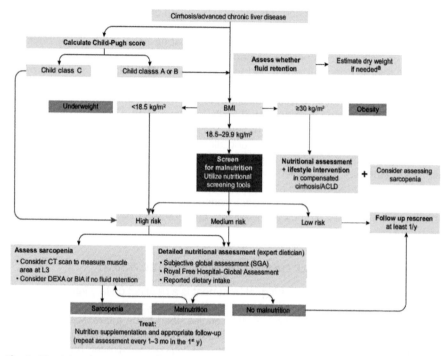

Fig. 1. Nutritional screening and assessment in patients with cirrhosis. [a]In cases of fluid retention, BW should be corrected by evaluating the patient's dry weight by post-paracentesis BW or weight recorded before fluid retention if available or by subtracting a percentage of weight based on severity of ascites (mild, 5%; moderate, 10%; and severe, 15%), with an additional 5% subtracted if bilateral pedal edema is present. ACLD, advanced chronic liver disease; BIA, bioelectrical impedance analysis; BW, body weight; DEXA, dual-energy X-ray absorptiometry. (*From* European Association for the Study of the Liver. EASL Clinical Practice Guidelines on nutrition in chronic liver disease. *J Hepatol.* 2019;70(1):172-193.)

of sarcopenia was more pronounced in patients with MELD score less than 15 or CPS class A or class B.[19]

Body mass assessment by simple bedside anthropometric methods of midarm muscle circumference is low cost and not affected by fluid retention. Whole-body dual-energy x-ray absorptiometry (DEXA) allows the measurement of bone mineral density, fat mass, and fat-free mass, but cost and availability limit its use. Tetrapolar bioelectrical impedance analysis (BIA) is a low-cost, portable modality; however, it is inaccurate in the presence of fluid retention.[1]

A reduction in muscle function has been used as an indirect measure of sarcopenia. The new European consensus on definition and diagnosis of sarcopenia states that sarcopenia is considered a muscle disease, with low muscle strength overtaking the role of low muscle mass as the principal determinant. This change is expected to facilitate prompt identification of sarcopenia in practice because in contrast to muscle mass and muscle quality (eg, myosteatosis), which are technically difficult to measure, muscle strength easily can be measured using simple tools.[20] Handgrip strength is a simple, inexpensive, and reliable method to detect reduction of muscle function. In cirrhotic patients, it can be used to detect malnutrition and predict major complications and mortality.[21,22]

Frailty, defined as a patient's vulnerability to stress and decreased physiologic reserve, also can be used for assessment of cirrhotic patients.[23,24] The Short Physical

Performance Battery, which consists of timed repeated chair stands, balance testing, and a timed 4 meters walk, is a predictor of LT waiting list mortality.[22]

The Liver Frailty Index, derived specifically to capture the construct of physical frailty in LT candidates, consists of handgrip strength, chair stands, and balance testing. In a large cohort, it was found to strongly predict waiting list mortality more accurately than the MELD sodium score.[25] The American Society of Transplantation advocates for longitudinal assessments of the Liver Frailty Index in LT candidates, aiming at standardizing incorporation of frailty into transplant decision making.[23]

The RFH–Global Assessment,[26] based on dry weight–based body mass index (BMI), midarm muscle circumference, and dietary intake, is reproducible and correlates with other measures of body composition in determining nutritional status in patients with cirrhosis. The RFH–Global Assessment stratifies patients as adequately nourished, moderately malnourished (or suspected to be), and severely malnourished. It predicts pretransplant survival and post-transplant complications, but its wide application might be limited by time requirements and the need for trained personnel for consistent results.

NUTRITIONAL AND LIFESTYLE SUPPORT OF THE CIRRHOTIC PATIENT

The first step of a productive nutritional treatment is a detailed dietary interview, identifying what and how much a patient is willing to eat and capable of eating as well as determining whether specific nutrient deficiencies need to be addressed. A detailed dietary intake assessment should include food, fluids, supplements, and number of meals and their timing throughout the day (eg, intervals between meals and if a patient follows recommendations regarding eating breakfast and late-evening snacks [LES]). It also should include barriers to eating: nausea, vomiting, specific food aversion, change in taste, low-sodium diet, early satiety, abdominal pain or discomfort, and diarrhea or constipation.[27] Evaluation of the dietary intake is time consuming, requires skilled personnel, and relies on patient recall and cooperation. At a minimum, patients should be asked about changes in their relative food intake, including quantity (eg, reduced by half) and over what period of time.

Cirrhosis is a state of accelerated starvation in which protein synthesis is decreased and gluconeogenesis from amino acids is increased. The accelerated starvation is aggravated by reduced dietary intake due to a variety of factors, including dysgeusia, anorexia of chronic disease, dislike for salt-restricted food, portal hypertension that contributes to impaired gut motility, decreased nutrient absorption, and protein-losing enteropathy.[28] Additional factors that result in decreased dietary intake include inappropriate dietary protein restriction, hospitalization with periods of fasting for diagnostic and therapeutic procedures, encephalopathy, and gastrointestinal bleeding.[1]

A meta-analysis of 13 randomized controlled trials (RCTs), including both enteral and parenteral nutritional interventions among patients with cirrhosis and alcoholic hepatitis, suggested a beneficial effect on morbidity and mortality. The data were not sufficiently strong, however, to conclude any treatment recommendations.[29] Because nutritional intervention improves survival and quality of life,[30] dietary management should be implemented for every malnourished patient, with regular follow-up to evaluate response, preferably by a dedicated nutritional team.[1,31] The EASL clinical practice guidelines on nutrition in chronic liver disease provide a comprehensive review of the recommended nutritional intake.[1] The approach of the majority of nutritional interventions in cirrhosis is to supply at least 35 kcal/kg/body weight (BW)/d, with a daily recommended protein intake of 1.2 g/kg/BW/d to 1.5 g/

kg/BW/d to prevent muscle mass loss and reverse it in those who are sarcopenic. Similar recommendations also were provided by the European Society for Clinical Nutrition and Metabolism (ESPEN) 2019 guidelines[2] and by the International Society for Hepatic Encephalopathy and Nitrogen Metabolism (ISHEN) 2013 consensus[32] (**Table 1**).

Obesity is an independent risk factor for clinical decompensation in cirrhotic patients.[12] In the obese patient with compensated cirrhosis, a reduction in BW through lifestyle interventions, including nutritional therapy and supervised moderate-intensity physical exercise, may prevent clinical decompensation and improve portal pressure.[12,33]

All recent guidelines provide specific recommendations for the obese cirrhotic patients, indicating that moderate caloric restriction to promote weight loss should be encouraged in obese patients with compensated cirrhosis (see **Table 1**). Nevertheless, over-restriction can result in endogenous muscle breakdown. In the ISHEN 2013 consensus, Amodio and colleagues[32] recommend careful monitoring alongside increased physical activity and caloric intake of 25 kcal/kg/d to 35 kcal/kg/d in obese patients (30–40 kg/m^2) and not less than 20 kcal/kg/d to 25 kcal/kg/d in morbidly obese patients (>40 kg/m^2).

The importance of substantial daily protein intake for sustaining adequate muscle mass has become clear, and tolerance of proteins is higher than previously believed.[32,34] Cordoba and colleagues[34] showed that administration of a low-protein diet (0.5 g/kg/d) worsened HE and exacerbated protein breakdown compared with a daily protein intake of 1.2 g/kg/d. Currently, the recommended daily protein intake is 1.2 g/kg/d to 1.5 g/kg/d.[1,2,32] For obese cirrhotic patients, the moderately hypocaloric diet must include adequate amounts of protein (1.2–1.5 g/kg/d) in order to achieve weight loss without muscle or lean mass depletion.[32] The EASL guidelines suggest a greater intake of protein of greater than 1.5 g/kg ideal BW (IBW) for obese patients undergoing caloric restriction for weight reduction (meaning a caloric reduction mostly from fat and carbohydrates)[1] (see **Table 1**).

In a small fraction of cirrhotic patients, there may be a variable tolerance to different dietary proteins according to their source. Some uncontrolled studies showed better tolerance to vegetable protein over meat protein and to dairy protein over mixed sources protein.[35–38] In an RCT among 120 patients with MHE treated with a 6-month, high-protein diet based on vegetable and dairy protein (1.0–1.5 g/kg ideal BW/d) versus nutrition education, a higher proportion of patients in the nutritional therapy group had reversal of MHE (71.1% vs 22.8%, respectively), and a lower proportion developed OHE (10% vs 21.7%, respectively). In addition, the nutritional therapy group had greater improvement in skeletal muscle mass and handgrip strength, correlating with MHE improvement.[39]

Branched-chain amino acids (BCAAs) supplementation can induce tolerability to meat protein and enable adequate protein intake.[40] Moreover, substituting meat with dairy or vegetable protein along with BCAA supplements is better than reducing total protein intake.[32] In a meta-analysis of 16 RCTs, BCAAs had a beneficial effect on HE compared with placebo or best supportive care (diet, lactulose, or neomycin); however, no conclusions could be drawn regarding its nutritional effects.[41]

Physical activity and exercise are anabolic stimuli that can improve muscle mass and function. The pathogenesis of sarcopenia and frailty in cirrhotic patients includes a low level of physical activity.[23] Despite the lack of robust evidence, consistent benefits of exercise in these patients include reversal of sarcopenia and improvements in aerobic capacity, muscle mass and strength, health-related quality of life, and hepatic

Table 1
Summary of protein and energy, sodium, and dietary pattern recommendations for patients with cirrhosis, as indicated by different associations

Society/ association	ISHEN, 2013,[32] and AASLD and EASL, 2014[73] for hepatic encephalopathy; and AASLD for ascites, 2012[69]			EASL, 2019[1]		ESPEN, 2019[2]	
BMI status[a]	Normal/overweight BMI (20–30 kg/m²)	Obese (30–40 kg/m²)	Morbid Obese (>40 kg/m²)	Mixed BMIs	Obese (BMI > 30 kg/m²)	Mixed BMIs	Obese (BMI > 30 kg/m²)
Daily energy	35–40 kcal/kg IBW	25–35 kcal/kg IBW	20–25 kcal/kg IBW	35 kcal/kg ABW (in nonobese individuals)	>5%–10% WR, moderately hypocaloric diet (−500–800 kcal/d)	30–35 kcal/kg only for DC Regular energy requirements in CC	WR No need for increased energy intake
Daily protein	1.2–1.5 g/kg IBW	1.2–1.5 g/kg IBW	1.2–1.5 g/kg IBW	1.2–1.5 g/kg ABW	>1.5 g/kg IBW	1.2 (for nonmalnourished patients with CC) −1.5 (to malnourished and/or sarcopenic cirrhotic patients)	—
Meal patterns	Small frequent meals throughout the waking hours			Split food intake into 3 main meals and 3 snacks		Three to 5 meals a day and LES	
LES	50 g of complex carbohydrate			No specific composition		No specific composition	
Dietary protein source in cases of HE	High protein intake per patient preference. Substitution of milk-based or vegetable protein is preferable to reduction of total protein intake.			Patients may tolerate animal protein (meat) less well than vegetable protein (beans, peas, etc.) and dairy proteins		In patients who are protein "intolerant," vegetable proteins should be used.	
Sodium restriction in cases of ascites	88 mmol/d, although the evidence is poor and debated. Intakes should not be reduced below 60 mmol/d because the diet becomes unpalatable.			80 mmol/d = 2 g of sodium, corresponding to 5 g of salt Take care to improve diet palatability.		When prescribing a low sodium diet, the increased risk of even lower food consumption should be balanced against its moderate advantage.	

Abbreviations: AASLD, American Association for the Study of Liver Diseases; ABW, actual BW; BW, body weight; CC, compensated cirrhosis; DC, decompensated cirrhosis; EASL, European Association for the Study of the Liver; ESPEN, European Society for Clinical Nutrition and Metabolism; HE, hepatic encephalopathy; IBW, ideal BW; ISHEN, International Society for Hepatic Encephalopathy and Nitrogen Metabolism; LC, liver cirrhosis; LES, late-evening snack; WR, weight reduction.
[a] In cases of fluid retention, BW should be corrected by evaluating the patient's dry weight.

venous pressure gradient.[33,42–44] Exercise must be tailored to a patient's ability, beginning with moderate intensity and maintained for the long term.[1] Two recent comprehensive reviews and meta-analyses on exercise in cirrhotics generally agree on the importance, benefit, safety, and applicability of moderate-intensity exercise and provide practical advice.[31,45,46] In a recent RCT, patients with cirrhosis (CPS class A or class B; ages 62 y ± 7 y) who performed 1-hour sessions of supervised resistance training (1 h, 3 times/wk, for 12 weeks) compared with no change in daily activity level had increased muscle strength and mass alongside beneficial effects on general performance measures.[47] Patients with cirrhosis on the transplant waiting list are advised, if possible, to perform 30-minute to 60-minute exercise sessions, combining both aerobic and resistance training, to achieve greater than or equal to 150 min/wk, along with a parallel increase in activities of daily living.[31]

Recommended Eating Pattern and Late-Evening Snack

One of the most important strategies to prevent accelerated starvation and the related proteolysis is to shorten fasting intervals between meals by eating every 4 hours to 6 hours.[1] Because the longest intermeal duration is at night, the efficacy of a LES has been studied extensively. An LES containing complex carbohydrates as well as protein reduces lipid oxidation, improves nitrogen balance, reduces skeletal muscle proteolysis, increases muscle mass, reduces HE, and improves quality of life; however, a reduction in mortality or need for transplantation has not been reported.[48,49] Although an LES containing at least 50 g of complex carbohydrate[32] was suggested by the ISHEN 2013 consensus article, a variety of night meal compositions appear to be effective as long as they include a reasonable amount of complex carbohydrates and protein (in most studies, the LES contained approximately 200–250 kcal and approximately 13.5 g protein) (**Table 2**), thus suggesting that the meal compositions can be decided according to patient preferences.

Micronutrients Requirements in the Cirrhotic Patient

Specific evidence regarding the beneficial effect of micronutrients and vitamin supplementation in cirrhotic patients is lacking. EASL guidelines suggest that clinically suspected or confirmed deficiency should be treated based on accepted general recommendations and common practice.[1] Because vitamin status is not assessed easily and multivitamin supplements are cheap and largely free of side effects, a course of oral multivitamin supplementation could be justified in decompensated patients.[1]

As for specific micronutrients, the most relevant ones with up-to-date literature are described. Vitamin D insufficiency, defined as less than 30 ng/mL, can be found in most patients.[50] Vitamin D deficiency (VDD), defined as less than 20 ng/mL, is the most common deficiency, affecting 70% to 90% of patients with liver disease.[50–52] Moreover, VDD severity corresponds with the severity of liver disease,[53–55] whether expressed as CPS class A, B or C, MELD score, or liver stiffness evaluated by transient elastography.[54,56,57] In a prospective study, including more than 300 cirrhotic patients, severe VDD at baseline was an independent risk factor for hepatic decompensation during 3 months to 12 months of follow-up (OR 3.25; 95% CI, 1.30–8.2).[58] The patients with severe VDD also had elevated inflammatory markers (eg, C-reactive protein and interleukin-6).[58] More so, in a cross-sectional study, vitamin D levels in hospitalized cirrhotic patients inversely correlated with the presence of infection, regardless of CPS class A,B or C or MELD score (OR 0.93; 95% CI, 0.894–0.959).[59] VDD also is a general predictor of liver disease–related mortality. In a prospective study spanning 22 years, higher serum 25(OH) vitamin D levels were associated with lower rates of chronic liver disease–related mortality, regardless of the

Table 2
Description of studies testing a variety of late-evening snacks in cirrhotic patients, indicating efficacy in improved survival, liver metabolism, muscle volume and strength, and quality of life; reduction of protein catabolism; and abnormal fuel metabolism

First Author, Year	Study Design	Study Population	Intervention	Late-evening Snack Nutritional Composition			
				Energy (kcal/meal)	Protein (g/meal)	Carbohydrate (g/meal)	Fat (g/meal)
Hanai et al,[74] 2020	Retrospective cohort study	523 cirrhotic patients (CPS classes A–C)	Daily use of a BCAA-enriched supplement (Aminoleban) before bedtime or as LES Follow-up of 2.4 y	213	13.5 protein, including 6.1 g BCAA	31.5	3.7
Maki et al,[75] 2019	Randomized crossover trial	10 cirrhotic patients	BCAA-enriched supplement (Aminoleban) as LES vs BCAA-enriched supplement (Aminoleban) during daytime vs no supplement (control) for 1 mo	210	13.5 protein, including 6.1 g BCAA	31.05	3.5
Hiraoka et al,[76] 2017	Noncontrolled trial	33 cirrhotic patients (CPS classes A–B)	BCAA-enriched supplement (Aminoleban) (average period 2.7 mo ± 0.7 mo) and walking exercise (additional 2000 steps/d)	210	13.5	31.5	3.5
Hidaka et al,[77] 2013	RCT	40 cirrhotic patients (CPS classes A–B)	BCAA granules (Livact) supplement after breakfast (4 g) + as LES (8 g) vs BCAA granules (Livact) supplement after each meal (4 g) for 3 mo	NM	L-isoleucine 952 mg, L-leucine 1904 mg, L-valine 1144 mg per 4 g of BCAA granules	NM	NM

Study	Design	Patients	Intervention				
Koreeda et al,[78] 2011	Noncontrolled trial	17 cirrhotic patients (CPS classes A–C)	Low-protein diet with 2 BCAA-enriched supplement (Aminoleban): 1 during daytime and 1 as LES for 6 mo	210	13.5 (BCAA 6 g)	NM	3.5
Yamanaka-Okumura et al,[79] 2010	RCT	39 cirrhotic patients (CPS class A)	High-CHO LES (rice ball, rice cake, sweet potato, cup of noodles, roll, crackers, banana, or 1 slice of bread with strawberry jam) vs controls without LES for 12 mo	149	3.6	NM	NM
Plank et al,[48] 2008	RCT	103 cirrhotic patients (CPS classes A–C)	2 cans of Ensure Plus or diabetic formula as LES vs during the day for 12 mo	710 (or 500 in the diabetic formula)	26 (or 30 g in the diabetic formula)	94 (or 45 in the diabetic formula)	25 (or 22.2 in the diabetic formula)
Nakaya et al,[80] 2007	RCT	48 cirrhotic patients (CPS classes A–C)	BCAA-enriched supplement as LES (Aminoleban) vs ordinary food as LES (rice ball, bread, or cookies) for 3 mo	210	13.5 vs 9 in the ordinary food	NM	3.5 vs 5 in the ordinary food
Yamanaka-Okumura et al,[81] 2006	Randomized crossover trial	21 hospitalized cirrhotic patients (CPS class A)	3 meals/d + LES (rice ball) vs 3 regular meals/d for 1 wk	200	4.3	44	0.9

(continued on next page)

Table 2
(continued)

First Author, Year	Study Design	Study Population	Intervention	Late-evening Snack Nutritional Composition			
				Energy (kcal/meal)	Protein (g/meal)	Carbohydrate (g/meal)	Fat (g/meal)
Sakaida et al,[82] 2004	Noncontrolled trial	11 hospitalized cirrhotic patients	2 packs of BCAA-enriched supplement (Aminoleban): 1 as LES and the other during daytime for 1 wk	210	13.7	NM	3.5
Sako,[83] 2003	Noncontrolled trial	8 cirrhotic patients (CPS classes B–C)	BCAA-enriched supplement (Aminoleban) for 3 mo	210	13.7	NM	3.5
Fukushima et al,[84] 2003	Randomized crossover trial	12 cirrhotic patients (CPS classes A–B)	BCAA granules after breakfast (4 g) + as LES (8 g) vs BCAA granules after each meal (4 g) vs no supplement for 1 wk	320	8 g amino acids	NM	NM
Nakaya et al,[85] 2002	Noncontrolled trial	30 cirrhotic patients (CPS classes A–C)	2 BCAA-enriched supplement (Aminoleban): 1 during daytime and 2 as LES for 1 wk	210	13.5	31.1	3.5
Yamauchi et al,[86] 2001	Randomized crossover trial	14 hospitalized cirrhotic patients (CPS classes A–C)	BCAA-enriched supplements (Aminoleban) as LES (22:30) days vs after dinner (19:00) for 14 d	210	13.7	NM	3.5

Study	Study design	Patients	Intervention				
Miwa et al,[87] 2000	Noncontrolled trial	12 hospitalized cirrhotic patients (CPS classes A–C)	250 mL liquid nutrient (Ensure Liquid) at bedtime for 1 d	250	14% of meal kcal	54.5% of meal kcal	31.5% of meal kcal
Chang et al,[88] 1997	Noncontrolled trial	16 hospitalized cirrhotic patients (CPS classes A–C)	Two slices of bread with strawberry jam as LES (intervention duration is NM)	Approximately 200	NM	50	NM
Verboeket-van de Venne et al,[89] 1995	Randomized crossover trial	8 cirrhotic patients (CPS classes A–B)	4 meals at 07:30, 12:00, 18:00, and 22:30 (considered as LES) vs 2 meals at 12:00 and 18:00 for 2 d	20% of daily kcal	12% of LES kcal	50% of LES kcal	38% of LES kcal
Zillikens et al,[90] 1993	RCT	8 cirrhotic patients	100 g polymeric glucose as LES vs water (control) for 2 d	Approximately 400	NM	100	NM
Swart et al,[91] 1989	Randomized crossover trial	9 cirrhotic patients (CPS class B)	4 or 6 meals/d, including LES vs 3 meals/d for 5 d. The LES was designed to contain approximately 20% of the total daily energy and protein intake.	349 (17% of total kcal)	13.2 g (20% of total daily protein)	NM	NM

Abbreviations: BCAA, branched-chain amino acids; CHO, carbohydrates; CPS, Child-Pugh score; LES, late evening snack; NM, not mentioned; RCT, randomized controlled trial.

presence of hepatitis B.[60] A meta-analysis of 1339 patients with cirrhosis found increased risk of mortality in the presence of severe VDD (relative risk 1.79; 95% CI, 1.44–2.22).[61]

Despite this evidence, the efficacy of vitamin D supplementation in cirrhosis has not been demonstrated convincingly. Among advanced decompensated cirrhotic patients (CPS score $\geq$10) randomly assigned to vitamin D treatment compared with standard care for 6 months, survival rates as well as CPS and MELD scores were comparable between the groups.[62] In a Cochrane review of 15 RCTs, including 1034 adult participants, vitamin D supplementation for chronic liver diseases had no beneficial or harmful effects on all-cause mortality (OR 0.69; 95% CI, 0.09–5.40), and the investigators' conclusion was that there is no convincing evidence for a therapeutic benefit in patients with chronic liver disease as a result of vitamin D supplementation.[63] Selected recent studies describing vitamin D in patients with chronic liver disease are summarized in **Table 3**. The ESPEN guidelines[2] conclude that according to the currently available evidence, micronutrients supplementation, including vitamin D, has no proved benefit aside from correction of deficiency state, similar to the general population. The EASL recommends assessment of plasma 25(OH) vitamin D levels in all patients with chronic liver disease, especially in advanced disease, cholestatic liver disease, or fatty liver disease.[1] Oral vitamin D supplementation is recommended in all patients with chronic liver disease who have vitamin D levels below 20 ng/mL until reaching a serum vitamin D level above 30 ng/mL. No specific dosage was recommended.[1]

Vitamin E is a lipid-soluble antioxidant that mainly prevents peroxidation of lipids. The dietary reference intakes for adult men and women is 15 mg/d (35 μmol/d or 22.4 IU/d) of α-tocopherol.[64] In a cross-sectional study of approximately 800 patients, there was an inverse association between reaching the recommended vitamin E intake and presence of nonalcoholic fatty liver disease (NAFLD) on ultrasound and NASH serum marker.[65] In a propensity score–adjusted study of patients with advanced liver fibrosis and cirrhosis, a dose of 800 IU/d for greater than or equal to 2 years was associated with reduced risk for mortality, LT, and hepatic decompensation.[66] In an RCT, 800 IU/d of vitamin E given to NASH patients, without diabetes or cirrhosis, reduced steatosis and lobular inflammation but not fibrosis.[67] According to the ESPEN, vitamin E supplement (800 IU/d) should be prescribed to nondiabetic adults with histologically confirmed NASH,[2] but there is no recommendation with regard to patients with cirrhosis.

The evidence regarding sodium restriction in cirrhotic patients is limited and conflicting. For example, in an RCT of cirrhotic patients with ascites, 98 patients were on a sodium-unrestricted diet and 102 patients on a sodium-restricted diet for 10 days, resulting in low blood sodium and renal impairment only in the restricted group. Furthermore, the time for ascites resolution was significantly shorter in the unrestricted group compared to the sodium-restricted group (30.24 d $\pm$ 3.12 d vs 47.19 d $\pm$ 9.22 d, respectively).[68] Nevertheless, the EASL recommends a reduction in dietary sodium intake in patients with ascites: 80 mmol/d of sodium, which corresponds to 2 g/d of sodium and a total of 5 g/d of salt, and not below 60 mmol/d, because this may render the diet unpalatable, compromising energy and protein intake.[1] The American Association for the Study of Liver Diseases (AASLD) recommendation regarding daily salt intake is similar.[69] The ESPEN does not specify the recommended intake but rather states that a moderate dietary sodium intake (60 mmol/d) usually is recommended[2] (see **Table 1**). In reality, following the recommendations is difficult and adherence is poor. In a prospective cohort study among 120 outpatients with cirrhosis and ascites, approximately 70% did not follow a moderately low-salt diet in practice, whereas 65% of them thought that they were following it.[70] The adherent patients had a 20% reduction in their mean daily calorie intake compared with nonadherent patients,

Table 3
Selected recent published studies describing vitamin D serum levels in patients with chronic liver disease

Authors, Year	Study Design	Study Population	Results Summary
Ramadan et al,[59] 2019	Cross-sectional	87 hospitalized cirrhotic patients (45 with infection/42 without infection)	• 71.4% with sufficient vitamin D levels in the group without infection and 11.1% in the group with infection • VDD was an independent predictor of infection in cirrhotic patients regardless of the CPS or MELD
Khan et al,[56] 2019	Case-control study	75 cirrhotic patients/75 controls	• 18.7% of patients and 45.3% of controls with sufficient vitamin D levels • Cirrhosis, CPS and MELD score associated with a low level of vitamin D adjusted for age, gender, BMI, residence, and education level
Buonomo et al,[92] 2019	Prospective cohort	345 cirrhotic patients (23/345 with active HCC)	• In cirrhotic patients severe VDD associated with poor survival irrespective of the presence of HCC
Kubesch et al,[58] 2018	Prospective cohort	338 patients with advanced liver fibrosis or cirrhosis	• 39% with sufficient vitamin D levels • Severe VDD an independent risk factor for hepatic decompensation • Inflammatory markers higher among patients with severe VDD
Jamil et al,[57] 2018	Prospective cohort	125 cirrhotic patients	• 12.8% with sufficient vitamin D levels • Age, female sex, MELD and CPS predictors of low vitamin D levels
Putz-Bankuti et al,[54] 2012	Prospective cohort	75 cirrhotic patients	• 71% of patients with vitamin D levels <20 ng/mL • Vitamin D levels inversely correlated with MELD score and CPS
Skaaby et al,[55] 2014	Prospective cohort	2649 subjects with a median follow-up of 16.5 y	• Vitamin D levels inversely associated with incident liver disease

Abbreviation: BMI, body mass index; CPS, Child-Pugh score; HCC, hepatocellular carcinoma; MELD, Model for End-Stage Liver Disease; VDD, Vitamin D deficiency.

without any difference in hyponatremia occurrence.[70] Besides nutritional intake, sodium can be found in substantial amounts in intravenous solutions, in particular antibacterial and antifungal treatments commonly used in hospitalized patients with liver cirrhosis and active infection, reaching up to 8 g of sodium per day.[71]

SUMMARY

Sarcopenia is a common complication of cirrhosis, which also may occur in obese patients. Dietary and moderate exercise interventions in patients with cirrhosis are consistently beneficial and safe, but large long-term studies are needed to test potential reversibility of sarcopenia and improved survival. Structured nutritional counseling should be performed in cirrhotic patients with malnutrition and all patients should be encouraged to avoid hypomobility and try exercise. The exercise should be practical, appropriate to their abilities, and always accompanied by nutritional intervention. Lifestyle intervention aiming at moderate weight reduction can be offered to compensated obese cirrhotic patients, with diet consisting of reduced caloric intake, achieved by reduction of carbohydrate and fat intake, while maintaining high protein intake. In practical terms, when addressing the topic of nutrition with patients with cirrhosis, it is advisable to keep it simple and combine nutritional education, motivation, and behavioral skills. Dedicated education around nutrition empowers patients to take control of their health and increases patient engagement.[72]

CLINICS CARE POINTS

- The first step of a productive nutritional treatment is a detailed dietary interview, to identify the type and quantity of foods the patient can eat, and if unintentional weight reduction has occurred.
- A detailed dietary intake assessment should include the timing and number of meals, meal composition (food, fluids, and supplements) and barriers for eating.
- Eating breakfast and late-evening snack is a relatively easy way to improve nutritional status, compliance may improve if the logic behind this recommendation is shared with the patient.
- Malnutrition and sarcopenia should be considered in every cirrhotic patient, including those with obesity.
- Regardless of the patient's BMI or recommended caloric intake (even if restricted to achieve weight reduction), high protein intake should be maintained.

CASE STUDY

A case study of nutritional advice provided for cirrhotic patient

The patient is a 55-year-old man with liver cirrhosis. Previously, he had an episode of HE approximately 1 month ago; he has no ascites and no varices. His anthropometrics are height 175 cm, weight 76 kg, and BMI 25 kg/m^2. He has a good appetite.

Treatment plan: optimal daily energy intake should be no less than the recommended 35 kcal/kg/actual BW/d (for nonobese individuals). Optimal daily protein intake should be no less than the recommended 1.2 g/kg/actual BW/d to 1.5 g/kg/actual BW/d.[1]

76 × 1.2 = 91 g protein

76 × 35 = 2660 kcal

General instructions (partially adopted from EASL guidelines[1])

- Split the food intake into 3 main meals (breakfast, lunch, and dinner) and 3 snacks (midmorning, midafternoon, and late evening). The LES is the most important one, because it covers the long interval between dinner and breakfast.
- If there are recurrent episodes of HE, it may be advised to eat less meat and instead to increase the intake of plant-sourced protein (beans, peas, etc.) and dairy-based proteins. The total protein intake should not be reduced. Any changes to the protein intake always should be discussed with a doctor or dietician.
- Eat a variety of vegetables on a daily basis and try keep a healthy diet in general. This includes preferring unprocessed food that is rich in fiber and low in added sugars and sodium.

Sample menu (this menu in provided as example; specific menu and instructions should be tailored to individual patients, according to their health status and preferences)

Energy: 2553 kcal

Protein: 99 g (1.3 g/kg)

Carbohydrate: 181 g

Fat: 154 g

Saturated fat: 29 g (10% total kcal)

Sodium: approximately 2000 mg

Breakfast

Two slices of whole grain bread, cucumber, and tomato (eat as many vegetables as desired) with 1 spoon of olive oil, 2 spoons of cheese, and 1 egg (18 g protein)

Midmorning snack

1 pear or apple + 5 walnuts

(4 g protein)

Lunch

100 g salmon with olive oil and garlic in the oven

0.5 cup of rice and 0.5 cup of lentils (majadra)

1 cup of cauliflower with 1 zucchini sautéed with olive oil and 1 spoon of sesame seeds

(38 g protein)

Midlunch snack

Smoothie: 1 banana + 0.5 cup of milk + 1 spoon of almond spread or 5 almonds

(6 g protein)

Dinner

2 tortillas with guacamole (0.5 avocado and 1 tomato)

Tofu (100 g) in marinade (1 spoon of sesame oil, 1 teaspoon ginger, and 1 spoon of lemon juice)

Cabbage and carrot salad with and 1 spoon of sesame

(20 g protein)

LES

Muesli: 1 yogurt + 10 strawberries + 1 teaspoon of honey + 1 spoon of natural peanut butter

(13 g protein)

Hot beverages can be consumed, such as coffee or tea, throughout the day, but added sugar should be restricted as much as possible.

DISCLOSURE

No commercial or financial conflicts of interest and any funding sources to declare.

REFERENCES

1. European Association for the Study of the Liver. EASL Clinical Practice Guidelines on nutrition in chronic liver disease. J Hepatol 2019;70(1):172–93.
2. Plauth M, Bernal W, Dasarathy S, et al. ESPEN guideline on clinical nutrition in liver disease. Clin Nutr 2019;38(2):485–521.
3. Lattanzi B, Giusto M, Albanese C, et al. The effect of 12 weeks of β-hydroxy-β-methyl-butyrate supplementation after liver transplantation: a pilot randomized controlled study. Nutrients 2019;11(9):2259.
4. Tsien C, Garber A, Narayanan A, et al. Post-liver transplantation sarcopenia in cirrhosis: a prospective evaluation. J Gastroenterol Hepatol 2014;29(6):1250–7.
5. van Vugt JLA, Alferink LJM, Buettner S, et al. A model including sarcopenia surpasses the MELD score in predicting waiting list mortality in cirrhotic liver transplant candidates: a competing risk analysis in a national cohort. J Hepatol 2018;68(4):707–14.
6. Montano-Loza AJ, Meza-Junco J, Baracos VE, et al. Severe muscle depletion predicts postoperative length of stay but is not associated with survival after liver transplantation. Liver Transpl 2014;20(6):640–8.
7. Kalafateli M, Mantzoukis K, Choi Yau Y, et al. Malnutrition and sarcopenia predict post-liver transplantation outcomes independently of the model for end-stage liver disease score. J Cachexia Sarcopenia Muscle 2017;8(1):113–21.
8. Carias S, Castellanos AL, Vilchez V, et al. Nonalcoholic steatohepatitis is strongly associated with sarcopenic obesity in patients with cirrhosis undergoing liver transplant evaluation. J Gastroenterol Hepatol 2016;31(3):628–33.
9. Choudhary NS, Saigal S, Saraf N, et al. Sarcopenic obesity with metabolic syndrome: a newly recognized entity following living donor liver transplantation. Clin Transplant 2015;29(3):211–5.
10. Montano-Loza AJ, Angulo P, Meza-Junco J, et al. Sarcopenic obesity and myosteatosis are associated with higher mortality in patients with cirrhosis. J Cachexia Sarcopenia Muscle 2016;7(2):126–35.
11. Dasarathy S. Posttransplant sarcopenia: an underrecognized early consequence of liver transplantation. Dig Dis Sci 2013;58(11):3103–11.
12. Berzigotti A, Garcia-Tsao G, Bosch J, et al. Obesity is an independent risk factor for clinical decompensation in patients with cirrhosis. Hepatology 2011;54(2):555–61.
13. Nishikawa H, Nishiguchi S. Sarcopenia and sarcopenic obesity are prognostic factors for overall survival in patients with cirrhosis. Intern Med 2016;55(8):855–6.
14. Merli M, Giusto M, Lucidi C, et al. Muscle depletion increases the risk of overt and minimal hepatic encephalopathy: results of a prospective study. Metab Brain Dis 2013;28(2):281–4.
15. Tandon P, Raman M, Mourtzakis M, et al. A practical approach to nutritional screening and assessment in cirrhosis. Hepatology 2017;65(3):1044–57.
16. Borhofen SM, Gerner C, Lehmann J, et al. The royal free hospital-nutritional prioritizing tool is an independent predictor of deterioration of liver function and survival in cirrhosis. Dig Dis Sci 2016;61(6):1735–43.
17. Carey EJ, Lai JC, Wang CW, et al. A multicenter study to define sarcopenia in patients with end-stage liver disease. Liver Transpl 2017;23(5):625–33.
18. van Vugt JL, Levolger S, de Bruin RW, et al. Systematic review and meta-analysis of the impact of computed tomography-assessed skeletal muscle mass on outcome in patients awaiting or undergoing liver transplantation. Am J Transplant 2016;16(8):2277–92.

19. Kang SH, Jeong WK, Baik SK, et al. Impact of sarcopenia on prognostic value of cirrhosis: going beyond the hepatic venous pressure gradient and MELD score. J Cachexia Sarcopenia Muscle 2018;9(5):860–70.

20. Cruz-Jentoft AJ, Bahat G, Bauer J, et al. Sarcopenia: revised European consensus on definition and diagnosis. Age Ageing 2019;48(4):601.

21. Tandon P, Tangri N, Thomas L, et al. A rapid bedside screen to predict unplanned hospitalization and death in outpatients with cirrhosis: a prospective evaluation of the clinical frailty scale. Am J Gastroenterol 2016;111(12):1759–67.

22. Wang CW, Feng S, Covinsky KE, et al. A comparison of muscle function, mass, and quality in liver transplant candidates: results from the functional assessment in liver transplantation study. Transplantation 2016;100(8):1692–8.

23. Kobashigawa J, Dadhania D, Bhorade S, et al. Report from the American Society of Transplantation on frailty in solid organ transplantation. Am J Transplant 2019; 19(4):984–94.

24. Lai JC, Feng S, Terrault NA, et al. Frailty predicts waitlist mortality in liver transplant candidates. Am J Transplant 2014;14(8):1870–9.

25. Lai JC, Covinsky KE, Dodge JL, et al. Development of a novel frailty index to predict mortality in patients with end-stage liver disease. Hepatology 2017;66(2):564–74.

26. Morgan MY, Madden AM, Soulsby CT, et al. Derivation and validation of a new global method for assessing nutritional status in patients with cirrhosis. Hepatology 2006;44(4):823–35.

27. Gabrielson DK, Scaffidi D, Leung E, et al. Use of an abridged scored Patient-Generated Subjective Global Assessment (abPG-SGA) as a nutritional screening tool for cancer patients in an outpatient setting. Nutr Cancer 2013;65(2):234–9.

28. Dasarathy S, Merli M. Sarcopenia from mechanism to diagnosis and treatment in liver disease. J Hepatol 2016;65(6):1232–44.

29. Fialla AD, Israelsen M, Hamberg O, et al. Nutritional therapy in cirrhosis or alcoholic hepatitis: a systematic review and meta-analysis. Liver Int 2015;35(9): 2072–8.

30. Iwasa M, Iwata K, Hara N, et al. Nutrition therapy using a multidisciplinary team improves survival rates in patients with liver cirrhosis. Nutrition 2013;29(11):1418–21.

31. Duarte-Rojo A, Ruiz-Margain A, Montano-Loza AJ, et al. Exercise and physical activity for patients with end-stage liver disease: improving functional status and sarcopenia while on the transplant waiting list. Liver Transpl 2018;24(1): 122–39.

32. Amodio P, Bemeur C, Butterworth R, et al. The nutritional management of hepatic encephalopathy in patients with cirrhosis: International Society for Hepatic Encephalopathy and Nitrogen Metabolism Consensus. Hepatology 2013;58(1):325–36.

33. Berzigotti A, Albillos A, Villanueva C, et al. Effects of an intensive lifestyle intervention program on portal hypertension in patients with cirrhosis and obesity: the SportDiet study. Hepatology 2017;65(4):1293–305.

34. Cordoba J, Lopez-Hellin J, Planas M, et al. Normal protein diet for episodic hepatic encephalopathy: results of a randomized study. J Hepatol 2004;41(1): 38–43.

35. Bessman AN, Mirick GS. Blood ammonia levels following the ingestion of casein and whole blood. J Clin Invest 1958;37(7):990.

36. Fenton J, Knight E, Humpherson P. Milk-and-cheese diet in portal-systemic encephalopathy. Lancet 1966;287(7430):164–6.

37. Greenberger NJ, Carley J, Schenker S, et al. Effect of vegetable and animal protein diets in chronic hepatic encephalopathy. Dig Dis Sci 1977;22(10):845–55.

38. Gheorghe L, Iacob R, Vadan R, et al. Improvement of hepatic encephalopathy using a modified high-calorie high-protein diet. Rom J Gastroenterol 2005; 14(3):231–8.
39. Maharshi S, Sharma BC, Sachdeva S, et al. Efficacy of nutritional therapy for patients with cirrhosis and minimal hepatic encephalopathy in a randomized trial. Clin Gastroenterol Hepatol 2016;14(3):454–60.e3 [quiz: e433].
40. Dam G, Ott P, Aagaard NK, et al. Branched-chain amino acids and muscle ammonia detoxification in cirrhosis. Metab Brain Dis 2013;28(2):217–20.
41. Gluud LL, Dam G, Les I, et al. Branched-chain amino acids for people with hepatic encephalopathy. Cochrane Database Syst Rev 2017;5:CD001939.
42. Kruger C, McNeely ML, Bailey RJ, et al. Home exercise training improves exercise capacity in cirrhosis patients: role of exercise adherence. Sci Rep 2018; 8(1):99.
43. Berzigotti A, Saran U, Dufour JF. Physical activity and liver diseases. Hepatology 2016;63(3):1026–40.
44. Zenith L, Meena N, Ramadi A, et al. Eight weeks of exercise training increases aerobic capacity and muscle mass and reduces fatigue in patients with cirrhosis. Clin Gastroenterol Hepatol 2014;12(11):1920–6.e2.
45. Tandon P, Ismond KP, Riess K, et al. Exercise in cirrhosis: translating evidence and experience to practice. J Hepatol 2018;69(5):1164–77.
46. Aamann L, Dam G, Rinnov AR, et al. Physical exercise for people with cirrhosis. Cochrane Database Syst Rev 2018;12:CD012678.
47. Aamann L, Dam G, Borre M, et al. Resistance training increases muscle strength and muscle size in patients with liver cirrhosis. Clin Gastroenterol Hepatol 2020; 18(5):1179–87.e6.
48. Plank LD, Gane EJ, Peng S, et al. Nocturnal nutritional supplementation improves total body protein status of patients with liver cirrhosis: a randomized 12-month trial. Hepatology 2008;48(2):557–66.
49. Tsien CD, McCullough AJ, Dasarathy S. Late evening snack: exploiting a period of anabolic opportunity in cirrhosis. J Gastroenterol Hepatol 2012;27(3):430–41.
50. Kitson MT, Roberts SK. D-livering the message: the importance of vitamin D status in chronic liver disease. J Hepatol 2012;57(4):897–909.
51. Hansen KE, Johnson MG. An update on vitamin D for clinicians. Curr Opin Endocrinol Diabetes Obes 2016;23(6):440–4.
52. Stokes CS, Krawczyk M, Reichel C, et al. Vitamin D deficiency is associated with mortality in patients with advanced liver cirrhosis. Eur J Clin Invest 2014;44(2): 176–83.
53. Arteh J, Narra S, Nair S. Prevalence of vitamin D deficiency in chronic liver disease. Dig Dis Sci 2010;55(9):2624–8.
54. Putz-Bankuti C, Pilz S, Stojakovic T, et al. Association of 25-hydroxyvitamin D levels with liver dysfunction and mortality in chronic liver disease. Liver Int 2012;32(5):845–51.
55. Skaaby T, Husemoen LL, Borglykke A, et al. Vitamin D status, liver enzymes, and incident liver disease and mortality: a general population study. Endocrine 2014; 47(1):213–20.
56. Khan MA, Dar HA, Baba MA, et al. Impact of Vitamin D status in chronic liver disease. J Clin Exp Hepatol 2019;9(5):574–80.
57. Jamil Z, Arif S, Khan A, et al. Vitamin D deficiency and its relationship with child-pugh class in patients with chronic liver disease. J Clin Transl Hepatol 2018;6(2): 135–40.

58. Kubesch A, Quenstedt L, Saleh M, et al. Vitamin D deficiency is associated with hepatic decompensation and inflammation in patients with liver cirrhosis: a prospective cohort study. PLoS One 2018;13(11):e0207162.

59. Ramadan HK, Makhlouf NA, Mahmoud AA, et al. Role of vitamin D deficiency as a risk factor for infections in cirrhotic patients. Clin Res Hepatol Gastroenterol 2019; 43(1):51–7.

60. Wang JB, Abnet CC, Chen W, et al. Association between serum 25(OH) vitamin D, incident liver cancer and chronic liver disease mortality in the Linxian Nutrition Intervention Trials: a nested case-control study. Br J Cancer 2013;109(7): 1997–2004.

61. Yang F, Ren H, Gao Y, et al. The value of severe vitamin D deficiency in predicting the mortality risk of patients with liver cirrhosis: a meta-analysis. Clin Res Hepatol Gastroenterol 2019;43(6):722–9.

62. Jha AK, Jha SK, Kumar A, et al. Effect of replenishment of vitamin D on survival in patients with decompensated liver cirrhosis: a prospective study. World J Gastrointest Pathophysiol 2017;8(3):133–41.

63. Bjelakovic G, Nikolova D, Bjelakovic M, et al. Vitamin D supplementation for chronic liver diseases in adults. Cochrane Database Syst Rev 2017;11: CD011564.

64. Institute of Medicine (US) Panel on Dietary Antioxidants and Related Compounds. Dietary reference intakes for vitamin C, vitamin E, selenium, and carotenoids. Washington, DC: The National Academies Press; 2000.

65. Ivancovsky-Wajcman D, Fliss-Isakov N, Salomone F, et al. Dietary vitamin E and C intake is inversely associated with the severity of nonalcoholic fatty liver disease. Dig Liver Dis 2019;51(12):1698–705.

66. Vilar-Gomez E, Vuppalanchi R, Gawrieh S, et al. Vitamin E improves transplant-free survival and hepatic decompensation among patients with nonalcoholic steatohepatitis and advanced fibrosis. Hepatology 2020;71(2):495–509.

67. Sanyal AJ, Chalasani N, Kowdley KV, et al. Pioglitazone, vitamin E, or placebo for nonalcoholic steatohepatitis. N Engl J Med 2010;362(18):1675–85.

68. Gu XB, Yang XJ, Zhu HY, et al. Effect of a diet with unrestricted sodium on ascites in patients with hepatic cirrhosis. Gut Liver 2012;6(3):355–61.

69. Runyon BA, AASLD. Introduction to the revised American Association for the Study of Liver Diseases Practice Guideline management of adult patients with ascites due to cirrhosis 2012. Hepatology 2013;57(4):1651–3.

70. Morando F, Rosi S, Gola E, et al. Adherence to a moderate sodium restriction diet in outpatients with cirrhosis and ascites: a real-life cross-sectional study. Liver Int 2015;35(5):1508–15.

71. Maimone S, Mazzeo AT, Squadrito G, et al. Sodium load and intravenous antimicrobials in patients with cirrhosis. Dig Liver Dis 2019;51(10):1490–2.

72. Lai JC, Tandon P. How I approach it: improving nutritional status in patients with cirrhosis. Am J Gastroenterol 2018;113(11):1574–6.

73. Vilstrup H, Amodio P, Bajaj J, et al. Hepatic encephalopathy in chronic liver disease: 2014 practice guideline by the American Association for the Study of Liver Diseases and the European Association for the Study of the Liver. Hepatology 2014;60(2):715–35.

74. Hanai T, Shiraki M, Imai K, et al. Late evening snack with branched-chain amino acids supplementation improves survival in patients with cirrhosis. J Clin Med 2020;9(4):1013.

75. Maki H, Yamanaka-Okumura H, Katayama T, et al. Late evening snacks with branched-chain amino acids improve the Fischer ratio with patients liver cirrhosis at fasting in the next morning. Clin Nutr ESPEN 2019;30:138–44.

76. Hiraoka A, Michitaka K, Kiguchi D, et al. Efficacy of branched-chain amino acid supplementation and walking exercise for preventing sarcopenia in patients with liver cirrhosis. Eur J Gastroenterol Hepatol 2017;29(12):1416.

77. Hidaka H, Nakazawa T, Kutsukake S, et al. The efficacy of nocturnal administration of branched-chain amino acid granules to improve quality of life in patients with cirrhosis. J Gastroenterol 2013;48(2):269–76.

78. Koreeda C, Seki T, Okazaki K, et al. Effects of late evening snack including branched-chain amino acid on the function of hepatic parenchymal cells in patients with liver cirrhosis. Hepatol Res 2011;41(5):417–22.

79. Yamanaka-Okumura H, Nakamura T, Miyake H, et al. Effect of long-term late-evening snack on health-related quality of life in cirrhotic patients. Hepatol Res 2010; 40(5):470–6.

80. Nakaya Y, Okita K, Suzuki K, et al. BCAA-enriched snack improves nutritional state of cirrhosis. Nutrition 2007;23(2):113–20.

81. Yamanaka-Okumura H, Nakamura T, Takeuchi H, et al. Effect of late evening snack with rice ball on energy metabolism in liver cirrhosis. Eur J Clin Nutr 2006;60(9):1067–72.

82. Sakaida I, Tsuchiya M, Okamoto M, et al. Late evening snack and the change of blood glucose level in patients with liver cirrhosis. Hepatol Res 2004;30S:67–72.

83. Sako K. Branched-chain amino acids supplements in the late evening decrease the frequency of muscle cramps with advanced hepatic cirrhosis. Hepatol Res 2003;26(4):327–9.

84. Fukushima H, Miwa Y, Ida E, et al. Nocturnal branched-chain amino acid administration improves protein metabolism in patients with liver cirrhosis: comparison with daytime administration. JPEN J Parenter Enteral Nutr 2003;27(5):315–22.

85. Nakaya Y, Harada N, Kakui S, et al. Severe catabolic state after prolonged fasting in cirrhotic patients: effect of oral branched-chain amino-acid-enriched nutrient mixture. J Gastroenterol 2002;37(7):531–6.

86. Yamauchi M, Takeda K, Sakamoto K, et al. Effect of oral branched chain amino acid supplementation in the late evening on the nutritional state of patients with liver cirrhosis. Hepatol Res 2001;21(3):199–204.

87. Miwa Y, Shiraki M, Kato M, et al. Improvement of fuel metabolism by nocturnal energy supplementation in patients with liver cirrhosis. Hepatol Res 2000;18(3): 184–9.

88. Chang WK, Chao YC, Tang HS, et al. Effects of extra-carbohydrate supplementation in the late evening on energy expenditure and substrate oxidation in patients with liver cirrhosis. J Parenter Enteral Nutr 1997;21(2):96–9.

89. Verboeket-van de Venne W, Westerterp K, Van Hoek B, et al. Energy expenditure and substrate metabolism in patients with cirrhosis of the liver: effects of the pattern of food intake. Gut 1995;36(1):110–6.

90. Zillikens M, Van den Berg J, Wattimena J, et al. Nocturnal oral glucose supplementation: the effects on protein metabolism in cirrhotic patients and in healthy controls. J Hepatol 1993;17(3):377–83.

91. Swart G, Zillikens M, Van Vuure J, et al. Effect of a late evening meal on nitrogen balance in patients with cirrhosis of the liver. BMJ 1989;299(6709):1202–3.

92. Buonomo AR, Scotto R, Zappulo E, et al. Severe Vitamin D deficiency increases mortality among patients with liver cirrhosis regardless of the presence of HCC. In Vivo 2019;33(1):177–82.

Diagnosis and Management of Hepatic Encephalopathy

Marika Rudler, MD, PhD[a,b], Nicolas Weiss, MD, PhD[a,c,d], Charlotte Bouzbib, MD[a,b], Dominique Thabut, MD, PhD[a,b,d],*

KEYWORDS

- Cirrhosis • Minimal hepatic encephalopathy • Hepatic encephalopathy
- Transjugular intrahepatic portosystemic shunt • Ammonemia

KEY POINTS

- Hepatic encephalopathy is a very common, life-threatening complication of cirrhosis.
- Clinicians become more and more interested in this clinical situation with the widespread use of TIPS in the management of portal hypertension-related complications.
- Liver transplantation should be discussed in case of refractory hepatic encephalopathy; in this setting, differential diagnosis have to be ruled out in order to maximize the chance of complete recovery.

INTRODUCTION

The prevalence and cumulative incidence of hepatic encephalopathy (HE) are difficult to state precisely. Thirty percent to 45% of cirrhotic patients could be affected by overt hepatic encephalopathy (OHE), and the prevalence of minimal hepatic encephalopathy (MHE) may be as high as 85% in some case series.[1] The joint American-European guidelines[2] define HE as "a brain dysfunction caused by liver insufficiency and/or portosystemic shunts." This definition highlights the importance of the causal relation between neurologic abnormalities, from subtle neuropsychological abnormalities to coma, and liver dysfunction and/or portosystemic shunts.

Conflict-of-interest statement: M. Rudler: speaker for Gore, Gilead, Abbvie; C. Bouzbib: speaker for Gilead, Abbvie; N. Weiss: consultancy for MedDay Pharmaceuticals; D. Thabut: consultancy for Gore, Alfasigma, Gilead, MSD, AbbVie, MedDay Pharmaceuticals.
a Brain Liver Salpêtrière Study Group, Sorbonne Université, INSERM UMR_S 938, Centre de Recherche Saint-Antoine & Institute of Cardiometabolism and Nutrition (ICAN), Paris 75013, France; b AP-HP, Sorbonne Université, Liver Intensive Care Unit, Hepatogastroenterology Department, Pitié-Salpêtrière Hospital, 47-83 Boulevard de l'Hôpital, Paris 75013, France; c AP-HP, Sorbonne Université, Neurological Intensive Care Unit, Neurology Department, Pitié-Salpêtrière Hospital, 47-83 Boulevard de l'Hôpital, Paris 75013, France; d Sorbonne Université, Paris F-75005, France
* Corresponding author. Intensive Care Unit, Hepatology Department, Pitié-Salpêtrière Hospital, 47-83 Boulevard de l'Hôpital, Paris 75013, France.
E-mail address: dominique.thabut@aphp.fr

According to the underlying liver disease, HE is divided into type A (resulting from acute liver disease), type B (resulting from portosystemic shunting without any liver disease), and type C (resulting from cirrhosis).[1] This review focuses on type C HE. The clinical impact of HE is of major importance for both the patient and their caregivers. A first episode of OHE is associated with a survival rate at 1 year of 35% to 45%.[3] HE is also associated with altered work capacity, an increase in falls, more car accidents, and poor quality of life.[4,5] After an episode of OHE, cognitive status often remains impaired, and patients display MHE. Thus, this condition represents a major burden for affected families/caregivers and health care systems.[6]

The peculiar medical presentation of HE, encompassing the specialties of both hepatology and neurology, renders a multidisciplinary approach to the disease very useful both to better describe the neurologic presentation and to rule out differential diagnoses. With this in mind, in 2012, the authors created a unique study group dedicated to the neurologic complications of liver diseases at the Pitié-Salpêtrière University Hospital in Paris: The Brain Liver Pitié-Salpêtrière Study (BLIPS) group. This group, which includes hepatologists, neurologists, liver surgeons, liver transplant specialists, neuroradiologists, neurophysiologists, neuropsychologists, pharmacists, biochemists, immunologists, and sleep medicine specialists, follows both outpatients and inpatients, from patients with MHE to patients with OHE in the intensive care unit (ICU). This multidisciplinary approach to HE patients appears to be fundamental in the diagnosis and management of both the patients and their caregivers.

In this review, the authors first focus on the pathophysiology of HE in cirrhosis and the diagnosis of HE and discuss the different therapeutic options. They summarize the available recommendations and suggest an algorithm based on the clinical experience of the BLIPS group.

Pathophysiology of Hepatic Encephalopathy in Cirrhosis

The pathophysiology of HE in cirrhotic patients is still not totally understood. Even if its correlation with the importance of neurologic impairment is regularly challenged, the implication of hyperammonemia has been well established for decades.[7,8] Recent works have highlighted the synergic effect of hyperammonemia and systemic inflammation[9,10] (Fig. 1). Only patients with systemic inflammation, signs of systemic inflammatory response syndrome, and/or elevated levels of proinflammatory cytokines (tumor necrosis factor-α [TNF-α], interleukin-6 [IL-6]) were found to develop HE in the presence of hyperammonemia. Hyperammonemia is the result not only of the increased intestinal production of ammonia by the enterocytes but also of liver failure responsible for decreased urea cycle function and/or the presence of portosystemic shunting. Once the liver metabolism of ammonia is impaired, only muscle cells and astrocytes can metabolize ammonia into glutamine through the glutamine synthase enzyme. This pathophysiological aspect probably explains why HE is more frequent in patients with major sarcopenia.[11,12] Astrocytes extrude osmotic compounds, such as myoinositol and taurine, to compensate for glutamine osmotic power in order to prevent swelling.[13] Of note, this is not the case in the setting of acute liver failure, whereby such compensatory mechanisms have no time to be initiated, thereby generating brain edema.[14] Whereas the presence of systemic inflammation is clearly established in HE, the existence and the pattern of neuro-inflammation are less understood. Microglial activation is incriminated, which could be associated with other pathophysiologic mechanisms. An increase in glutamine levels associated with neuroinflammation leads to an increase in the glutamatergic and GABAergic tones.[15,16] The accumulation of other substances in the central nervous system has been found in HE: aromatic amino acids, mercaptans, manganese, benzodiazepine-like

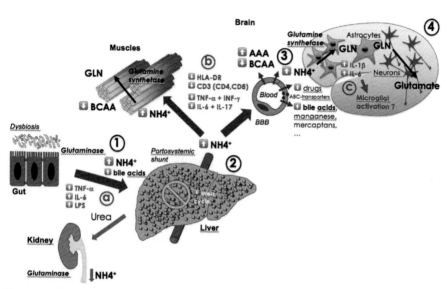

Fig. 1. Pathophysiology of HE. Intestinal microbiota dysbiosis and increased intestinal ammonia production through the enterocytes lead to hyperammonemia, increased secondary to primary bile acids (1), and increased inflammatory markers (lipopolysaccharide [LPS], IL-6, TNF-α) in the portal vein (A). Liver failure responsible for a decreased urea cycle function and the presence of portosystemic shunting will worsen hyperammonemia (2), systemic inflammation (with increased levels of IL-6, IL-17, TNF-α, and decreased expression of HLA-DR and T-lymphocytes count), (B) but also in several other substances that cannot be any longer metabolized by the liver. Ammonia can be metabolized in muscle cells into glutamine through glutamine synthetase but has a side effect to decrease BCAA levels. Ammonia and most of the inflammatory markers cross the blood-brain barrier (3) and can thus be metabolized into glutamine through glutamine synthetase in astrocytes cytosol. Glutamine osmotic power is compensated by the extrusion of other osmotic compounds (myoinositol and taurine) outside the astrocytes. Whereas the presence of systemic inflammation is clearly established in HE, the existence and the pattern of neuroinflammation are less well understood (C). Microglial activation is incriminated, which could be associated with other pathophysiologic mechanisms. Taken together, an increase in glutamine levels associated with neuro-inflammation led to both an increase in the glutamatergic and GABAergic tones that explain neurologic symptoms (4). Several substances accumulate in the central nervous system: aromatic amino acids, mercaptans, manganese, benzodiazepine-like compounds, and drugs (3). Some are due to impaired liver metabolism (mercaptans, manganese), whereas others are due to an abnormal imbalance in transport through the blood-brain barrier (aromatic amino acids) or modulation of ABC-transporters efflux pump associated with impaired liver metabolism. GLN, glutamine; IFN-γ, interferon-γ.

compounds, or xenobiotics.[8,17] In particular, the accumulation of bile acids brings some new insights to HE pathophysiology and accounts for the link between intestinal microbiota dysbiosis and neuroinflammation.[18] Whether the accumulation of xenobiotics is part of HE pathophysiology or a feature of drug-induced encephalopathy is still unclear.[17] The implication of dysbiosis in the pathophysiology of HE is outlined by the recent randomized control trial of fecal microbiota transplantation (FMT) compared with standard of care or placebo.[19,20] This trial showed that FMT was able to lower inflammatory cytokines levels, hyperammonemia, and the secondary/primary bile acid ratio.[19]

Diagnosis of Hepatic Encephalopathy

The diagnosis of OHE is relatively standardized and includes a wide range of clinical manifestations according to the severity of HE. Other diagnoses should be ruled out. The diagnosis of MHE is more complicated, as there is no applicable gold standard, and there are many differential diagnoses. Accurately phenotyping neurocognitive disorders is particularly important when liver transplantation is being considered.

Diagnosis of overt hepatic encephalopathy

Clinical diagnosis. The clinical presentation of OHE ranges from asterixis to coma. The most frequent/typical symptoms of OHE are asterixis, which is the first manifestation of OHE, and psychomotor slowing.[21] Lethargy, extrapyramidal syndrome,[22] seizures,[23] and coma[24] are less frequently observed. Of note, the clinical manifestations of OHE fluctuate over time, and this explains why the diagnosis is sometimes not easy to make and not always reproducible in a given patient.

Paraclinical diagnosis. Some tests are useful to support the diagnosis of HE, especially on initial presentation and when a differential diagnosis is difficult. In the authors' team, they tend to perform a complete workup as often as possible. This workup includes measurement of the plasma ammonia level, electroencephalogram (EEG), and cerebral imaging, especially MRI (Appendix 1).

The role of the plasma ammonia level in HE has been largely debated for decades. As discussed earlier, it is known that a high plasma ammonia level plays a crucial role in the pathophysiology of HE.[25,26] The American Association for the Study of Liver Diseases and the European Association for the Study of the Liver guidelines,[2] as well as the recent French guidelines,[20] recommend reconsideration of the diagnosis of HE if the plasma ammonia level is normal,[1] with the negative predictive value being approximately 80%. However, the positive predictive value of the ammonia level is still debated in the setting of cirrhosis, and the plasma ammonia level is not useful for a positive diagnosis. The prognostic value of a high plasma ammonia is still debated in the setting of cirrhosis.[26–29] Recently, in a large retrospective series of patients who were included prospectively in 3 different cohorts, some investigators pointed out that ammonia level was an independent prognostic factor of mortality in patients with or without OHE.[30] This finding suggests that normalization of ammonemia should be a therapeutic target. Outside of the acute setting, it has been suggested that the fasting plasma ammonia level predicted the risk and frequency of HE episodes.[31] This phenomenon was shown in the past in a very different setting also implicating ammonia overload, that is, urea cycle disorders.[32] A recent retrospective study of more than 100 patients reported that inpatient management of OHE with lactulose was not influenced by either the presence or the level of ammonia, suggesting that ammonia levels do not presently guide physicians in clinical practice.[33] In the authors' opinion, the issue of ammonia response-guided therapy has to be solved in the future. Appendix 2 delineates the pros and cons of the measurement of the plasma ammonia level.

The real issue with ammonia measurement is that this test is unreliable. It is not routinely performed in every center, and some conditions need to be fulfilled for it to be interpretable. Recommendations include collecting the blood sample with no venous stasis (ie, ideally without use of a tourniquet), completely filling the tube, transporting it quickly to the laboratory on ice, and cautiously interpreting the measurement (for example, it may be distorted if hemolysis or severe jaundice was present) (see Appendix 2). The only risk incurred when the test is not correctly performed is abnormally high values (>100 μmol/L). In this case, the most likely diagnosis is false hyperammonemia. After control, if the ammonia values stay very high, inborn errors of metabolism, especially urea cycle disorders, should be ruled out.[34] The authors' team performs ammonia measurements at each episode of encephalopathy in a cirrhotic patient.

EEG typically displays a slowing of basic rhythmic activity with triphasic waves and anterior-predominant abnormalities in HE (**Fig. 2**A). These abnormalities may be observed in OHE or MHE and correlate with the severity of HE and the severity of cirrhosis.[35] EEG enables one to rule out epilepsy, which may be useful when patients have abnormal movements or coma. EEG reading needs to be performed by experienced neurophysiologists to ensure an accurate diagnosis.[36–38] Moreover, EEG abnormalities are sometimes missing and, above all, are not specific to HE; these abnormalities may be present in any metabolic encephalopathy, including sepsis, hypercapnia, or drug-induced encephalopathy.[2,39] Last, the issue of EEG availability is a major obstacle to its use in general practice.

Cerebral imaging is mostly useful to rule out other disease processes. It should be performed at least for the first episode of HE and should be repeated for each episode of HE with atypical symptoms, especially if focal central nervous system symptoms

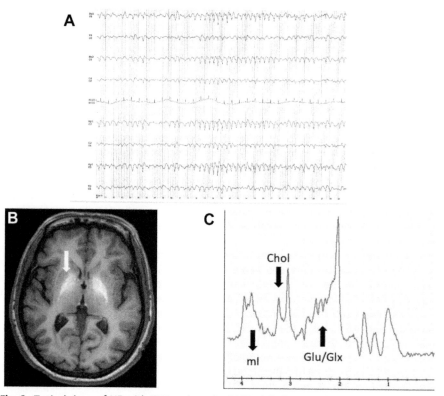

Fig. 2. Typical signs of HE with EEG and cerebral MRI. (*A*) The EEG shows a slowing of basic rhythmic activity, triphasic waves, anterior-predominant abnormalities, and worsening if hearing or painful stimulation. (*B*) Cross-section of cerebral MRI, T1 acquisition: spontaneous hypersignal in basal ganglia (*arrow*). (*C*) Magnetic resonance spectroscopy of corona radiata: increase of glutamine + glutamate (Glu/Glx), decrease of myoinositol (mI), and decrease of choline (Chol).

are present. Brain imaging cannot be done in some patients displaying confusion, except under anesthesia, and this is a major concern. This limitation considerably hampers the diagnostic process, at least in the acute phase. Cerebral MRI is the best test option, but cerebral computed tomographic (CT) scan should be done if MRI is not available. Cerebral MRI typically shows spontaneous T1 hypersignal in the basal ganglia, probably because of manganese overload (**Fig. 2**B), but this may reflect portosystemic shunting more than HE.[40,41] Performing magnetic resonance spectroscopy, which analyzes metabolic spectra in specific areas of cerebral tissue, may be useful to reinforce the diagnosis of HE.[42–45] It typically shows an increase in glutamine and glutamate, a decrease in myoinositol, and a decrease in choline in the corona radiata (**Fig. 2**C). However, brain spectroscopy is only available in a few centers. Its diagnostic and prognostic values have not been studied; thus, its use cannot be recommended in clinical practice. In the authors' experience, if a typical profile is seen, particularly an increase in glutamine and glutamate, this can suggest ammonia hypermetabolism in the astrocytes and may be of interest in cases whereby ammonia levels are not constantly increased. Conversely, if spectroscopy is normal, the diagnosis of HE should be reconsidered.

In summary, the need for a paraclinical workup will depend on the clinical presentation (typical or not), medical history (first bout or not), and protocols of the center. The usefulness of different paraclinical testing is shown in Appendix 1.

Differential diagnosis. The main differential diagnosis of HE types and their characteristics is presented in **Table 1**. In the authors' experience, in the absence of any focal sign, the main differential diagnoses of OHE are other causes of metabolic encephalopathy, alcohol withdrawal, and, more rarely, nonconvulsive status epilepticus.

When nonconvulsive status epilepticus is suspected, EEG is very useful to confirm or rule out the diagnosis and to avoid overprescribing benzodiazepines, which may worsen HE. Other causes of metabolic encephalopathy include sepsis,[46] drug-induced encephalopathy, dysnatremia, hyperuricemia, and hypercapnia. The relationship between sepsis and encephalopathy in the setting of cirrhosis has been known for years.[46] Numerous medications are neurotoxic, and this is of even more concern in cirrhotic patients, as the blood-brain barrier is probably more permeable. As a matter of fact, in a study of the cerebrospinal fluid in cirrhotic patients with encephalopathy, the authors showed the presence of several compounds that are known to be neurotoxic, such as antibiotics.[18]

Other differential diagnoses must be investigated, especially if patients have focal central nervous system signs (see **Table 1**). In some situations, encephalopathy may reveal inborn errors of metabolism, with urea cycle defects occurring frequently.[34,47,48] Although rare, these diagnoses are essential because they lead to specific treatments in an emergency, such as protein restriction, hypercaloric carbohydrate and lipid intake, the use of ammonia-scavenging drugs, and sometimes renal replacement therapy. Inborn errors of metabolism should particularly be considered in cases of severe neurologic symptoms with high hyperammonemia (>150 μmol/L), subnormal hepatic blood tests, and family history of hepatic or neurologic disease. In **Fig. 3**, the authors suggest an algorithm in case of suspicion of OHE.

Diagnosis of minimal hepatic encephalopathy

Clinical diagnosis of minimal hepatic encephalopathy. MHE is still difficult to diagnose in many cases because of (1) the absence of a diagnostic gold standard that can be

Table 1
Main differential diagnosis of hepatic encephalopathy

	Differential Diagnosis	Circumstances	Neurologic Signs and Diagnosis Confirmation	Comments
OHE	Epilepsy/status epilepticus	Sometimes due to alcohol or drug withdrawal, sometimes due to a focalized cerebral lesion, sometimes spontaneous	Seizures Sometimes coma if nonconvulsing: diagnosis with EEG	
	Metabolic cause of delirium			
	Drug-induced encephalopathy	Several drugs, HIV	Drug dosage in the blood	Possible in the absence of an obvious drug known to be neurotoxic and with drugs concentrations in the normal ranges in the blood
	Other metabolic encephalopathies (uremic or hypercapnic or septic encephalopathy, hyponatremia or hypernatremia)	Renal failure, respiratory insufficiency, sepsis	Blood tests (urea level, blood gases, inflammatory syndrome), known identified infection Same EEG as HE (slowing and triphasic waves)	
	Alcohol withdrawal	Sometimes due to hospitalization	History Tip tremor, sweat, hallucinations, seizures	
	Benzodiazepines withdrawal	Sometimes due to hospitalization	History Seizures Urinary toxic analysis	Treatment with benzodiazepines despite the risk of worsening HE
	Carential encephalopathy (Gayet-Wernicke-Korsakoff syndrome, folic acid or vitamin B12 deficiency, vitamin PP deficiency)	Severe undernourishment and alcohol intake, autoimmune disease, hematologic disease, or overweight surgery	Oculomotor abnormalities, nystagmus, amnesia, false recognition, delirium, hypothermia, paraesthesia Specific vitamin dosage Normal ammonia level	Progressive worsening most frequently, but acute onset is possible, little fluctuation, associated systemic signs

(continued on next page)

Table 1
(continued)

Differential Diagnosis	Circumstances	Neurologic Signs and Diagnosis Confirmation	Comments
Osmotic demyelination syndrome (formerly centropontine or extrapontine myelinolysis)	Rapid fluctuation of natremia	Tetraparesis and/or facial palsy FLAIR hypersignal in cerebral MRI (pontine in the case of centropontine myelinolysis, diffuse if extrapontine)	Large interindividual sensitivity
Focal cerebral lesion			
Subdural or epidural haematoma Cerebral thrombophlebitis	Falls with head injury, Thrombophilia	Hyperdensity on brain CT scan Vein obstruction on brain CT scan with contrast-enhancement agent injection or on brain MRI angiogram	Do not hesitate to perform a cerebral imaging if atypical clinic signs of HE
Ischemic or hemorrhagic stroke	Arterial hypertension, cardiovascular risk factor, male sex	Cerebral MRI	
Miscellaneous			
Reversible posterior leukoencephalopathy syndrome	Especially when immunosuppression (post-liver transplantation) in the context of arterial hypertension and renal function impairment	Delirium, headache, seizures, cortical blindness White matter vasogenic edema affecting the posterior occipital and parietal lobes of the brain on MRI	
Autoimmune or paraneoplastic encephalitis	Known cancer or autoimmune disease	Delirium, seizures, mouth and face dyskinesia Lymphocytic meningitis on lumbar puncture Autoimmune antibodies specific for encephalitis (anti-NMDA-R, anti-LGI-1, anti-Caspr-2, anti-Hu)	

Inborn error of metabolism (urea cycle disorders are the most frequent)	Family history	Highly elevated ammonia levels; Blood amino acid chromatography; Urinary organic acid, including urinary orotic acid	High value of ammonemia discordant with the absence of icterus and low level of transaminases; Treatment with diet rules
MHE *Neurocognitive disorders* Vascular dementia	Metabolic cause of cirrhosis	Brain imaging (vascular leukopathy on cerebral MRI), neuropsychologic testing, neurodegenerative biomarkers (normal), normal ammonia level	Progressive worsening, absence of fluctuation
Alcoholic dementia	Chronic alcohol intake	Neuropsychologic assessment, atrophy on brain imaging with important cerebellar atrophy, normal ammonia level	Progressive worsening, absence of fluctuation
Carential encephalopathy (Gayet-Wernicke-Korsakoff syndrome, folic acid or vitamin B12 deficiency, vitamin PP deficiency)	Severe undernourishment and alcohol intake, autoimmune disease, haematological disease or overweight surgery	Oculomotor abnormalities, nystagmus, amnesia, false recognition, delirium, hypothermia, paraesthesia; Specific vitamin dosage; Normal ammonia level	Progressive worsening, little fluctuation, associated systemic signs
Neurodegenerative disorder (Alzheimer disease or frontotemporal dementia)	Family history sometimes	Neuropsychologic assessment, hippocampus atrophy on cerebral MRI, neurodegenerative biomarkers in lumbar puncture, PET-FDG scanning; Normal ammonia level	Progressive worsening, absence of fluctuation
Endocrinal encephalopathies (Hashimoto encephalopathy, Addison disease) (rare) *Psychiatric disorders*	Thyroiditis, autoimmune disease, tuberculosis	TSH, T4, cortisol; Normal ammonia level	Rapid response to corticosteroids in the case of Hashimoto encephalopathy
Depression	Previous history of mental or depressive disorder, anxiety	Elimination diagnosis	Sometimes in the context of Wilson disease

(continued on next page)

Table 1
(continued)

Differential Diagnosis	Circumstances	Neurologic Signs and Diagnosis Confirmation	Comments
Toxic encephalopathies			
Over-the-counter use of sedatives (opioids, benzodiazepines)	Several prescription drugs, previous history of addiction	Urinary or blood testing, normal ammonia level	Possible despite the theoretic counterindication of cirrhosis
Alcohol intake	History of alcohol addiction	Blood testing, normal ammonia level	Some fluctuation, importance of the discussion with relatives
CNS infection (rare)			
Syphilis	Hepatitis C or B cirrhosis	Specific blood and cerebrospinal fluid testing	Reversible with antibiotics
HIV	Hepatitis C or B cirrhosis	HIV serology	Slowly progressive
Lyme disease	Specific regions, outdoor activities or work	Specific blood and cerebrospinal fluid serology and Western blot	Other organ involvement
Hepatitis B and C	Hepatitis B or C cirrhosis	Possible abnormalities on MR spectroscopy	Discussed
Miscellaneous (rare)			
Obstructive sleep apnea syndrome and other sleep disorders	Frequently associated with obesity and arterial hypertension	Headache, need for naps Hypercapnia Apnea-hypopnea Index >5 if obstructive sleep apnea	Questioning relatives may be helpful
Autoimmune disease with neurologic involvement (lupus, sarcoidosis, Gougerot-Sjogren, Behçet disease)	Autoimmune disease	Specific blood abnormalities, meningitis on lumbar puncture	
Autoimmune or paraneoplastic encephalitis	Known cancer or autoimmune disease	Autoimmune antibodies specific for encephalitis (anti-NMDA-R, anti-LGI-1, anti-Caspr-2, anti-Hu)	Rare in the context, other organ involvement

Abbreviations: CNS, central nervous system; FLAIR, fluid-attenuated inversion recovery; HIV, human immunodeficiency virus; TSH, thyroid-stimulating hormone.

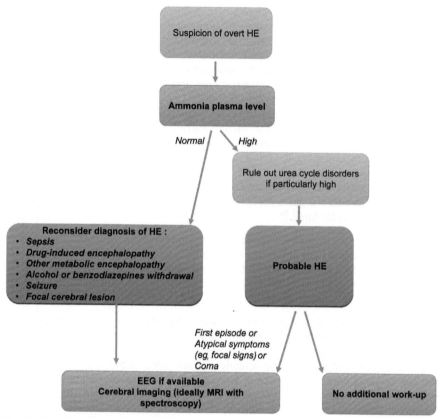

Fig. 3. Algorithm if suspicion of OHE.

performed routinely in clinical practice, (2) the fluctuating character of symptoms, and (3) the fact that many patients are not aware of (anosognosia) or tend to hide their symptoms. Special attention should be paid to the caregivers, as they often relay subtle abnormalities not mentioned by the patients. Of major importance is comparison with the previous cognitive status. Indeed, to diagnose MHE when seeing a patient with cognitive symptoms, it is mandatory to assess a deterioration of cognitive status over time along with worsening of liver disease, and fluctuation of symptoms. Last, one must be aware of the many differential diagnoses of cognitive disorders (see later discussion under the differential diagnosis section). Among the differential diagnoses, only seizures could present with fluctuating symptoms. Thus, in the absence of any fluctuations, MHE should be suspected.

MHE includes psychometric or neuropsychological alterations of tests exploring psychomotor speed/executive functions or neurophysiologic alterations without clinical evidence of mental change. Clinical presentation can also include a trivial lack of awareness, euphoria or anxiety, shortened attention span, impairment of addition or subtraction, and altered sleep rhythm. These symptoms are sometimes outlined by the caregiver. In this case, it is recommended by some experts to classify HE as stage 1 and not MHE (see later discussion under classification).

A neuropsychological assessment is necessary to confirm the diagnosis of MHE. The psychometric hepatic encephalopathy score[48] is considered by many the gold standard. It includes 5 tests that enable one to assess psychomotor speed and visuo-spatial ability. Other tests may be used,[2,49] such as the critical flicker frequency test, which assesses the patient's ability to discriminate a discontinuous light with decreasing frequency[50–52]; the inhibitory control test[53]; the scan test[54]; and the Stroop test.[55] Two abnormal tests are usually considered to diagnose MHE.[1,2] However, all those tests are time-consuming. These tests are dependent on the level of education, which renders their interpretation difficult.

Recently, the animal naming test has been suggested to screen easily and quickly for MHE.[56] This test only requires a timer, and the practitioner has to count the number of animals that the patient can name in 1 minute (Appendix 3). In 1 prospective series, naming more than 20 animals in 1 minute could rule out MHE with a negative predictive value of 76% and a specificity of 78%.[57] Of note, cutoffs may differ between languages, and this test must be validated among different countries. The animal naming test can be considered a good screening test and is recommended by the French guidelines to screen for MHE.[58]

Paraclinical diagnosis of minimal hepatic encephalopathy. Some studies suggest that EEG is more sensitive than psychometric tests[59–61] for the diagnosis of MHE. Moreover, some EEG features may predict OHE occurrence at 1 year.[62] Other paraclinical tests, such as ammonemia and brain imaging, can be useful for the diagnosis of MHE. Their indications and interpretation are the same as for OHE.

Differential diagnosis of minimal hepatic encephalopathy. The differential diagnosis of MHE can be cumbersome. Differential diagnoses are displayed in **Table 1**. Distinguishing between MHE and neurodegenerative disorders at the stage of minimal cognitive impairment (MCI) is particularly difficult. Among the diagnoses, MCI of vascular origin is frequent because of the growing incidence of metabolic cirrhosis. Alcoholic neurotoxicity, Gayet-Wernicke-Korsakoff encephalopathy, and neurodegenerative diseases also must be suspected, especially if patients display persistent temporospatial disorientation, anterograde amnesia, dyspraxia, or speech disorders. In such situations, caregivers often describe progressive worsening of symptoms and little fluctuation. Moreover, distinction between MHE and depression is sometimes difficult. A focal cerebral lesion should be ruled out if there is any doubt in the diagnosis.

If MHE is suspected, 2 options can be proposed: either perform a rather complete workup, or in some centers like the authors' center, perform a therapeutic test. In **Fig. 4**, the authors propose an algorithm in the case of suspicion of MHE.

Classifications

Many classifications of HE have been used over the years, and many revisions have taken place. The authors describe here the latest classification, modified from West Haven, and it includes the different ways of characterizing HE. All the following items should be provided when discussing a patient: type of HE, stage of HE, time course, and precipitating factors.

According to the clinical presentation (see earlier discussion under previous sections). Symptoms depend on the severity of HE, usually described with the West Haven classification (**Table 2**).[2] When the classical neurologic examination is normal, HE is defined as minimal or stage I HE. In stage I HE, the relatives can point out symptoms, whereas in MHE, only neuropsychological/physiologic testing supports symptoms. In the last proposed version of the West Haven classification, covert hepatic encephalopathy (CHE) brings MHE and stage I HE together; in fact,

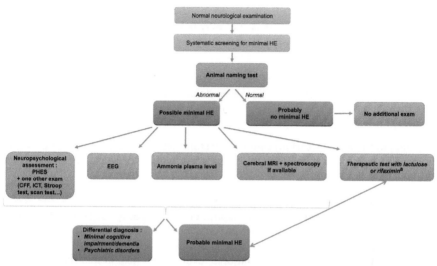

Fig. 4. Algorithm for the diagnosis of MHE. CFF, critical flicker frequency test; ICT, inhibitory control test; PHES, Psychometric Hepatic Encephalopathy Score. [a]Validated in France as first-line treatment of MHE.

Table 2
West Haven classification

	Stage of HE	Symptoms
CHE	Minimal	Psychometric or neuropsychologic alterations of tests exploring psychomotor speed/executive functions or neurophysiologic alterations without clinical evidence of mental change
	I	• Trivial lack of awareness • Euphoria or anxiety • Shortened attention span • Impairment of addition or subtraction • Altered sleep rhythm
OHE	II	• Lethargy or apathy • Disorientation for time • Obvious personality change • Inappropriate behavior • Dyspraxia • Asterixis
	III	• Somnolence to semistupor • Responsive to stimuli • Confused • Gross disorientation • Bizarre behavior
	IV	Coma

Adapted from Ferenci P, Lockwood A, Mullen K, et al. Hepatic encephalopathy-definition, nomenclature, diagnosis, and quantification: final report of the working party at the 11th World Congresses of Gastroenterology, Vienna, 1998 Hepatology 2002; 35(3)716-21 ; with permission.

whether minimal and stage I HE should be merged into a unique category is still a matter of debate, as the outcome is probably not the same between the 2 entities. However, the distinction between MHE and stage I HE can be cumbersome in clinical practice.

According to time course. Symptoms of HE are classically fluctuant and interspersed with remission phases (episodic HE). HE is defined as recurrent when patients have more than 2 episodes of OHE within 6 months and persistent if behavioral alterations are always present and interspersed with relapses of OHE.

According to the existence of precipitating factors. HE is sometimes contemporary to another insult. Some of those factors can be either triggers or causes of encephalopathy (see later discussion).

Diagnosis of hepatic encephalopathy: remaining issues

Precipitating factor/trigger vs cause of hepatic encephalopathy. Sepsis and medications can induce encephalopathy in patients outside of the setting of cirrhosis/portosystemic shunts. Hence, both can be considered as differential diagnoses or as precipitating factors of HE. Ammonia levels could help in this matter: hyperammonemia in the context of encephalopathy suggests HE with a precipitating factor.

Brain reserve. Cirrhotic patients often display other causes of brain damage than HE, either related to the cause of their liver disease (metabolic syndrome, for example, with vascular risk factors, alcohol abuse) or related to other diseases and age. Hence, HE should, in some cases, be envisioned as an explanation of only part of the neurologic symptoms. This aspect is particularly important when discussing liver transplantation, as "complete neurologic recovery" is a goal that is not always attainable.

Treatment of Clinical Hepatic Encephalopathy

General management of hepatic encephalopathy

The general management of HE is based on several principles: (1) exclusion of other conditions mimicking HE (see later discussion under algorithm for the diagnosis of HE), (2) evaluation of the severity of HE in order to manage patients with altered consciousness in the ICU, (3) identification and treatment of precipitating factors, (4) empirical ammonia-lowering treatment, and (5) prevention of HE recurrence (**Fig. 5**).

Treatment of precipitating factors

Precipitating factors include gastrointestinal bleeding, infection, dehydration/hyponatremia/renal failure, constipation, and use of medications. These factors may precede HE or be contemporary to HE. Identifying and treating the precipitating factors of HE is mandatory, as treatment of the precipitating factors has been shown to improve HE in 90% of cases. Moreover, prevention of HE relies on the elimination of precipitating factors.

Gastrointestinal bleeding. HE is often linked to gastrointestinal bleeding and is related, in this situation, to deteriorating liver function, inflammation, infection, and hyperammonemia. A primary prophylaxis of HE with lactulose is required in cases of gastrointestinal bleeding[63] (see later discussion).

Hyponatremia. Hyponatremia is associated with an increased risk of HE,[64] and there is a correlation between hyponatremia and HE severity. It seems therefore crucial to

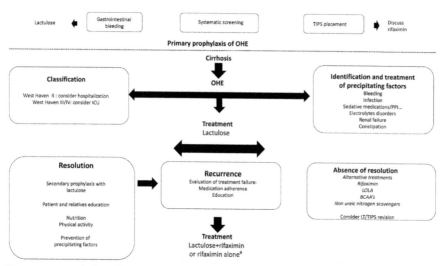

Fig. 5. Proposed algorithm for the prophylaxis and treatment of HE. LT, liver transplantation. [a]In case of lactulose intolerance.

maintain a sodium level greater than 130 mmol/L. Moreover, hyponatremia is associated with a lower response to HE therapy, including lactulose.

Constipation. Patients with cirrhosis often complain of constipation, which is accompanied by ascites, dysautonomia, and prolonged bed rest. Constipation may lead to HE through bacterial overgrowth.

Medications. Several retrospective studies have suggested a link between proton pump inhibitor (PPI) use and HE.[65] PPI cause alterations in gut microbiota. The elimination of the gastric acid barrier may facilitate dysbiosis, leading to bacterial overgrowth. Another hypothesis relies on drug-drug interaction with the blood-brain barrier.[66] In 1 recent prospective series of more than 300 patients, PPI use was associated with MHE, OHE, and increased mortality in patients with cirrhosis.[67] It seems therefore appropriate to regularly evaluate the balance between benefits and risks in such situations. The same results are observed with the use of sedative medications, such as benzodiazepines; several retrospective studies suggested a link between HE and benzodiazepines,[68] which should be considered precipitating factors. Therefore, such medications should not be prescribed to patients with cirrhosis except in cases of delirium tremens, a situation in which the efficacy of benzodiazepines has been clearly demonstrated.[69]

Available therapeutics
Nonabsorbable disaccharides. Lactulose and lactitol are nonabsorbable disaccharides that reduce the intestinal production/absorption of ammonia by different mechanisms[70]: (1) a laxative effect, resulting in an overall decrease in transit time; (2) a reduction in intraluminal pH, leading to increased formation of NH_4^+ from NH_3, with NH_4^+ not being absorbed; and (3) a decrease in bacteria-producing ammonia.

Recently, a meta-analysis including 31 randomized controlled trials (RCTs)[71] showed that lactulose improved the resolution of HE episodes (relative risk [RR] = 0.62, 95% confidence interval [CI]: 0.39–0.99), as well as survival (RR = 0.49, 95% CI: 0.23–1.05) when compared with placebo/no intervention. Lactulose is also superior to placebo in secondary prophylaxis of HE,[72,73] in primary prophylaxis in patients with gastrointestinal bleeding,[63] and in MHE.[71] Lactulose is approved for the treatment of OHE episodes, secondary prophylaxis, and primary prophylaxis in cases of gastrointestinal bleeding. The French guidelines also recommend lactulose for the treatment of MHE.[58] Clinical tolerance remains the main issue.

Polyethylene glycol (PEG) is an osmotic laxative that increases ammonia excretion. PEG has been studied in 2 RCTs in OHE alone[74] or in association with lactulose.[75] PEG was associated with improvement of HE at 24 hours, faster resolution or greater improvement of HE versus placebo at 24 hours, and shorter hospitalization duration versus lactulose alone. Nevertheless, these RCTs were conducted in a small series of patients with a short follow-up.

Rifaximin. Rifaximin is a broad-spectrum, poorly absorbed antibiotic that is thought to reduce ammonia production by eliminating ammonia-producing colonic bacteria. In a recent meta-analysis[76] comparing rifaximin and placebo or lactulose, rifaximin improved the probability of HE resolution (RR = 1.34, 95% CI: 1.11–1.62) and survival (RR = 0.64, 95% CI: 0.43–0.94). Noteworthy, this meta-analysis included studies published more than 15 years ago with fewer than 65 patients. It is therefore not indicated to treat an episode of OHE with rifaximin alone. More recently, an RCT[77] demonstrated the efficacy of rifaximin in combination with lactulose versus lactulose alone in OHE grades 2 to 4. The combination showed a higher probability of achieving the resolution of HE, a shorter length of hospitalization, and improvement in survival when compared with lactulose alone. However, the use of rifaximin in the treatment of HE needs further confirmation. Regarding secondary prophylaxis, the efficacy of rifaximin was first evaluated in 1 RCT with 299 patients who were treated with lactulose and suggested that rifaximin reduced the probability of developing HE by 58% when compared with placebo and reduced the rate of hospitalization.[78] Maintenance therapy with rifaximin for 24 months was also associated with better prevention of HE recurrence and with a good safety profile. Two RCTs evaluated the efficacy of rifaximin versus placebo or lactulose in MHE.[79,80] The first RCT found a significant improvement when compared with placebo, whereas the second RCT showed comparable results between the 2 treatment groups. Tolerance was significantly better in the rifaximin group.

Rifaximin is approved for secondary prophylaxis of HE, when lactulose is ineffective (then associated with lactulose), or alone in the case of lactulose intolerance. The French guidelines also recommend rifaximin for the treatment of MHE.[58]

L-Ornithine L-aspartate. L-Ornithine L-aspartate (LOLA) is the salt of the natural amino acids ornithine and aspartate. LOLA demonstrated the capacity to increase ammonia removal by residual hepatocytes and skeletal muscle of patients with cirrhosis. More than 30 studies have been published in the setting of HE that compare LOLA to placebo, lactulose, antibiotics, probiotics, or branched-chain amino acids (BCAAs). The results have been pooled in a meta-analysis of 33 RCTs,[81] and they did not reveal any beneficial effect of LOLA over the other treatments mainly because of bias related to the studies.

Flumazenil. Flumazenil is a specific GABA receptor antagonist. Its efficacy has been suggested in several RCTs and 2 meta-analyses.[82,83] In the first meta-analysis, flumazenil was associated with significant improvement in OHE and in electroencephalographic abnormalities, and in the second meta-analysis, flumazenil significantly improved the resolution of HE without any improvement in survival.

Probiotics. Probiotics have been studied in several small series that have been analyzed in a meta-analysis (21 studies, 1420 patients). Only 2 RCTs evaluated the efficacy of probiotics in OHE and did not reveal any improvement when compared with placebo.

Branched-chain amino acids. BCAAs, that is, valine, leucine, and isoleucine, are reduced in patients with cirrhosis and impair the conversion of ammonia into glutamine in the skeletal muscle. A Cochrane review of 16 RCTs comparing BCAAs and placebo/no intervention/diet/neomycin or lactulose[84] showed that BCAAs have a beneficial effect on the symptoms of HE but no effect on mortality, quality of life, or nutritional parameters. Data on the prevention of HE are more convincing, as 4 studies suggested a reduction in the number of bouts of HE. The main issue regarding BCAAs is their availability/reimbursement in several countries.

Nonpharmacologic therapeutics. Malnutrition is common in cirrhosis and is associated with an increased risk of sarcopenia. Muscle tissue plays a major role in nitrogen metabolism. Therefore, a low protein diet is not recommended, and optimal daily energy or protein intake should be similar to that of non-HE patients (35–40 kcal/kg/d and 1.2–1.5 g/kg/d, respectively). Physical exercise should be encouraged.

Education of patients with HE and of their relatives or caregivers is a key factor in reducing HE recurrence and, as a consequence, hospital admissions. It includes the effects of medication and potential side effects, the importance of compliance, the recognition of early signs of recurrence, and appropriate actions.

Perspectives in management
Medications
Fecal microbiota transplantation The rationale for the use of FMT in HE is the modulation of gut microbiota composition and function. This treatment was investigated by Bajaj and colleagues,[20] who performed an RCT comparing its efficacy in terms of cognitive improvement, adverse events, microbiota, and metabolic changes versus standard of care in patients with recurrent HE. After 150 days of follow-up, there was cognitive improvement in the FMT group, together with increased microbial diversity and expansion of beneficial taxa. No severe adverse events were registered. Long-term data confirmed sustained clinical improvement and the safety of FMT.[19]

Nonureic nitrogen scavengers Nonureic nitrogen scavengers include sodium benzoate, sodium phenylbutyrate, glycerol phenylbutyrate, and ornithine phenylacetate. Preliminary data suggest that scavengers could be effective in HE; sodium phenylbutyrate was effective in patients with HE who were hospitalized in the ICU in terms of clinical improvement and reduction of ammonemia.[85] Ornithine phenylacetate stimulates glutamine synthetase activity in peripheral organs. One phase 2b RCT compared ornithine phenylacetate to placebo in OHE and suggested clinical improvement in patients with hyperammonemia, although the primary endpoint addressing all the patients was not reached. A phase 3 study will be conducted soon in patients with hyperammonemia.

Other measures
Telemedicine Telehealth and mobile health technologies have been used in several chronic diseases, including liver diseases. Closely monitoring symptoms is part of the management of HE. In a preliminary study,[86] after discharge, home monitoring was done using an iPad with the patient buddy app (monitoring cognition, among other things). This study suggested that many potential readmissions related to HE were prevented via early outpatient interventions.

Shunt obturation/ligation Shunt obturation or ligation can be considered in patients with demonstrated and accessible portosystemic shunts. Current available data are restricted to retrospective studies. This technique should be discussed on a case-by-case basis.

Liver transplantation Liver transplantation is considered the ultimate therapeutic option for refractory HE. Issues regarding HE and liver transplantation are described elsewhere.[87] Prioritization of these patients is currently based on liver function and could therefore underestimate their risk of mortality and hospitalization. Hence, it is important to adequately weight the prognostic impact of persistent/highly recurrent HE in patients on the waiting list for transplantation, possibly adding a quantitative or clinical HE parameter to the available scoring systems.

Proposed algorithm for the prophylaxis and treatment of hepatic encephalopathy
The avoidance of any precipitating factor is part of treatment of HE (see **Fig. 5**). MHE should be screened for in all patients with cirrhosis.

All patients should receive lactulose as a first-line treatment of OHE. Alternative therapeutics may also be attempted. Flumazenil may be an interesting therapeutic option in patients with HE related to benzodiazepine use and in patients with stage IV HE to avoid orotracheal intubation. Secondary prophylaxis of HE includes lactulose and then rifaximin + lactulose or rifaximin alone in cases of lactulose intolerance.

Particular Situation: Hepatic Encephalopathy and Transjugular Intrahepatic Portosystemic Shunt Placement

Prevention of hepatic encephalopathy in patients who are candidates for transjugular intrahepatic portosystemic shunt placement
HE occurs in approximately 35% of cases after transjugular intrahepatic portosystemic shunt (TIPS) placement. Many studies have described the risk factors of HE after TIPS[88,89]: age greater than 65 years, a high model for end-stage liver disease or Child-Pugh score, a previous episode of HE, MHE, and sarcopenia. The best prevention for HE after TIPS is to properly select good candidates for TIPS placement. The authors strongly recommend discussing TIPS placement and liver transplantation at the same time to anticipate the patient's management in the case of TIPS failure or HE after TIPS. Whether pharmacologic treatments should be used as a primary prophylaxis of HE before TIPS placement was investigated. Two RCTs have been published, and they did not reveal any efficacy of lactulose, rifaximin, or LOLA. Recently, 1 RCT[90] evaluated rifaximin and placebo 2 weeks before and then 6 months after TIPS placement: the probability of remaining free of HE was higher in the rifaximin group. Rifaximin will probably be indicated for the primary prophylaxis of OHE before TIPS.

Hepatic encephalopathy management in patients with transjugular intrahepatic portosystemic shunt
In the case of refractory HE after TIPS, reduction or occlusion of the shunt can be attempted, but liver transplantation should always be discussed in this situation.

SUMMARY

HE is the most common complication of cirrhosis and is even life-threatening when progressing to coma. Diagnostic issues remain, especially in the setting of MHE. New pharmacologic therapeutic options are under study. There is growing evidence that telemedicine and mobile health could effectively address unmet needs, especially for therapeutic guidance and monitoring. Most of the patients can be managed with lactulose or rifaximin, education, and the control of precipitating factors. Nevertheless, liver transplantation should be considered in patients with refractory HE or with poor liver function.

CLINICS CARE POINTS

- The diagnosis of HE should be reconsidered if ammonia in normal.
- The animal naming test is an easy tool for the screening of MHE.
- A differential diagnosis has to be ruled out in case of refractory HE and if liver transplantation is envisioned.

REFERENCES

1. Ferenci P, Lockwood A, Mullen K, et al. Hepatic encephalopathy-definition, nomenclature, diagnosis, and quantification: final report of the working party at the 11th World Congresses of Gastroenterology, Vienna, 1998. Hepatology 2002;35(3):716–21.
2. Vilstrup H, Amodio P, Bajaj J, et al. Hepatic encephalopathy in chronic liver disease: 2014 practice guideline by the American Association for the Study of Liver Diseases and the European Association for the Study of the Liver. Hepatol Baltim Md 2014;60(2):715–35.
3. Jepsen P, Ott P, Andersen PK, et al. Clinical course of alcoholic liver cirrhosis: a Danish population-based cohort study. Hepatology 2010;51:1675–82.
4. Román E, Córdoba J, Torrens M, et al. Minimal hepatic encephalopathy is associated with falls. Am J Gastroenterol 2011;106(3):476–82.
5. Shaw J, Bajaj JS. Covert hepatic encephalopathy: can my patient drive? J Clin Gastroenterol 2017;51(2):118–26.
6. Elsaid M, John T, Li Y, et al. The health care burden of hepatic encephalopathy. Clin Liver Dis 2020;24(2):263–75.
7. Romero-Gómez M, Montagnese M, Jalan R. Hepatic encephalopathy in patients with acute decompensation of cirrhosis and acute-on-chronic liver failure. J Hepatol 2015;62(2):437–47.
8. Weiss N, Jalan R, Thabut D. Understanding hepatic encephalopathy. Intensive Care Med 2018;44(2):231–4.
9. Shawcross DL, Davies NA, Williams R, et al. Systemic inflammatory response exacerbates the neuropsychological effects of induced hyperammonemia in cirrhosis. J Hepatol 2004;40(2):247–54.
10. Shawcross DL, Wright G, Olde Damink SW, et al. Role of ammonia and inflammation in minimal hepatic encephalopathy. Metab Brain Dis 2007;22(1):125–38.
11. Wijarnpreecha K, Werlang M, Panjawatanan P, et al. Association between sarcopenia and hepatic encephalopathy: a systematic review and meta-analysis. Ann Hepatol 2020;19(3):245–50.
12. Nardelli S, Lattanzi B, Merli M, et al. Muscle alterations are associated with minimal and overt hepatic encephalopathy in patients with liver cirrhosis. Hepatology 2019;70(5):1704–13.
13. Kato M, Hughes RD, Keays RT, et al. Electron microscopic study of brain capillaries in cerebral edema from fulminant hepatic failure. Hepatology 1992;15:1060–6.
14. Romero-Gómez M. Role of phosphate-activated glutaminase in the pathogenesis of hepatic encephalopathy. Metab Brain Dis 2005;20:319–25.

15. Groiss SJ, Butz M, Baumgarten TJ, et al. GABA-ergic tone hypothesis in hepatic encephalopathy - revisited. Clin Neurophysiol 2019;130(6):911–6.
16. Palomero-Gallagher N, Bidmon HJ, Cremer M, et al. Neurotransmitter receptor imbalances in motor cortex and basal ganglia in hepatic encephalopathy. Cell Physiol Biochem 2009;24(3–4):291–306.
17. Weiss N, Junot C, Rudler M, et al. Hepatic vs. drug-induced encephalopathy in cirrhotic patients? Liver Int 2016;36(8):1233–4.
18. Weiss N, Barbier Saint Hilaire P, Colsch B, et al. Cerebrospinal fluid metabolomics highlights dysregulation of energy metabolism in overt hepatic encephalopathy. J Hepatol 2016;65(6). 1120-V.
19. Bajaj JS, Fagan A, Gavis EA, et al. Long-term outcomes of fecal microbiota transplantation in patients with cirrhosis. Gastroenterology 2019;156(6):1921–3.e3.
20. Bajaj JS, Kassam Z, Fagan A, et al. Fecal microbiota transplant from a rational stool donor improves hepatic encephalopathy: a randomized clinical trial. Hepatology 2017;66(6):1727–38.
21. Harris MK, Elliott D, Schwendimann RN, et al. Neurologic presentations of hepatic disease. Neurol Clin 2010;28(1):89–105.
22. Weissenborn K, Ehrenheim C, Hori A, et al. Pallidal lesions in patients with liver cirrhosis: clinical and MRI evaluation. Metab Brain Dis 1995;10(3):219–31.
23. Newey CR, George P, Sarwal A, et al. Electro-radiological observations of grade III/IV hepatic encephalopathy patients with seizures. Neurocrit Care 2018;28(1):97–103.
24. Mouri S, Tripon S, Rudler M, et al. FOUR score, a reliable score for assessing overt hepatic encephalopathy in cirrhotic patients. Neurocrit Care 2015;22(2):251–7.
25. Ong JP, Aggarwal A, Krieger D, et al. Correlation between ammonia levels and the severity of hepatic encephalopathy. Am J Med 2003;114(3):188–93.
26. Lockwood AH. Blood ammonia levels and hepatic encephalopathy. Metab Brain Dis 2004;19(3–4):345–9.
27. Nicolao F, Efrati C, Masini A, et al. Role of determination of partial pressure of ammonia in cirrhotic patients with and without hepatic encephalopathy. J Hepatol 2003;38(4):441–6.
28. Mallet M, Weiss N, Thabut D, et al. Why and when to measure ammonemia in cirrhosis? Clin Res Hepatol Gastroenterol 2018;42(6):505–11.
29. Gundling F, Zelihic E, Seidl H, et al. How to diagnose hepatic encephalopathy in the emergency department. Ann Hepatol 2013;12(1):108–14.
30. Shalimar, Sheikh MF, Mookerjee RP, et al. Prognostic role of ammonia in patients with cirrhosis. Hepatology 2019;70(3):982–94.
31. Vierling JM, Mokhtarani M, Brown RS Jr, et al. Fasting blood ammonia predicts risk and frequency of hepatic encephalopathy episodes in patients with cirrhosis. Clin Gastroenterol Hepatol 2016;14(6):903–6.e1.
32. Lee B, Diaz GA, Rhead W, et al. Glutamine and hyperammonemic crises in patients with urea cycle disorders. Mol Genet Metab 2016;117(1):27–32.
33. Haj M, Rockey DC. Ammonia levels do not guide clinical management of patients with hepatic encephalopathy caused by cirrhosis. Am J Gastroenterol 2020;115(5):723–8.
34. Weiss N, Mochel F, Rudler M, et al. Peak hyperammonemia and atypical acute liver failure: the eruption of an urea cycle disorder during hyperemesis gravidarum. J Hepatol 2017. https://doi.org/10.1016/j.jhep.2017.09.009. S0168-8278(17)32289-4.

35. Marchetti P, D'Avanzo C, Orsato R, et al. Electroencephalography in patients with cirrhosis. Gastroenterology 2011;141(5):1680–9.e1-2.
36. Amodio P, Pellegrini A, Ubiali E, et al. The EEG assessment of low-grade hepatic encephalopathy: comparison of an artificial neural network-expert system (ANNES) based evaluation with visual EEG readings and EEG spectral analysis. Clin Neurophysiol 2006;117(10):2243–51.
37. Rudler M, Marois C, Weiss N, et al. Status epilepticus in patients with cirrhosis: how to avoid misdiagnosis in patients with hepatic encephalopathy. Seizure 2017;45:192–7.
38. Karanfilian BV, Cheung M, Dellatore P, et al. Laboratory abnormalities of hepatic encephalopathy. Clin Liver Dis 2020;24(2):197–208.
39. Guerit J-M, Amantini A, Fischer C, et al. Neurophysiological investigations of hepatic encephalopathy: ISHEN practice guidelines. Liver Int Off 2009;29(6):789–96.
40. Rudler M, Weiss N, Perlbarg V, et al. Combined diffusion tensor imaging and magnetic resonance spectroscopy to predict neurological outcome before transjugular intrahepatic portosystemic shunt. Aliment Pharmacol Ther 2018;48(8):863–74.
41. Uchino A, Noguchi T, Nomiyama K, et al. Manganese accumulation in the brain: MR imaging. Neuroradiology 2007;49(9):715–20.
42. Kreis R, Ross BD, Farrow NA, et al. Metabolic disorders of the brain in chronic hepatic encephalopathy detected with H-1 MR spectroscopy. Radiology 1992;182(1):19–27.
43. Kreis R, Farrow N, Ross BD. Localized 1H NMR spectroscopy in patients with chronic hepatic encephalopathy. Analysis of changes in cerebral glutamine, choline and inositols. NMR Biomed 1991;4(2):109–16.
44. Hermann B, Rudler M, Galanaud D, et al. Magnetic resonance spectroscopy: a surrogate marker of hepatic encephalopathy? J Hepatol 2019;71(5):1055–7.
45. Zeng G, Penninkilampi R, Chaganti J, et al. Meta-analysis of magnetic resonance spectroscopy in the diagnosis of hepatic encephalopathy. Neurology 2020;94(11):e1147–56.
46. Sharshar T, Annane D, de la Grandmaison GL, et al. The neuropathology of septic shock. Brain Pathol 2004;14(1):21–33.
47. Laemmle A, Gallagher RC, Keogh A, et al. Frequency and pathophysiology of acute liver failure in ornithine transcarbamylase deficiency (OTCD). PLoS One 2016;11(4):e0153358.
48. Weissenborn K, Ennen JC, Schomerus H, et al. Neuropsychological characterization of hepatic encephalopathy. J Hepatol 2001;34(5):768–73.
49. Tapper EB, Parikh ND, Waljee AK, et al. Diagnosis of minimal hepatic encephalopathy: a systematic review of point-of-care diagnostic tests. Am J Gastroenterol 2018;113(4):529–38.
50. Kircheis G, Hilger N, Häussinger D. Value of critical flicker frequency and psychometric hepatic encephalopathy score in diagnosis of low-grade hepatic encephalopathy. Gastroenterology 2014;146(4):961–9.
51. Kircheis G, Wettstein M, Timmermann L, et al. Critical flicker frequency for quantification of low-grade hepatic encephalopathy. Hepatol Baltim Md 2002;35(2):357–66.
52. Romero-Gómez M, Córdoba J, Jover R, et al. Value of the critical flicker frequency in patients with minimal hepatic encephalopathy. Hepatol Baltim Md 2007;45(4):879–85.

53. Bajaj JS, Hafeezullah M, Franco J, et al. Inhibitory control test for the diagnosis of minimal hepatic encephalopathy. Gastroenterology 2008;135(5): 1591–600.e1.

54. Mardini H, Saxby BK, Record CO. Computerized psychometric testing in minimal encephalopathy and modulation by nitrogen challenge and liver transplant. Gastroenterology 2008;135(5):1582–90.

55. Bajaj JS, Thacker LR, Heuman DM, et al. The Stroop smartphone application is a short and valid method to screen for minimal hepatic encephalopathy. Hepatol Baltim Md 2013;58(3):1122–32.

56. Campagna F, Montagnese S, Ridola L, et al. The animal naming test: an easy tool for the assessment of hepatic encephalopathy. Hepatol Baltim Md 2017;66(1): 198–208.

57. Labenz C, Beul L, Toenges G, et al. Validation of the simplified animal naming test as primary screening tool for the diagnosis of covert hepatic encephalopathy. Eur J Intern Med 2019;60:96–100.

58. Recommandations formalisées d'experts. Association Française pour l'Étude du Foie. Diagnostic et prise en charge de l'encéphalopathie hépatique sur cirrhose. Available at: https://afef.asso.fr/wp-content/uploads/2019/10/RECO_AFEF_2019_DEF.pdf.

59. Quero JC, Hartmann IJ, Meulstee J, et al. The diagnosis of subclinical hepatic encephalopathy in patients with cirrhosis using neuropsychological tests and automated electroencephalogram analysis. Hepatol Baltim Md 1996;24(3): 556–60.

60. Ucar F, Erden G, Ozdemir S, et al. First data on the biological variation and quality specifications for plasma ammonia concentrations in healthy subjects. Clin Chem Lab Med 2016;54(5):857–63.

61. Saxena N, Bhatia M, Joshi YK, et al. Electrophysiological and neuropsychological tests for the diagnosis of subclinical hepatic encephalopathy and prediction of overt encephalopathy. Liver 2002;22(3):190–7.

62. Amodio P, Del Piccolo F, Pettenò E, et al. Prevalence and prognostic value of quantified electroencephalogram (EEG) alterations in cirrhotic patients. J Hepatol 2001;35(1):37–45.

63. Sharma P, Agrawal A, Sharma BC, et al. Prophylaxis of hepatic encephalopathy in acute variceal bleed: a randomized controlled trial of lactulose versus no lactulose. J Gastroenterol Hepatol 2011;26:996–1003.

64. Guevara M, Baccaro ME, Torre A, et al. Hyponatremia is a risk factor of hepatic encephalopathy in patients with cirrhosis: a prospective study with time-dependent analysis. Am J Gastroenterol 2009;104:1382–9.

65. Tsai CF, Chen MH, Wang YP, et al. Proton pump inhibitors increase risk for hepatic encephalopathy in patients with cirrhosis in a population study. Gastroenterology 2017;152(1):134–41.

66. Assaraf J, Weiss N, Thabut D. Proton pump inhibitor administration triggers encephalopathy in cirrhotic patients by modulating blood-brain barrier drug transport. Gastroenterology 2017;152(8):2077.

67. Nardelli S, Gioia S, Ridola L, et al. Proton pump inhibitors are associated with minimal and overt hepatic encephalopathy and increased mortality in patients with cirrhosis. Hepatology 2019;70(2):640–9.

68. Lee PC, Yang YY, Lin MW, et al. Benzodiazepine-associated hepatic encephalopathy significantly increased healthcare utilization and medical costs of Chinese cirrhotic patients: 7-year experience. Dig Dis Sci 2014;59:1603–16.

69. Amato L, Minozzi S, Vecchi S, et al. Benzodiazepines for alcohol withdrawal. Cochrane Database Syst Rev 2010;(3):CD005063.
70. Riggio O, Varriale M, Testore GP, et al. Effect of lactitol and lactulose administration on the fecal flora in cirrhotic patients. J Clin Gastroenterol 1990;12(4): 433–6.
71. Gluud LL, Vilstrup H, Morgan MY. Nonabsorbable disaccharides for hepatic encephalopathy: a systematic review and meta-analysis. Hepatology 2016;64: 908–22.
72. Agrawal A, Sharma BC, Sharma P, et al. Secondary prophylaxis of hepatic encephalopathy in cirrhosis: an open-label, randomized controlled trial of lactulose, probiotics, and no therapy. Am J Gastroenterol 2012;107:1043–50.
73. Sharma BC, Sharma P, Agrawal A, et al. Secondary prophylaxis of hepatic encephalopathy: an open-label randomized controlled trial of lactulose versus placebo. Gastroenterology 2009;137:885–91, 891.e1.
74. Naderian M, Akbari H, Saeedi M, et al. Polyethylene glycol and lactulose versus lactulose alone in the treatment of hepatic encephalopathy in patients with cirrhosis: a non-inferiority randomized controlled trial. Middle East J Dig Dis 2017;9:12–9.
75. Rahimi RS, Singal AG, Cuthbert JA, et al. Lactulose vs polyethylene glycol 3350–electrolyte solution for treatment of overt hepatic encephalopathy: the HELP randomized clinical trial. JAMA Intern Med 2014;174:1727–33.
76. Kimer N, Krag A, Moller S, et al. Systematic review with meta-analysis: the effects of rifaximin in hepatic encephalopathy. Aliment Pharmacol Ther 2014;40: 123–32.
77. Sharma BC, Sharma P, Lunia MK, et al. A randomized, double-blind, controlled trial comparing rifaximin plus lactulose with lactulose alone in treatment of overt hepatic encephalopathy. Am J Gastroenterol 2013;108:1458–63.
78. Bass NM, Mullen KD, Sanyal A, et al. Rifaximin treatment in hepatic encephalopathy. N Engl J Med 2010;362:1071–81.
79. Sidhu SS, Goyal O, Mishra BP, et al. Rifaximin improves psychometric performance and health-related quality of life in patients with minimal hepatic encephalopathy (the RIME trial). Am J Gastroenterol 2011;106:307–16.
80. Sidhu SS, Goyal O, Parker RA, et al. Rifaximin vs. lactulose in treatment of minimal hepatic encephalopathy. Liver Int 2016;36:378–85.
81. Goh ET, Stokes CS, Sidhu SS, et al. L-ornithine L-aspartate for prevention and treatment of hepatic encephalopathy in people with cirrhosis. Cochrane Database Syst Rev 2018;(5):Cd012410.
82. Goulenok C, Bernard B, Cadranel JF, et al. Flumazenil vs. placebo in hepatic encephalopathy in patients with cirrhosis: a meta-analysis. Aliment Pharmacol Ther 2002;16:361–72.
83. Goh ET, Andersen ML, Morgan MY, et al. Flumazenil versus placebo or no intervention for people with cirrhosis and hepatic encephalopathy. Cochrane Database Syst Rev 2017;(8):Cd002798.
84. Gluud LL, Dam G, Les I, et al. Branched-chain amino acids for people with hepatic encephalopathy. Cochrane Database Syst Rev 2017;(5):Cd001939.
85. Weiss N, Tripon S, Lodey M, et al. Treating hepatic encephalopathy in cirrhotic patients admitted to ICU with sodium phenylbutyrate: a preliminary study. Fundam Clin Pharmacol 2018;32(2):209–15.
86. Ganapathy D, Acharya C, Lachar J, et al. The patient buddy app can potentially prevent hepatic encephalopathy-related readmissions. Liver Int 2017;37: 1843–51.

87. Weiss N, Thabut D. Neurological complications occurring after liver transplantation: role of risk factors, hepatic encephalopathy, and acute (on chronic) brain injury. Liver Transpl 2019;25(3):469–87.
88. Salerno F, Cammà C, Enea M, et al. Transjugular intrahepatic portosystemic shunt for refractory ascites: a meta-analysis of individual patient data. Gastroenterology 2007;133(3):825–34.
89. Bai M, Qi X, Yang Z, et al. Predictors of hepatic encephalopathy after transjugular intrahepatic portosystemic shunt in cirrhotic patients: a systematic review. J Gastroenterol Hepatol 2011;26(6):943–51.
90. Bureau C, Jézéquel C, Thabut D, et al. Rifaximin reduces hepatic encephalopathy risk after TIPS. Hepatology 2019;70(S1):10A.

APPENDIX 1: USEFUL WORKUP FOR THE DIAGNOSIS AND DIFFERENTIAL DIAGNOSIS OF HEPATIC ENCEPHALOPATHY

Examinations	Usefulness
Measurement of ammonia plasma level	• Suggests a differential diagnosis if normal • Prognostic value is high (severity of HE, recurrence of HE, other organ failure, mortality)
Electroencephalogram	• May strengthen the diagnosis of HE but may be normal without ruling out HE • May have a better sensitivity than psychometric tests for MHE • Predictive of OHE at 1 y • May diagnose seizures as a differential diagnosis
Cerebral CT scan	• Reveals a differential diagnosis, such as expansive intracranial process
Cerebral MRI + spectroscopy	• Reveals a differential diagnosis, such as vascular leukoencephalopathy, vasculitis, expansive intracranial process, or other metabolic disorders • Spectroscopy acknowledges high glutamine brain content. Normal spectroscopy suggests a differential diagnosis

Appendix 2

APPENDIX 2: PROS AND CONS OF MEASUREMENT OF AMMONIA PLASMA LEVEL

Pros	Cons
• Based on a simple blood test • Available • Inexpensive • Easily interpretable, as opposed to EEG or cerebral MRI and spectroscopy • Diagnostic value: the diagnosis of HE should be reconsidered if the plasma ammonia level is normal • Prognostic value: a high ammonia plasma level is associated with the severity of HE, recurrence of HE, other organ failure, and mortality • Therapeutic target?	• Needs specific conditions of blood collection to be interpretable: 　○ No venous stasis (ie, ideally without use of tourniquet) 　○ Completely fill the EDTA tube and immediately homogenize by spinning 　○ Bring the tube quickly to the laboratory on ice at +4°C 　○ Interferes with hemolysis, severe jaundice, physical exercise, tobacco, or high protein diet • Measurement may vary according to laboratories • Correlation with psychometric tests is debated in MHE • Therapeutic target?

Appendix 3

APPENDIX 3: ANIMAL NAMING TEST INSTRUCTIONS

REQUIRED TIME: less than 2 minutes

REQUIRED EQUIPMENT: paper, pen, timer

INSTRUCTION: "Tell me the names of as many animals as you can think of, as quickly as possible, in 1 minute." If the person says nothing for 15 seconds, say "A dog is an animal. Can you tell me more animals?" If the person stops before 60 seconds, say "Any more animals?"

SCORING: Count the total number of animals (not including repetitions or nonanimal words)

INTERPRETATION: A cutoff of 15 to 20 animals in 1 minute seems reasonable to rule out MHE, and MHE is possible below this cutoff. Cutoffs depend on validation studies according to language.

Acute Decompensation and Acute-on-Chronic Liver Failure

Philip Ferstl, Dr med[a], Jonel Trebicka, Dr med, PhD[a,b],*

KEYWORDS

- Cirrhosis • Portal hypertension • Systemic inflammation • Metabolic dysfunction
- Immune paralysis • Bacterial infection • Organ failure

KEY POINTS

- Acute decompensation is a heterogenous syndrome characteristic of end-stage liver disease.
- Throughout the various stages of acute decompensation, portal hypertension, systemic inflammation, and metabolic dysfunction are progressively aggravated.
- Acute-on-chronic liver failure is the final and most fatal stage of acute decompensation and is characterized by massive systemic inflammation.

CIRRHOSIS, ACUTE DECOMPENSATION, AND ACUTE-ON-CHRONIC LIVER FAILURE

Liver cirrhosis is the common end stage of all chronic liver diseases. Acute decompensation (AD) and its maximal form acute-on-chronic liver failure (ACLF) are a major cause of death in these patients.[1–3] Accounting for 14,544,000 disability-adjusted life-years worldwide, cirrhosis has become a major health care problem.[4] AD is by far the main reason for repeated hospitalization in patients with cirrhosis.[5] Treatment of AD and ACLF primarily aims at organ support.[6,7] Therapies are therefore unspecific, difficult, and expensive, and the clinical risk assessment and stratification of these patients are gaining paramount importance.[8]

The main precipitants leading to the occurrence of AD are proven bacterial infections, severe alcoholic hepatitis, gastrointestinal bleeding with shock, and toxic encephalopathy.[9] The onset and severity of AD correlate with the extent of systemic inflammation (SI); hence, it is assumed that the precipitating insult must cross a certain threshold to cause AD.[8–10] Among the various stages of AD, pre-ACLF is the condition that precedes to ACLF.[11] AD and ACLF will become more severe upon precipitants

[a] Department for Internal Medicine I, University Hospital, Goethe University, Theodor-Stern-Kai 7, Frankfurt am Main 60590, Germany; [b] European Foundation for the Study of Chronic Liver Failure, Travesera de Gracia 11, 08021 Barcelona, Spain
* Corresponding author. Medizinische Klinik 1, Theodor-Stern-Kai 7, Frankfurt am Main 60590, Germany.
E-mail address: Jonel.trebicka@kgu.de

Clin Liver Dis 25 (2021) 419–430
https://doi.org/10.1016/j.cld.2021.01.009
1089-3261/21/© 2021 The Author(s). Published by Elsevier Inc. This is an open access article under the CC BY-NC-ND license (http://creativecommons.org/licenses/by-nc-nd/4.0/).
liver.theclinics.com

with concomitant organ failure (OF), and in the case of multiple precipitants.[9] ACLF is now considered the most severe form of AD, but their clinical phenotype as well as their inflammatory signature differs notably. SI is the hallmark of both AD and ACLF.

DEFINITION AND PATHOPHYSIOLOGY OF ACUTE DECOMPENSATION
Four Phenotypes of Acute Decompensation

AD is very common in end-stage liver disease, and it encompasses a variety of decompensating events.[12] A decompensating event is defined as any of the following 4 events: ascites, gastrointestinal bleeding, hepatic encephalopathy, or bacterial infection.[13] The course of end-stage cirrhosis is complicated by these decompensating events, which occur in an unanticipated and repeated manner.[14] Bacterial infections often lead to further decompensation events.[15] Gastrointestinal bleeding is significantly associated with new onset of spontaneous bacterial peritonitis and other bacterial infections.[12] Therefore, in patients with ascites, gastrointestinal bleeding, or hepatic encephalopathy, a decompensation event may cause another within the course of the disease.[14,16,17] Once patients with cirrhosis develop a first episode of AD, the median survival drops from 12 to less than 2 years.[18,19] For patients, the transition from compensated to decompensated cirrhosis is a "prognostic watershed," and it spotlights the clinical significance of AD.[12]

Four Different Trajectories of Acute Decompensation

Stable decompensated cirrhosis
Because decompensated cirrhosis is a polymorphic and dynamic process rather than a steady state, a concise sequence of severity grades of AD has been proposed.[11] This classification comprises four distinguished stages. Stable decompensated cirrhosis (SDC) is characterized by complications of cirrhosis, lower SI, and the possibility of timely recompensation.[20–22] Patients with SDC are therefore not readmitted because of further AD events. OFs are very rarely observed in SDC; however, brain or liver dysfunction does occur in 23% and 14% of patients, respectively. In many instances, SDC is preceded or accompanied by bacterial infections, which resolve however, and the patients may return to the stage of recompensation. The 1-year mortality is 10% in SDC.[11]

Unstable decompensated cirrhosis
Unstable decompensated cirrhosis (UDC) is associated with significant portal hypertension (PHT), shows a remarkably increased incidence of bacterial infections, and thus spawns further decompensation events.[11,20,23] Upon AD at the initial hospital admission, UDC is characterized by the necessity of at least 1 readmission owing to further decompensation events, but ACLF does not occur in these patients. Although organ dysfunctions occur more often than in SDC (29%, 19%, and 16% for brain, circulatory, and liver dysfunction, respectively), OF are still not frequently observed in UDC. Patients with UDC have a 1-year mortality of 36%. Importantly, gastrointestinal bleeding is significantly more often observed in UDC than in pre-ACLF, which underlines the role of clinically significant PHT in UDC.[11]

Pre–acute-on-chronic liver failure
Pre-ACLF is defined as an episode of AD, during or upon which ACLF develops.[11] It is associated with significant SI, therefore distinguishing pre-ACLF from SDC and UDC. However, because the notion of pre-ACLF has been described in 2020, it is important to disambiguate that the past studies investigating SI did not explicitly mention the term pre-ACLF.[20,23] Pre-ACLF is clinically characterized with a significant increase

in renal dysfunction (23% compared with 7% in both UDC and SDC). Among the non-ACLF forms of AD, prognosis is worst in pre-ACLF patients, with a 1-year mortality of 67%.[11]

Acute-on-chronic liver failure

Patients who develop ACLF have OFs. This means that ACLF may be constituted by either any 2 nonrenal OFs, any non-renal OF together with brain dysfunction, or any cirrhotic patient with acute renal failure.[1] Further OFs are possible and will lead to a more severe ACLF grade. Varying definitions of ACLF have been proposed by the EASL (European Association for the Study of the Liver), NACSELD (North American Consortium for the Study of End-Stage Liver Disease), and APASL (Asian Pacific Association for the Study of the Liver), but all of them rely on clinical characteristics, including the deterioration of liver function in combination with OFs.[24–26] ACLF is a highly dynamic entity of AD, and complete deterioration may occur within days. This includes the "full-blown" clinical picture of multiorgan failure, and intensive care, including organ support, is often necessary. Among all ACLF stages, renal failure is observed most frequently, followed by liver and coagulation failure (56%, 44%, and 28%, respectively).[1] ACLF is associated with a 28-day mortality of 22% (ACLF-1) up to 77% (ACLF-3).[1,3,27,28]

Discrimination of Acute Decompensation from Acute-On-Chronic Liver Failure

The presence of 2 or more OFs in patients with cirrhosis, combined with signs of both hepatic and systemic inflammation (SI), defines the condition of ACLF.[8] Altogether, ACLF encompasses 6 entities of OFs: renal, cerebral, liver, coagulation, circulation, and/or respiratory OF. For each of these OFs, specific and concise thresholds have been defined, and the severity of ACLF is graded from 1 to 3, depending on the number of organ systems failing. Exceptions with less than 2 OFs that also constitute ACLF are (A) single kidney failure, since it was observed that patients with renal failure have a disproportional poor prognosis,[1] and (B) cerebral dysfunction together with any non-kidney OF. Considering these clear cutoffs, the pragmatic clinical diagnosis of ACLF is straightforward. Nevertheless, the presence of ACLF depends on the time and dynamic of decompensation. There is uncertainty whether kidney failure alone or single OF with kidney dysfunction is as relevant as 2 OFs, which is a matter of debate among the different societies. However, the CANONIC study, which defined ACLF based on the mortality, could be reproduced by different studies and even the PREDICT study.[1,8,9,11] Because in ACLF the most important issue is probably to improve survival, those effects are subject to further clinical research.

Pathophysiology of Acute Decompensation and Acute-On-Chronic Liver Failure

Portal hypertension

For the most part, decompensation events arise because of the existence of PHT. PHT is therefore a central element predisposing for AD and ACLF. In a nutshell, PHT is a condition of increased hydrostatic pressure in the portal vein. This state of hypertension leads to (A) a reflex dilation of splanchnic arteriolae, and via circulatory dysfunction to vasodilation of peripheral arteries[29]; (B) excessive collateral angiogenesis with the formation of esophageal, gastric, and rectal varices[30–32]; and (C) bacterial translocation owing to inflammation of the intestinal lymphatic tissue, dysfunctional intestinal innervation, and epithelial swelling, resulting in SI.[33–36] Importantly, significant bacterial translocation only occurs in cirrhotic PHT, and not in acute and/or noncirrhotic PHT.[37] As a consequence, gastrointestinal bleeding may occur because of the spontaneous rupture of a varix; ascites owing to hydrostatic pressure itself; or spontaneous bacterial peritonitis owing to a leaky intestinal barrier. Because PHT links bacterial translocation and SI, it also predisposes to the occurrence of ACLF.[28] It is noteworthy that SI can also be reduced by transjugular intrahepatic portosystemic shunt (TIPS), which is another strong hint pointing at the link between PHT and SI.[38,39] Furthermore, because of its hemodynamic derangements, PHT is a necessity for ACLF, for example, in the case of cirrhotic cardiomyopathy, which might lead to circulatory failure, and diminished effective arterial blood volume, leading to hepatorenal syndrome.[24,28,40]

Systemic inflammation

Interestingly enough, C-reactive protein (CRP) and leukocytes as biomarkers of SI are higher in patients with pre-ACLF than in patients with unstable or SDC (**Fig. 1**).[11] It was shown that patients with AD and an increased neutrophil-to-lymphocyte ratio especially tend to develop ACLF and die.[41] It was further observed that elevated levels of interleukin-6 (IL-6), IL-1RA, and HNA2 in patients with AD were independently associated with development of ACLF within 28 days.[23] IL-1α, IL-1β, plasma renin, and copeptin, as well as other cytokines, are further inflammation markers that may be elevated in AD and, importantly, are strongly associated with the development of ACLF.[22,42] These findings promote the hypothesis that the baseline inflammatory profile in AD may a priori discriminate patients with and without courses of ACLF, and only SI capable of inducing end-organ damage is therefore also be thought to be significant for the development of ACLF.[9,23]

In ACLF, the overall inflammatory response is much more pronounced than in SDC, UDC, or pre-ACLF.[42,43] Because a disproportionly high expression of humoral markers is observed but nevertheless bacterial infections occur at a breathtaking rate, it has to be assumed that the cellular immune system is dysfunctional or even paralyzed in ACLF.[27,44,45] Not only in bacterial infection but also in alcoholic ACLF and probably many other precipitators as well, the reason of leukocytosis lies in an increase of neutrophils, which putatively lose their ability to kill bacteria in ACLF.[27,41] Another important antimediator of ACLF is nitric oxide, a potent vasoconstrictor synthesized by the hepatic endothelium. It is capable of counterbalancing vasodilatory stimuli enacted by cytokines but loses its protective function because of ACLF-associated reactive oxygen species generated in the inflammatory portal and sinusoidal milieu.[46]

Metabolic dysfunction

SI in general and AD in particular predispose to hypermetabolic states in which micronutrients, such as glucose, amino acids, and fatty acids, are preferentially held

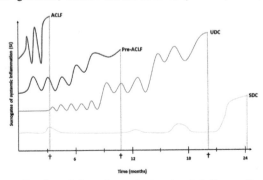

Fig. 1. Schematic visualization of time-dependent systemic inflammation in the four trajectories of acute decompensation.

available for immune cells with high metabolic demand.[47,48] The deprivation of nutrients combined with an inflammatory signature can lead to mitochondrial dysfunction in crucial organs, such as kidney, heart, and liver, thus facilitating the genesis of ACLF.[49,50] Moreover, recent research has shed light on lipid metabolism in ACLF. These lipids are a heterogenous group of inflammatory mediators in blood and tissue, and they are synthesized by the 3 enzymatic families of cyclooxygenases, lipoxygenases, and cytochrome P450 epoxygenases. These enzymes produce a broad array of lipid mediators promoting inflammation and driving neutrophilic bactericidal activity. A panel of these mediators specific for AD has been described, and moreover, leukotriene E4 is capable of differentiating healthy controls from patients with ACLF. On the other hand, LXA_5, which is an anti-inflammatory and proresolution mediator, was significantly underrepresented in ACLF patients.[47]

PRECIPITANTS OF ACUTE DECOMPENSATION
Unidentifiable Precipitants

It is extremely important to identify the precipitant at the pre-ACLF stage. In around 57% of patients with AD, no precipitant is detectable.[9] For many of these patients, it has to be assumed that bacterial translocation and SI cause these events.[28] Bacterial pathogens are translocated from a leaky gut into the blood in a continuous, discontinuous, or burstlike manner and could therefore initiate beginning organ dysfunction.[23,33–36] Indeed, SI is not only observed in UDC and pre-ACLF, but also in patients with compensated cirrhosis or SDC who, importantly, may also have beginning PHT.[20,23,51] It is furthermore noteworthy that SI can apparently be symptomatically treated with intravenous albumin, and survival benefits have been shown in subsets of cirrhotic patients.[52] However, in the other 43% of AD patients, a precipitant is identifiable, and these can therefore be treated more specifically.[9]

Proven Bacterial Infections

Proven infections are defined as bacterial infections with an identifiable source, meaning positive cultures, according to clinical and/or laboratory signs of bacterial infection in patients with cirrhosis, as described before.[53] Gut dysbiosis, loss of intestinal integrity, bacterial translocation, and portosystemic shunting make patients with cirrhosis prone to bacterial infection.[15] Proven infections are the major cause of AD, accounting for 58% of AD patients with an identifiable precipitant.[9] Furthermore, proven infections are equally distributed among SDC, UDC, and pre-ACLF.[11] Importantly, these 3 forms of AD may lead into one another, but they may also cause OFs, which again have a negative impact on the patient's outcome.[24] Routine surrogate markers of SI, such as leukocytes, CRP, and IL-6, are commonly and unspecifically increased in proven infections, making these parameters an insufficient discriminator between infection-triggered AD and infection-triggered ACLF.[23] Severe infections, such as spontaneous peritonitis or pneumonia, are more often found in ACLF, and severe sepsis almost inevitably leads to ACLF, suggesting that the severity of the event itself decides the course for the development and grade of ACLF.[53,54]

About one-half of patients with proven infections develops ACLF, and they develop positive sepsis criteria, most importantly, the SEPSIS-3 criteria and the quick sequential OF assessment, significantly more than patients without ACLF.[17] These patients are characterized by severe SI, most importantly, by elevated levels of leukocytes, CRP, and IL-6.[20,23,54] The 28-day mortality from proven infections in AD patients without ACLF is 5%, but in the case of ACLF amounts to 37%.[17] It is therefore absolutely mandatory to start antimicrobial treatment as early as possible.[9,55] Thereby, inappropriate antimicrobial therapy is associated with the development of ACLF, and mortality upon inappropriate initial antimicrobial treatment worsens 28-day mortality to 54%, compared with 29% in the case of appropriate treatment.[53] Moreover, broad empiric antimicrobial therapy, including coverage of multidrug-resistant organisms (MDRO), had a higher treatment response and is therefore recommended.[9] However, early deescalation of antimicrobial therapy after isolation of the causative pathogen is strongly recommended in order to minimize the antimicrobial selection pressure and occurrence of MDRO.[56] Therefore, microbiologic cultures should be obtained in every patient with clinically suspected bacterial or fungal infection.[12]

Multidrug-Resistant Infections

The prevalence of MDRO is increasing around the globe, with multidrug-resistant gram-negative bacteria resembling the most threatening class of pathogens.[57] On a general basis, cirrhotic patients with MDRO and extensively drug-resistant organisms (XDRO) are sicker as reflected by MELD (model for end-stage liver disease) and ACLF scores, have more complicated courses, and are admitted to the intensive care unit more often.[58] It is noteworthy that particularly in patients with ACLF, infection with XDRO can be observed more frequently.[17] In patients with cirrhosis, it was shown that severe sepsis and septic shock are associated with the development of ACLF, whereas infection without sepsis was more common in AD patients.[59] Obviously, because these infections are more difficult to treat and empiric therapies fail more often, a higher incidence of ACLF would be expected in the case of infection with MDRO and XDRO.[53,56,59] However, in-depth analyses of ACLF courses in these patients are still lacking. In any case, the finding that XDRO are associated with more severe infections and ACLF deserves further mechanistic investigation.

Severe Alcoholic Hepatitis

Around one-third of AD cases is precipitated by severe alcoholic hepatitis.[11] The clinical course and outcome are similar to patients with proven infections. These patients exhibit a broad array of dysfunctional components within the immune system, which, among others, are intrinsic immunosuppression,[60] a dysfunctional adaptive immune system,[61] dysfunctional neutrophils,[62–64] and oxidative burst mitigating in monocyte function.[65] Moreover, metabolic dysfunction in severe alcoholic hepatitis manifests through changes in mitochondrial function.[66] It was recently shown that the DNA-dependent protein kinase catalytic subunit facilitates the occurrence of alcohol-related liver disease by canonic activation of a pathway with the downstream target p53.[67] Mitochondrial function may therefore serve as a therapeutic target in alcoholic hepatitis.[66] Furthermore, alcohol intake mitigates the intestinal microflora and bile acid metabolism, and, via the gut-brain axis, thus has indirect impact on brain function.[68,69] However, as of now, clinically established treatment of severe alcoholic hepatitis is limited to corticosteroids, which have been shown to improve short-term survival, but not the intermediate or long-term prognosis.

Toxic Encephalopathy

Drug-induced liver injury has long been considered a trigger of AD because of hepatotoxic, nephrotoxic, or neurotoxic effects.[70] However, the PREDICT-2 investigation proved solely neurotoxic drugs administered within the past month to be capable of inducing AD, which were also significantly associated with development ACLF. Neurotoxic drugs precipitating AD were exclusively opioids and benzodiazepines; however, no significant effect was detected in patients upon administration of hepatotoxic and nephrotoxic drugs.

Gastrointestinal Bleeding with Shock

As was shown in the PREDICT-1 and PREDICT-2 investigations, AD patients who present with gastrointestinal bleeding are significantly more often attributed to "mild" AD stages, that is, SDC and UDC.[9,11] Also, patients with ACLF have a more significant history of bleeding than patients without ACLF.[71] These observations might be explained by the fact that patients with bleeding have significantly less SI than patients with ascites or other decompensation events, and fewer patients with gastrointestinal bleeding without previous decompensation of cirrhosis should therefore develop ACLF, compared with patients with, for example, ascites.[20,71] Of note, bacterial translocation, which is the most important driver of SI, is reliant on the existence of ascites.[28,35]

However, once patients with gastrointestinal bleeding are in circulatory shock, they are at risk of developing AD and ACLF.[9] Furthermore, likelihood of rebleeding doubles in patients with ACLF and history of bleeding, and in that case, these patients are at very high risk of death.[71] However, they do benefit significantly from preemptive or early transjugular intrahepatic portosystemic shunt (pTIPS), compared with ACLF patients who did not receive pTIPS (42-day mortality: 13.6% vs 51.0%; 1-year mortality: 22.7% vs 56.5%; $P = .002$).[71] These observations came in line with previous findings showing that pTIPS could significantly improve survival in severely decompensated patients with variceal hemorrhage and Child C cirrhosis up to 13 points.[72,73] These patients are often on the verge of death, but treatment of PHT with pTIPS has been shown to be a significant relief and is therefore recommended by current international and Baveno guidelines.[12,74,75]

Multiple and Other Precipitants

Some factors, which had been considered putative precipitators in the past, were further elucidated by the second investigation of the PREDICT-2. Among supposed precipitants that were earlier thought to cause AD, drug-induced liver injury is now recognized as a coincidental factor in the pathogenesis of AD.[9] The PREDICT-2 study also significantly contributed to the notion that therapeutic paracenteses, TIPS implantation, and major surgical procedures are not significantly associated with development of AD or ACLF. Importantly, reactivation of viral hepatitis B leads among triggers in many Asian countries, but is only of minor importance in the western world.[26] However, the course of AD becomes much more severe in the case of multiple precipitants, and the inflammatory signature is also drastically enhanced.[9]

SUMMARY

AD is a condition responsible for many deaths in cirrhosis. AD may have different courses from SDC to ACLF, which is the most deadly syndrome in cirrhosis and is characterized by a 3-month mortality of 51%. In absence of OF, SI and PHT determine the course of disease. Significant research must be performed in order to stratify care and develop treatment strategies for AD patients.

CLINICS CARE POINTS

- The severity of acute decompensation is reflected by the degree of systemic inflammation, while the grade of acute-on-chronic liver failure is defined by the numbers of failing organs.

- Precipitants of acute decompensation and acute-on-chronic liver failure must be identified and treated, if possible.
- Patients with variceal bleeding and acute-on-chronic liver failure do benefit from preemptive TIPS placement.
- In patients with bacterial infection, early and adequate antimicrobial treatment may prevent acute-on-chronic liver failure.
- Patients with ACLF-3 should immediately be admitted to intensive care unit for organ support.

DISCLOSURE

P. Ferstl: Consultancies, SNIPR Biome. J. Trebicka, PhD: Speaker's fees and/or consultancies: Gore, Bayer, Alexion, MSD, Gilead, Intercept, Norgine, Grifols, Versantis, and Martin Pharmaceutical.

Financial support: J. Trebicka is supported by grants from the Deutsche Forschungsgemeinschaft (SFB TRR57 to P18), European Union's Horizon 2020 Research and Innovation Programme (Galaxy, No. 668031, MICROB-PREDICT, No. 825694, and DECISION No. 84794), Societal Challenges-Health, Demographic Change, and Well-Being (No. 731875), and Cellex Foundation (PREDICT).

REFERENCES

1. Moreau R, Jalan R, Gines P, et al. Acute-on-chronic liver failure is a distinct syndrome that develops in patients with acute decompensation of cirrhosis. Gastroenterology 2013;144(7):1426–37, 1437.e1-9.
2. Perricone G, Jalan R. Acute-on-chronic liver failure: a distinct clinical syndrome that has reclassified cirrhosis. Clin Liver Dis (Hoboken) 2019;14(5):171–5.
3. Sundaram V, Jalan R, Wu T, et al. Factors associated with survival of patients with severe acute-on-chronic liver failure before and after liver transplantation. Gastroenterology 2019;156(5):1381–91.e3.
4. Murray CJ, Barber RM, Foreman KJ, et al. Global, regional, and national disability-adjusted life years (DALYs) for 306 diseases and injuries and healthy life expectancy (HALE) for 188 countries, 1990-2013: quantifying the epidemiological transition. Lancet 2015;386(10009):2145–91.
5. Bajaj JS, Reddy KR, Tandon P, et al. The three-month readmission rate remains unacceptably high in a large North American cohort of cirrhotic patients. Hepatology 2015. https://doi.org/10.1002/hep.28414.
6. Olson JC. Acute-on-chronic liver failure: management and prognosis. Curr Opin Crit Care 2019;25(2):165–70.
7. Karvellas CJ, Bagshaw SM. Advances in management and prognostication in critically ill cirrhotic patients. Curr Opin Crit Care 2014;20(2):210–7.
8. Arroyo V, Moreau R, Jalan R. Acute-on-chronic liver failure. N Engl J Med 2020;382(22):2137–45.
9. Trebicka J, Fernandez J, Papp M, et al. PREDICT identifies precipitating events associated with the clinical course of acutely decompensated cirrhosis. J Hepatol 2020. https://doi.org/10.1016/j.jhep.2020.11.019.
10. Arroyo V, Moreau R, Kamath PS, et al. Acute-on-chronic liver failure in cirrhosis. Nat Rev Dis Primers 2016;2:16041.

11. Trebicka J, Fernandez J, Papp M, et al. The PREDICT study uncovers three clinical courses of acutely decompensated cirrhosis that have distinct pathophysiology. J Hepatol 2020. https://doi.org/10.1016/j.jhep.2020.06.013.
12. Angeli P, Bernardi M, Villanueva C, et al. EASL Clinical Practice Guidelines for the management of patients with decompensated cirrhosis. J Hepatol 2018;69(2):406–60.
13. Jalan R, Gines P, Olson JC, et al. Acute-on chronic liver failure. J Hepatol 2012;57(6):1336–48.
14. Garcia-Tsao G. Current management of the complications of cirrhosis and portal hypertension: variceal hemorrhage, ascites, and spontaneous bacterial peritonitis. Dig Dis 2016;34(4):382–6.
15. Jalan R, Fernandez J, Wiest R, et al. Bacterial infections in cirrhosis: a position statement based on the EASL Special Conference 2013. J Hepatol 2014;60(6):1310–24.
16. Fernández J, Acevedo J, Prado V, et al. Clinical course and short-term mortality of cirrhotic patients with infections other than spontaneous bacterial peritonitis. Liver Int 2016. https://doi.org/10.1111/liv.13239.
17. Wong F, Piano S, Singh V, et al. Clinical features and evolution of bacterial infection-related acute-on-chronic liver failure. J Hepatol 2020. https://doi.org/10.1016/j.jhep.2020.07.046.
18. Ginés P, Quintero E, Arroyo V, et al. Compensated cirrhosis: natural history and prognostic factors. Hepatology 1987;7(1):122–8.
19. D'Amico G, Garcia-Tsao G, Pagliaro L. Natural history and prognostic indicators of survival in cirrhosis: a systematic review of 118 studies. J Hepatol 2006;44(1):217–31.
20. Costa D, Simbrunner B, Jachs M, et al. Systemic inflammation increases across distinct stages of advanced chronic liver disease and correlates with decompensation and mortality. J Hepatol 2020. https://doi.org/10.1016/j.jhep.2020.10.004.
21. Villanueva C, Aracil C, Colomo A, et al. Acute hemodynamic response to beta-blockers and prediction of long-term outcome in primary prophylaxis of variceal bleeding. Gastroenterology 2009;137(1):119–28.
22. Monteiro S, Grandt J, Uschner FE, et al. Differential inflammasome activation predisposes to acute-on-chronic liver failure in human and experimental cirrhosis with and without previous decompensation. Gut 2020. https://doi.org/10.1136/gutjnl-2019-320170.
23. Trebicka J, Amoros A, Pitarch C, et al. Addressing profiles of systemic inflammation across the different clinical phenotypes of acutely decompensated cirrhosis. Front Immunol 2019;10:476.
24. Bajaj JS, O'Leary JG, Reddy KR, et al. Survival in infection-related acute-on-chronic liver failure is defined by extrahepatic organ failures. Hepatology 2014;60(1):250–6.
25. O'Leary JG, Reddy KR, Garcia-Tsao G, et al. NACSELD acute-on-chronic liver failure (NACSELD-ACLF) score predicts 30-day survival in hospitalized patients with cirrhosis. Hepatology 2018;67(6):2367–74.
26. Sarin SK, Choudhury A, Sharma MK, et al. Acute-on-chronic liver failure: consensus recommendations of the Asian Pacific Association for the study of the Liver (APASL): an update. Hepatol Int 2019;13(4):353–90.
27. Gustot T, Jalan R. Acute-on-chronic liver failure in patients with alcohol-related liver disease. J Hepatol 2019;70(2):319–27.
28. Trebicka J, Reiberger T, Laleman W. Gut-liver axis links portal hypertension to acute-on-chronic liver failure. Visc Med 2018;34(4):270–5.

29. Bernardi M, Moreau R, Angeli P, et al. Mechanisms of decompensation and organ failure in cirrhosis: from peripheral arterial vasodilation to systemic inflammation hypothesis. J Hepatol 2015;63(5):1272–84.

30. Morales-Ruiz M, Jiménez W. Neovascularization, angiogenesis, and vascular remodeling in portal hypertension. In: Sanyal AJ, Shah VH, editors. Portal hypertension - pathobiology, evaluation, and treatment. Totowa, (NJ): Humana Press; 2005. p. 99–112.

31. Tugues S, Fernandez-Varo G, Muñoz-Luque J, et al. Antiangiogenic treatment with sunitinib ameliorates inflammatory infiltrate, fibrosis, and portal pressure in cirrhotic rats. Hepatology 2007;46(6):1919–26.

32. Bosch J, Abraldes JG, Berzigotti A, et al. The clinical use of HVPG measurements in chronic liver disease. Nat Rev Gastroenterol Hepatol 2009;6(10):573–82.

33. Fernández J, Clària J, Amorós A, et al. Effects of albumin treatment on systemic and portal hemodynamics and systemic inflammation in patients with decompensated cirrhosis. Gastroenterology 2019;157(1):149–62.

34. Wiest R, Garcia-Tsao G. Bacterial translocation (BT) in cirrhosis. Hepatology 2005;41(3):422–33.

35. Wiest R, Lawson M, Geuking M. Pathological bacterial translocation in liver cirrhosis. J Hepatol 2014;60(1):197–209.

36. Schierwagen R, Alvarez-Silva C, Madsen MSA, et al. Circulating microbiome in blood of different circulatory compartments. Gut 2019;68(3):578–80.

37. Garcia-Tsao G, Albillos A, Barden GE, et al. Bacterial translocation in acute and chronic portal hypertension. Hepatology 1993;17(6):1081–5.

38. Berres ML, Asmacher S, Lehmann J, et al. CXCL9 is a prognostic marker in patients with liver cirrhosis receiving transjugular intrahepatic portosystemic shunt. J Hepatol 2015;62(2):332–9.

39. Berres ML, Lehmann J, Jansen C, et al. Chemokine (C-X-C motif) ligand 11 levels predict survival in cirrhotic patients with transjugular intrahepatic portosystemic shunt. Liver Int 2016;36(3):386–94.

40. Wong F. Recent advances in our understanding of hepatorenal syndrome. Nat Rev Gastroenterol Hepatol 2012;9(7):382–91.

41. Cai YJ, Dong JJ, Dong JZ, et al. A nomogram for predicting prognostic value of inflammatory response biomarkers in decompensated cirrhotic patients without acute-on-chronic liver failure. Aliment Pharmacol Ther 2017;45(11):1413–26.

42. Clària J, Stauber RE, Coenraad MJ, et al. Systemic inflammation in decompensated cirrhosis: characterization and role in acute-on-chronic liver failure. Hepatology 2016;64(4):1249–64.

43. Sen S, Davies NA, Mookerjee RP, et al. Pathophysiological effects of albumin dialysis in acute-on-chronic liver failure: a randomized controlled study. Liver Transpl 2004;10(9):1109–19.

44. Wasmuth HE, Kunz D, Yagmur E, et al. Patients with acute on chronic liver failure display "sepsis-like" immune paralysis. J Hepatol 2005;42(2):195–201.

45. Bernsmeier C, Pop OT, Singanayagam A, et al. Patients with acute-on-chronic liver failure have increased numbers of regulatory immune cells expressing the receptor tyrosine kinase MERTK. Gastroenterology 2015;148(3):603–15.e14.

46. Thabut D, Tazi KA, Bonnefont-Rousselot D, et al. High-density lipoprotein administration attenuates liver proinflammatory response, restores liver endothelial nitric oxide synthase activity, and lowers portal pressure in cirrhotic rats. Hepatology 2007;46(6):1893–906.

47. López-Vicario C, Checa A, Urdangarin A, et al. Targeted lipidomics reveals extensive changes in circulating lipid mediators in patients with acutely decompensated cirrhosis. J Hepatol 2020;73(4):817–28.
48. Ganeshan K, Nikkanen J, Man K, et al. Energetic trade-offs and hypometabolic states promote disease tolerance. Cell 2019;177(2):399–413.e12.
49. Van Wyngene L, Vandewalle J, Libert C. Reprogramming of basic metabolic pathways in microbial sepsis: therapeutic targets at last? EMBO Mol Med 2018;10(8). https://doi.org/10.15252/emmm.201708712.
50. Moreau R, Clària J, Aguilar F, et al. Blood metabolomics uncovers inflammation-associated mitochondrial dysfunction as a potential mechanism underlying ACLF. J Hepatol 2020;72(4):688–701.
51. Jachs M, Hartl L, Schaufler D, et al. Amelioration of systemic inflammation in advanced chronic liver disease upon beta-blocker therapy translates into improved clinical outcomes. Gut 2020. https://doi.org/10.1136/gutjnl-2020-322712.
52. Di Pascoli M, Fasolato S, Piano S, et al. Long-term administration of human albumin improves survival in patients with cirrhosis and refractory ascites. Liver Int 2019;39(1):98–105.
53. Fernández J, Acevedo J, Wiest R, et al. Bacterial and fungal infections in acute-on-chronic liver failure: prevalence, characteristics and impact on prognosis. Gut 2018;67(10):1870–80.
54. Gustot T, Durand F, Lebrec D, et al. Severe sepsis in cirrhosis. Hepatology 2009; 50(6):2022–33.
55. Piano S, Brocca A, Mareso S, et al. Infections complicating cirrhosis. Liver Int 2018;38(Suppl 1):126–33.
56. Ferstl PG, Müller M, Filmann N, et al. Noninvasive screening identifies patients at risk for spontaneous bacterial peritonitis caused by multidrug-resistant organisms. Infect Drug Resist 2018;11:2047–61.
57. Piano S, Singh V, Caraceni P, et al. Epidemiology and effects of bacterial infections in patients with cirrhosis worldwide. Gastroenterology 2019;156(5): 1368–80.e10.
58. Ferstl PG, Filmann N, Brandt C, et al. The impact of carbapenem resistance on clinical deterioration and mortality in patients with liver disease. Liver Int 2017. https://doi.org/10.1111/liv.13438.
59. Fernández J, Prado V, Trebicka J, et al. Multidrug-resistant bacterial infections in patients with decompensated cirrhosis and with acute-on-chronic liver failure in Europe. J Hepatol 2019;70(3):398–411.
60. O'Brien AJ, Fullerton JN, Massey KA, et al. Immunosuppression in acutely decompensated cirrhosis is mediated by prostaglandin E2. Nat Med 2014;20(5): 518–23.
61. Markwick LJ, Riva A, Ryan JM, et al. Blockade of PD1 and TIM3 restores innate and adaptive immunity in patients with acute alcoholic hepatitis. Gastroenterology 2015;148(3):590–602.e10.
62. Stadlbauer V, Mookerjee RP, Wright GA, et al. Role of Toll-like receptors 2, 4, and 9 in mediating neutrophil dysfunction in alcoholic hepatitis. Am J Physiol Gastrointest Liver Physiol 2009;296(1):G15–22.
63. Mookerjee RP, Stadlbauer V, Lidder S, et al. Neutrophil dysfunction in alcoholic hepatitis superimposed on cirrhosis is reversible and predicts the outcome. Hepatology 2007;46(3):831–40.

64. Boussif A, Rolas L, Weiss E, et al. Impaired intracellular signaling, myeloperoxidase release and bactericidal activity of neutrophils from patients with alcoholic cirrhosis. J Hepatol 2016;64(5):1041–8.

65. Vergis N, Khamri W, Beale K, et al. Defective monocyte oxidative burst predicts infection in alcoholic hepatitis and is associated with reduced expression of NADPH oxidase. Gut 2017;66(3):519–29.

66. Abdallah MA, Singal AK. Mitochondrial dysfunction and alcohol-associated liver disease: a novel pathway and therapeutic target. Signal Transduct Target Ther 2020;5(1):26.

67. Zhou H, Zhu P, Wang J, et al. DNA-PKcs promotes alcohol-related liver disease by activating Drp1-related mitochondrial fission and repressing FUNDC1-required mitophagy. Signal Transduct Target Ther 2019;4:56.

68. Bajaj JS. Alcohol, liver disease and the gut microbiota. Nat Rev Gastroenterol Hepatol 2019;16(4):235–46.

69. Lachar J, Bajaj JS. Changes in the microbiome in cirrhosis and relationship to complications: hepatic encephalopathy, spontaneous bacterial peritonitis, and sepsis. Semin Liver Dis 2016;36(4):327–30.

70. Jalan R, Saliba F, Pavesi M, et al. Development and validation of a prognostic score to predict mortality in patients with acute-on-chronic liver failure. J Hepatol 2014;61(5):1038–47.

71. Trebicka J, Gu W, Ibáñez-Samaniego L, et al. Rebleeding and mortality risk are increased by ACLF but reduced by pre-emptive TIPS. J Hepatol 2020;73(5):1082–91.

72. Hernández-Gea V, Procopet B, Giráldez Á, et al. Preemptive-TIPS improves outcome in high-risk variceal bleeding: an observational study. Hepatology 2019;69(1):282–93.

73. Kumar R, Kerbert AJC, Sheikh MF, et al. Determinants of mortality in patients with cirrhosis and uncontrolled variceal bleeding. J Hepatol 2020. https://doi.org/10.1016/j.jhep.2020.06.010.

74. Gerbes A, Labenz J, Appenrodt B, et al. Aktualisierte S2k-Leitlinie der Deutschen Gesellschaft für Gastroenterologie, Verdauungs- und Stoffwechselkrankheiten (DGVS) "Komplikationen der Leberzirrhose". Z Gastroenterol 2019;57:611–80.

75. de Franchis R, Faculty BV. Expanding consensus in portal hypertension: report of the Baveno VI Consensus Workshop: stratifying risk and individualizing care for portal hypertension. J Hepatol 2015;63(3):743–52.

Management of Severe and Refractory Ascites

Hélène Larrue, MD, Jean Pierre Vinel, MD, Christophe Bureau, MD, PhD*

KEYWORDS

- Ascites • Portal hypertension • Cirrhosis • Albumin • TIPS • Liver transplantation
- Large-volume paracentesis

KEY POINTS

- As soon as refractory ascites is diagnosed, LT must be considered as it is the only curative treatment.
- Special care must be given to control the underlying liver disease and to sodium restriction.
- TIPS is then proposed, both as a final treatment or as a waiting therapeutic in bridge to LT.
- Careful selection to each treatment is essential to avoid further decompensation but also to limit therapeutic complications.

INTRODUCTION

Ascites is one of the most common complications of cirrhosis, as 50% to 60% of cirrhotic patients will develop ascites within 10 years after diagnosis.[1] After a first episode of ascites, refractory ascites will develop in 10% of the patients.[2] The occurrence of refractory ascites is a milestone in the history of the disease, as it is associated with a 2-year mortality of 65%,[3] poor quality of life, and an increased risk of spontaneous bacterial peritonitis (SBP) and hepatorenal syndrome (HRS). It is for these reasons that any patient with refractory ascites should be considered for (LT). However, a minority of them are candidates for LT, and the waiting time on list could be very long. Therefore, other options must be considered. Choosing between the different therapeutic options must be done regarding the improvement in the prognosis and focusing on quality of life and nutritional status improvement. Ascites is uncomplicated when it is not infected, refractory, or associated with HRS.

In this review, the authors focus on the management of refractory ascites.

Service d'Hépatologie Hôpital Rangueil 1, Avenue Jean Poulhès CHU Toulouse France and Université Toulouse III-Paul Sabatier, France 31400
* Corresponding author.
E-mail address: bureau.c@chu-toulouse.fr

Clin Liver Dis 25 (2021) 431–440
https://doi.org/10.1016/j.cld.2021.01.010
1089-3261/21/© 2021 Elsevier Inc. All rights reserved.

Box 1
Classification of ascites stage

Grade 1 (mild): Ascites is only detectable by ultrasound examination

Grade 2 (moderate): Clinically perceptible

Grade 3 (large): Marked abdominal distention

DEFINITIONS

First-line treatment of patients with cirrhosis and moderate or large ascites (**Box 1** provides a classification of grading) consists of sodium restriction (80–120 mmol per day with diet education) and single morning doses of oral spironolactone and furosemide, beginning with 100 mg of the former and 40 mg of the latter.

According to the International Club of Ascites, diagnostic criteria of refractory ascites rely on lack of response to diuretic treatment, early ascites recurrence, or diuretic induced complications. They are summarized in **Box 2**.

Ascites is defined as refractory when it cannot be mobilized or whenever its early recurrence cannot be prevented by medical therapy. The definition encompasses 2 different situations:

- Diuretic-resistant ascites: Patients do not respond to sodium restriction at the maximum doses of diuretics (400 mg of spironolactone and 160 mg of furosemide).
- Diuretic-intractable ascites: Patients cannot be treated by diuretics because of diuretics-induced complications that preclude the use of an effective dosage.

Box 2
Diagnostic criteria of refractory ascites

- Diuretic-resistant ascites: patients do not respond to sodium restriction at the maximum doses of diuretics (400 mg of spironolactone and 160 mg of furosemide).
- Diuretic-intractable ascites: patients cannot be treated by diuretics because of diuretics-induced complications that preclude the use of an effective dosage.
  - Diuretic treatment duration:
    Spironolactone 400 mg per day and Furosemide 160 mg per day for at least 1 week, together with a low-sodium diet (<5.2 g per day)
  - Lack of response to diuretic treatment:
    Mean weight loss of less than 800 g over 4 days and urinary sodium output less than oral intake
  - Early ascites recurrence:
    Reappearance of grade 2 or 3 ascites within 4 weeks of initial mobilization
  - Diuretic-induced complications:
    Hepatic encephalopathy without any other precipitating factor
    Renal impairment with an increase of serum creatinine by greater than 100% to a value greater than 2 mg/dL
    Hyponatremia with a decrease of serum sodium by greater than 10 mmol/L to less than 125 mmol/L
    Hypokalemia or hyperkalemia to less than 3 mmol/L or greater than 6 mmol/L

Adapted from: Moore KP, Wong F, Gines P, Bernardi M, Ochs A, Salerno F, Angeli P, Porayko M, Moreau R, Garcia-Tsao G, Jimenez W, Planas R, Arroyo V. The management of ascites in cirrhosis: report on the consensus conference of the International Ascites Club. Hepatology. 2003 Jul;38(1):258-66. https://doi.org/10.1053/jhep.2003.50315. PMID: 12830009; with permission.

PATHOPHYSIOLOGY

Ascites results from both portal hypertension and liver insufficiency. Ascites generally develops when portal pressure gradient exceeds 10 mm Hg. In cirrhosis, portal pressure increases first because of an increased resistance to portal blood flow at the level of the liver vascular bed. Increased resistance is secondary to a mechanical component (modifications of the liver architecture) but also to a dynamic one (decrease of vasodilator agents and increase in vasoconstrictor agents) leading to an increased intrahepatic vascular tone.

Secondary portosystemic collateral develops, and splanchnic vasodilatation is responsible for an increase in blood flow. Vasodilatation results in a decrease of systemic vascular resistance and in an effective arterial hypovolemia. Increased cardiac output, activation of sympathetic, antidiuretic, and renin-angiotensin-aldosterone systems aim to counteract the effective hypovolemia but contribute to renal vasoconstriction and water and sodium retention.

Hypoalbuminemia owing to hepatic insufficiency is responsible for a decrease in oncotic pressure leading to a fluid leakage to interstitial sector.[4]

Moreover, advanced cirrhosis is an inflammatory state whereby there are higher levels of proinflammatory cytokines that increase arterial nitric oxide production and exacerbate splanchnic vasodilatation and subsequent effective arterial underfilling. Decreased effective volume predisposes to the development of refractory ascites. Bacterial translocation following intestinal dysbiosis and increased intestinal permeability is frequent and contributes to the release of proinflammatory cytokines.[5]

MANAGEMENT AND THERAPEUTIC OPTIONS
General Measures

One of the most important steps is to treat the underlying liver disease (abstinence of alcohol, antiviral therapy, and so forth). It can result in resolution of ascites, and it clearly demonstrates that refractory ascites can be transient. In randomized studies comparing transjugular intrahepatic portosystemic shunt (TIPS) to repeated paracenteses, up to 20% of the patients did not require further repeated large-volume paracenteses probably because of the control of the etiologic factor resulting in an improvement of portal hypertension and/or liver functions.

Diuretics have usually been discontinued in patients with refractory ascites. The European guideline recommends discontinuing diuretics if the urine sodium is less than 30 mmol per day during diuretic therapy.

A precipitating factor must be sought for hepatocellular carcinoma, portal vein thrombosis, acute alcoholic hepatitis, SBP, and similar.

The safety of nonselective beta-blockers in patients with refractory ascites has been recently questioned. A detrimentary effect could be due to their negative impact on arterial blood pressure, the increase rate of postparacentesis circulatory dysfunction (PPCD), and an impairment of renal function and of systolic function.[6] Blood pressure and renal function should be monitored closely, and consideration should be given to discontinuing or not initiating beta-blockers in patients or situations with decreased organ perfusion or hypotension (systolic blood pressure <90 mm Hg, mean arterial pressure <65 mm Hg, acute kidney injury, SBP). At Baveno VI, it was proposed that after discontinuation of beta-blockers, they should be carefully reinitiated after the resolution of the event. In those situations, doses greater than 80 mg should be avoided.

Other agents known to be deleterious for renal function in such patients should be avoided, such as nonsteroidal anti-inflammatory drugs, angiotensin-converting enzyme inhibitors, angiotensin receptor blockers, and aminoglycosides.

Large-Volume Paracentesis with Albumin Infusion

Large-volume paracentesis with albumin infusion (LVP + A; 8 g/L of ascites removed is the dose commonly used) is the standard and the first-line treatment of tense ascites.[7] It rapidly relieves abdominal distension, diminishing pain and discomfort, and can be performed in an outpatient setting. However, recurrence of ascites is the rule because this is a local treatment with no beneficial impact on any mechanism involved in the ascites formation. Furthermore, LVP is associated with a risk of PPCD defined as an increase in plasma renin activity of greater than 50% to greater than 4 ng/mL/h on the sixth day after the procedure. PPCD is associated with a rapid recurrence of ascites and a high risk of HRS.[8] Albumin infusion in LVP of more than 5 L reduces the incidence of PPCD, and a meta-analysis of 17 trials showed a reduction in mortality with an odds ratio of death of 0.64 (95% confidence interval, 0.41–0.98) when albumin was used compared with other plasma expanders.[9]

Transjugular Intrahepatic Portosystemic Shunt

TIPS is a side-to-side portocaval shunt inside the liver connecting a main portal branch with a large hepatic vein. It reduces ascites formation by decreasing portal pressure, increasing at least transiently the effective arterial blood volume and decompressing both the portal venous system and the hepatic microcirculation, leading to a decreased formation of lymph. A decrease in plasma renin activity, plasma aldosterone, and noradrenalin concentrations is observed following TIPS implantation. This leads to an improvement in renal perfusion.[10] Six randomized studies aiming to compare TIPS and LVP in the treatment of patients with refractory ascites were performed (**Table 1**). All these studies clearly showed that TIPS is more effective than LVP in preventing recurrence of ascites. However, patients treated with TIPS were consistently found to have an increased risk of encephalopathy. The results regarding survival are discrepant according to the different reports. Many meta-analyses have also been published. The first one found TIPS was more effective in preventing recurrence of ascites, but the risk of encephalopathy was increased, and survival was unchanged compared with LVP. However, in the sole meta-analysis with individual data performed by Salerno and colleagues,[18] the actuarial probability of transplant-free survival was better in patients allocated to the TIPS arm than to the LVP group (63% and 52% at 1 year, respectively). It suggests that some patients would benefit

Table 1
Randomized controlled trials comparing transjugular intrahepatic portosystemic shunt versus large-volume paracenteses in patients with recurrent ascites

Study	Stent	Patients (TIPS vs LVP + A)	Survival Rate (TIPS vs LVP + A)
Lebrec et al.[11] J Hepatol 1996	Bare	13 vs 12	29% vs 56% at 2 y[a]
Rössle et al.[12] N Engl J Med 2000	Bare	29 vs 31	58% vs 32% at 2 y
Ginès et al.[13] Gastroenterology 2002	Bare	20 vs 18	26% vs 30% at 2 y
Sanyal et al.[14] Gastroenterology 2003	Bare	52 vs 57	35% vs 33% at 2 y
Salerno et al.[15] Hepatology 2004	Bare	33 vs 33	59% vs 29% at 2 y[a]
Narahara et al.[16] J gastroenterol 2011	Bare	30 vs 30	64% vs 35% at 2 y[a]
Bureau et al.[17] Gastroenterology 2017	Covered	29 vs 33	93% vs 52% at 1 y[a]

[a] Significant difference.

from the procedure. The parameters associated with mortality in multivariate analysis were an older age, a higher bilirubin level, and a lower plasma sodium level and treatment allocation. In another study, it has been shown that bilirubin level and platelets count could be useful to select good candidates for the TIPS procedure. Finally, bare metallic stents were used in all the six first randomized controlled trials (RCT). The use of covered stents improves the primary patency of the shunt. The most recent RCT comparing TIPS using polytetrafluoroethylene-covered stents with LVP + A showed a better transplantation-free survival at 1 year (93% in the TIPS group vs 52% in the LVP + A group).[17]

As mentioned above, a careful selection of patients is crucial. TIPS creation is contraindicated in patients with advanced liver failure (Child Pugh > C11 or model for end-stage liver disease [MELD] >18), heart failure, or recurrent/chronic hepatic encephalopathy. A preprocedural assessment is needed, including liver function tests, cardiac evaluation (nt-pro BNP, transthoracic echocardiography [TTE] with diastolic dysfunction screening), and encephalopathy screening. Contraindications are listed in **Box 3**.[19]

Three main complications may develop after TIPS creation: liver failure, hepatic encephalopathy, and cardiac failure. Liver failure is now a rare event after a planned procedure when the selection of candidates is accurate. Hepatic encephalopathy occurs in 25% to 50% of cases, irrespective of the type of stent used.[20] In the RCT comparing covered TIPS versus standard of care (LVP + A), the 1-year probability of remaining free of overt hepatic encephalopathy was 65% in both groups.[17] Recent data suggest that underdilatation of a covered stent could lower the risk of hepatic encephalopathy.[21] However, underdilated stents have been reported to passively autoexpand to their nominal diameter some weeks after the procedure.[22] New controlled expansion stents have been introduced in 2016, but few data about their efficacy are available.[23] Preliminary results of a recent RCT comparing Rifaximin to placebo after TIPS creation found the occurrence of hepatic encephalopathy was lowered to 39% in the Rifaximin group versus 66% in the placebo group within the 6 months after TIPS creation.[24]

TIPS creation causes an increased cardiac preload, leading to an increased ventricular filling pressure, and can reveal an underlying cirrhotic cardiomyopathy. Cardiac failure occurs in up to 20% within the first year after TIPS, in a median of 30 days (2–210 days).[25] Pre-TIPS cardiac evaluation is therefore mandatory. Pulmonary

---

Box 3
Usual contraindications to transjugular intrahepatic portosystemic shunt placement in patients with refractory ascites

Advanced liver failure defined as:
    Child-Pugh greater than C11
    MELD greater than 18,
    Bilirubin greater than 50 μmol/L,
    INR greater than 2,
    Platelets less than 75 G/L

Recurrent overt hepatic encephalopathy

Cardiac dysfunction: Pulmonary hypertension (PAPm $\geq$ 45 mm Hg)
    Aortic stenosis
    Diastolic dysfunction (E/A > 1.5, E/E' > 10, LAVI > 34 mL/m^2)
    Systolic dysfunction (LVEF < 50%)

Abbreviations: LAVI, left atrial volume index; LVEF, left ventricular ejection fraction; INR, international normalized ratio; PAPM, mean pulmonary arterial pressure; RA, refractory ascites.

hypertension and aortic stenosis are contraindications for shunt creation. When the nt-pro BNP value is greater than 125 pg/mL, a complete TTE is needed. TTE parameters identified signs of diastolic dysfunction to predict cardiac failure after shunt creation: an E/A ratio greater than 1.5 or an E/e' ratio greater than 10 or a left atrial volume index greater than 34 mL/m^2.

Automated Low-Flow Ascites Pump

The automated low-flow ascites pump (alfapump system) consists of a subcutaneous implantable and rechargeable device, which diverts ascitic fluid from the peritoneal cavity to the urinary bladder, allowing a daily slow and continuous evacuation. The daily amount of ascitic fluid to be removed can be adjusted. An RCT showed that alfa-pump reduces the need for LVP, and this procedure was associated with an improvement of nutritional status and quality of life.[26] However, survival was similar in the group of patients treated by alfapump compared with those treated by LVP. That is the reason it should be indicated in patients who are ineligible for TIPS and LT, with an expected survival of greater than 3 months. Contraindications are renal failure with creatinine greater than 132 μmol/L or estimated glomerular filtration rate less than 30 mL/min/1.32 m^2, at least 2 or more systemic or local abdominal infections in the previous 6 months, recent intra-abdominal surgery, history of bladder cancer, previous solid organ transplantation, and bilirubin level greater than 85 μmol/L.[27]

Routine prophylactic antibiotic use (norfloxacin 400 mg/d or ciprofloxacin 750 mg/d) has reduced the incidence of bacterial infections.[28]

Even if the pump performs a continuous small paracentesis, it has been shown that the dispositive was associated with impairment of renal function by activating vasoconstrictors systems. Acute kidney injury was reported in 30% of patients, and creatinine levels increased by a mean of 23 μmol/L after pump insertion.[29] Whether albumin infusion should be systematic in all or in patients at high risk of renal failure requires further investigations.[30]

Liver Transplantation

It is worth noting that patients with refractory ascites should be evaluated for a LT as soon as the diagnosis is completed, as it is the only way to treat the underlying liver disease and to improve long-term prognosis. LT is the only curative option in patients with a high MELD score or a high Child-Pugh score and in patients with prior recurrent or chronic hepatic encephalopathy. Either TIPS or the alfapump system should be used while awaiting treatments.

Other Therapeutic Options

Albumin infusions

Albumin infusions could have several beneficial effects: they work as a plasma expander but also have homeostatic properties as a potent scavenger, anti-inflammatory, and antioxidant molecule. Recently, 2 randomized studies investigated the long-term use of albumin administration in patients with ascites. The ANSWER study enrolled 431 patients with persisting ascites, either in the standard of care group or in the albumin group (40 g twice a week for 2 weeks and then 40 g weekly) for 18 months.[31] The investigators observed a better control of ascites, a decreased rate of other cirrhosis-related complications, and a better overall survival in patients treated in the albumin group (survival 77% vs 66%). A prospective nonrandomized study including 70 patients with cirrhosis and refractory ascites (albumin 20 g twice a week) showed similar results.[32] However, a placebo-controlled trial in patients on the waiting list for LT failed to show any difference

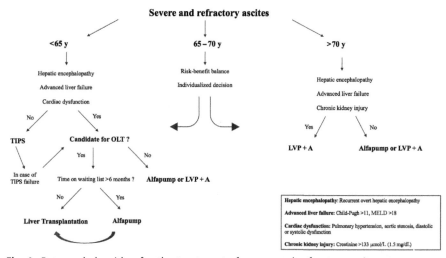

Fig. 1. Proposed algorithm for the treatment of severe and refractory ascites.

in clinical outcomes in patients treated by albumin infusion (40 g of albumin every 2 weeks + midodrine 15–30 mg/d) compared with placebo.[33] Many differences between the 2 studies can explain the different results observed (characteristics of patients, doses used, short follow-up in the latter), but perspectives could be to tailor the administration of albumin-to-serum albumin concentration.[34]

Vasopressors
Vasoconstrictors have been investigated in reducing the incidence of PPCD, but the data are controversial.

Oral midodrine (alpha-1-adrenergic agonist) 7.5 mg 3 times daily has been shown in a randomized trial to increase urine volume, urinary sodium, mean arterial pressure, and survival.

A randomized study found no significant difference between albumin infusions group and midodrine (for 2 days after LVP or for 30 days after LVP) in developing renal impairment, hyponatremia, or mortality at 1 month.[35]

Vasoconstrictors, mainly terlipressin, are used in variceal bleeding and HRS. Terlipressin could have a beneficial effect in patients with ascites by reducing splanchnic vasodilatation and by improving hyperdynamic state.[36] However, although some reports suggest that terlipressin reduces the need for paracenteses, the results of a double-blind randomized study failed to show any difference between patients treated by placebo or terlipressin.[37]

Vasopressin receptors antagonists
Vaptans are a selective oral vasopressin v2-receptor antagonist used in euvolemic or hypovolemic hyponatremia. In a large dedicated RCT in patients with cirrhosis and ascites, no benefit of satavaptan alone or in combination with diuretics was demonstrated. Moreover, the mortality was higher in the group treated by satavaptan.[38]

An RCT evaluating the effect of midodrine alone, tolvaptan alone, or midodrine + tolvaptan versus standard medical therapy (sodium restriction, diuretics, and LVP) showed midodrine alone and combination of midodrine and tolvaptan but not tolvaptan alone were better to control refractory ascites than standard medical therapy at 3 months ($P<.5$). The morbidity and mortality were the same in all groups.[39]

SUMMARY

Considering the poor prognosis, severe and refractory ascites is a milestone in cirrhotic patients. LT must be considered first. In the case of contraindication to LT or when the waiting period is estimated to be more than 6 months, TIPS should be discussed in eligible patients. When TIPS is contraindicated, either alfapump or LVP + A may be discussed regarding the risk-benefit balance and the quality of life. The place of albumin infusion must be specified. Regardless of the type of treatment, a careful selection of patients is crucial to avoid further decompensation and specific complications of each treatment (**Fig. 1**).

CONFLICT OF INTEREST

H. Larrue: none. J.P. Vinel: none. C. Bureau: Gore (speaker fees), Sequana Medical (participation to the European trial sponsored by Sequana Medical).

REFERENCES

1. Ginés P, Quintero E, Arroyo V, et al. Compensated cirrhosis: natural history and prognostic factors. Hepatology 1987;7(1):122–8.
2. Planas R, Montoliu S, Ballesté B, et al. Natural history of patients hospitalized for management of cirrhotic ascites. Clin Gastroenterol Hepatol 2006;4(11):1385–94.
3. D'Amico G, Morabito A, D'Amico M, et al. Clinical states of cirrhosis and competing risks. J Hepatol 2018;68(3):563–76.
4. Fortune B, Cardenas A. Ascites, refractory ascites and hyponatremia in cirrhosis. Gastroenterol Rep (Oxf) 2017;5(2):104–12.
5. Clària J, Stauber RE, Coenraad MJ, et al. Systemic inflammation in decompensated cirrhosis: characterization and role in acute-on-chronic liver failure. Hepatology 2016;64(4):1249–64.
6. Téllez L, Ibáñez-Samaniego L, Pérez Del Villar C, et al. Non-selective beta-blockers impair global circulatory homeostasis and renal function in cirrhotic patients with refractory ascites. J Hepatol 2020. https://doi.org/10.1016/j.jhep.2020.05.011.
7. European Association for the Study of the Liver, Electronic address: easloffice@easloffice.eu, European Association for the Study of the Liver. EASL clinical practice guidelines for the management of patients with decompensated cirrhosis. J Hepatol 2018;69(2):406–60.
8. Ginés P, Tító L, Arroyo V, et al. Randomized comparative study of therapeutic paracentesis with and without intravenous albumin in cirrhosis. Gastroenterology 1988;94(6):1493–502.
9. Bernardi M, Caraceni P, Navickis RJ, et al. Albumin infusion in patients undergoing large-volume paracentesis: a meta-analysis of randomized trials. Hepatology 2012;55(4):1172–81.
10. Rössle M, Gerbes AL. TIPS for the treatment of refractory ascites, hepatorenal syndrome and hepatic hydrothorax: a critical update. Gut 2010;59(7):988–1000.
11. Lebrec D, Giuily N, Hadengue A, et al. Transjugular intrahepatic portosystemic shunts: comparison with paracentesis in patients with cirrhosis and refractory ascites: a randomized trial. French Group of Clinicians and a Group of Biologists. J Hepatol 1996;25(2):135–44.
12. Rössle M, Ochs A, Gülberg V, et al. A comparison of paracentesis and transjugular intrahepatic portosystemic shunting in patients with ascites. N Engl J Med 2000;342(23):1701–7.

13. Ginès P, Uriz J, Calahorra B, et al. Transjugular intrahepatic portosystemic shunting versus paracentesis plus albumin for refractory ascites in cirrhosis. Gastroenterology 2002;123(6):1839–47.
14. Sanyal AJ, Genning C, Reddy KR, et al. The North American Study for the treatment of refractory ascites. Gastroenterology 2003;124(3):634–41.
15. Salerno F, Merli M, Riggio O, et al. Randomized controlled study of TIPS versus paracentesis plus albumin in cirrhosis with severe ascites. Hepatology 2004; 40(3):629–35.
16. Narahara Y, Kanazawa H, Fukuda T, et al. Transjugular intrahepatic portosystemic shunt versus paracentesis plus albumin in patients with refractory ascites who have good hepatic and renal function: a prospective randomized trial. J Gastroenterol 2011;46(1):78–85.
17. Bureau C, Thabut D, Oberti F, et al. Transjugular intrahepatic portosystemic shunts with covered stents increase transplant-free survival of patients with cirrhosis and recurrent ascites. Gastroenterology 2017;152(1):157–63.
18. Salerno F, Cammà C, Enea M, et al. Transjugular intrahepatic portosystemic shunt for refractory ascites: a meta-analysis of individual patient data. Gastroenterology 2007;133(3):825–34.
19. Fagiuoli S, Bruno R, Debernardi Venon W, et al. Consensus conference on TIPS management: techniques, indications, contraindications. Dig Liver Dis 2017; 49(2):121–37.
20. Riggio O, Nardelli S, Moscucci F, et al. Hepatic encephalopathy after transjugular intrahepatic portosystemic shunt. Clin Liver Dis 2012;16(1):133–46.
21. Schepis F, Vizzutti F, Garcia-Tsao G, et al. Under-dilated TIPS associate with efficacy and reduced encephalopathy in a prospective, non-randomized study of patients with cirrhosis. Clin Gastroenterol Hepatol 2018;16(7):1153–62.e7.
22. Pieper CC, Jansen C, Meyer C, et al. Prospective evaluation of passive expansion of partially dilated transjugular intrahepatic portosystemic shunt stent grafts-a three-dimensional sonography study. J Vasc Interv Radiol 2017;28(1): 117–25.
23. Miraglia R, Maruzzelli L, Di Piazza A, et al. Transjugular intrahepatic portosystemic shunt using the new Gore Viatorr controlled expansion endoprosthesis: prospective, single-center, preliminary experience. Cardiovasc Intervent Radiol 2019;42(1):78–86.
24. Bureau C, Thabut D, Jezequel C, et al. The use of rifaximin in the prevention of overt hepatic encephalopathy after transjugular intrahepatic portosystemic shunt: a randomized controlled trial. Ann Intern Med 2021. [Epub ahead of print].
25. Billey C, Billet S, Robic MA, et al. A prospective study identifying predictive factors of cardiac decompensation after transjugular intrahepatic portosystemic shunt: the Toulouse algorithm. Hepatology 2019;70(6):1928–41.
26. Bureau C, Adebayo D, Chalret de Rieu M, et al. Alfapump® system vs. large volume paracentesis for refractory ascites: a multicenter randomized controlled study. J Hepatol 2017;67(5):940–9.
27. Wong F, Bendel E, Sniderman K, et al. Improvement in quality of life and decrease in large-volume paracentesis requirements with the automated low-flow ascites pump. Liver Transpl 2020;26(5):651–61.
28. Bellot P, Welker M-W, Soriano G, et al. Automated low flow pump system for the treatment of refractory ascites: a multi-center safety and efficacy study. J Hepatol 2013;58(5):922–7.

29. Lepida A, Marot A, Trépo E, et al. Systematic review with meta-analysis: automated low-flow ascites pump therapy for refractory ascites. Aliment Pharmacol Ther 2019;50(9):978–87.

30. Solà E, Sanchez-Cabús S, Rodriguez E, et al. Effects of alfapump™ system on kidney and circulatory function in patients with cirrhosis and refractory ascites. Liver Transpl 2017;23(5):583–93.

31. Caraceni P, Riggio O, Angeli P, et al. Long-term albumin administration in decompensated cirrhosis (ANSWER): an open-label randomised trial. Lancet 2018; 391(10138):2417–29.

32. Di Pascoli M, Fasolato S, Piano S, et al. Long-term administration of human albumin improves survival in patients with cirrhosis and refractory ascites. Liver Int 2019;39(1):98–105.

33. Solà E, Solé C, Simón-Talero M, et al. Midodrine and albumin for prevention of complications in patients with cirrhosis awaiting LT. A randomized placebo-controlled trial. J Hepatol 2018;69(6):1250–9.

34. Caraceni P, Tufoni M, Zaccherini G, et al. On-treatment serum albumin level can guide long-term treatment in patients with cirrhosis and uncomplicated ascites. J Hepatol 2020. https://doi.org/10.1016/j.jhep.2020.08.021.

35. Yosry A, Soliman ZA, Eletreby R, et al. Oral midodrine is comparable to albumin infusion in cirrhotic patients with refractory ascites undergoing large-volume paracentesis: results of a pilot study. Eur J Gastroenterol Hepatol 2019;31(3):345–51.

36. Bai Z, An Y, Guo X, et al. Role of terlipressin in cirrhotic patients with ascites and without hepatorenal syndrome: a systematic review of current evidence. Can J Gastroenterol Hepatol 2020;2020:5106958.

37. Carbonell N, Louvet A, Rousseau A, et al. Terlipressine plus albumine versus albumine seule chez des patients atteints de cirrhose avec ascite réfractaire traités par paracentèse: essai prospectif multicentrique français randomisé contre placebo (essai TERAS). Résumé n°CO-034 AFEF 2017 Nice.

38. Wong F, Watson H, Gerbes A, et al. Satavaptan for the management of ascites in cirrhosis: efficacy and safety across the spectrum of ascites severity. Gut 2012; 61(1):108–16.

39. Rai N, Singh B, Singh A, et al. Midodrine and tolvaptan in patients with cirrhosis and refractory or recurrent ascites: a randomised pilot study. Liver Int 2017;37(3): 406–14.

Monitoring Renal Function and Therapy of Hepatorenal Syndrome Patients with Cirrhosis

Adrià Juanola, MD[a,b], Cristina Solé, MD, PhD[a,b,c],
David Toapanta, MD[a], Pere Ginès, MD, PhD[a,b,c,d,*],
Elsa Solà, MD, PhD[a,b,c,d]

KEYWORDS

- Cirrhosis • Acute kidney injury • Hepatorenal syndrome • Terlipressin • Biomarkers
- Liver transplantation

KEY POINTS

- Differential diagnosis of the causes of acute kidney injury (AKI) in cirrhosis is essential to start correct treatment as soon as possible and improve outcomes.
- The diagnostic criteria of HRS-AKI recently have been modified and the cutoff value of serum creatinine has been removed, thus leading to earlier identification and start of treatment.
- Vasoconstrictors, in particular terlipressin, together with intravenous albumin is the first-line pharmacologic treatment of patients with hepatorenal syndrome (HRS)-AKI and should be started as soon as possible after its diagnosis.
- Liver transplantation represents the definitive treatment of patients with HRS-AKI. Therefore, if there are no contraindications, all patients with HRS-AKI should be evaluated for liver transplantation.

Funding: Part of the work discussed in this article was supported by grant funding from Plan Nacional I+D+I and cofunded by ISCIII–Subdirección General de Evaluación and European Regional Development Fund FEDER (PI16/00043 and PI18/00727). The European Commission Horizon 2020 program, grant LIVERHOPE: 731875. Some of the investigators involved have been supported by the AGAUR 2017-SGR-01281. A.J. is funded by Contratos Río Hortega (CM19/00044) granted by Instituto de Salud Carlos III and by the Award 'Emili Letang' granted by Hospital Clínic de Barcelona.

[a] Liver Unit, Hospital Clínic de Barcelona, 08036 Barcelona, Catalonia, Spain; [b] Institut d'Investigacions Biomèdiques August Pi i Sunyer, Barcelona, Catalonia, Spain; [c] Centro de Investigación Biomédica en Red de Enfermedades Hepáticas y Digestivas, Barcelona, Spain; [d] Faculty of Medicine and Health Sciences, University of Barcelona, Barcelona, Catalonia, Spain
* Corresponding author. Liver Unit, Hospital Clínic de Barcelona, 08036 Barcelona, Catalonia, Spain.
E-mail address: pgines@clinic.cat

ACUTE KIDNEY INJURY IN CIRRHOSIS: RELEVANCE OF THE PROBLEM

Acute kidney injury (AKI) is a common complication of patients with cirrhosis, occurring in up to 20% to 50% of hospitalized patients for an acute decompensation of cirrhosis.[1–6] The development of AKI is associated with very high short-term and long-term mortality that directly correlates with the severity of AKI.[2,3,7] A systematic review of 74 studies showed that the overall median mortality in patients with cirrhosis and AKI was 67%, 30-day mortality was 58%, and at 1 year mortality was 63%.[8] In addition, there is accumulating evidence showing that AKI predisposes to development of chronic kidney disease (CKD) in patients with cirrhosis, which is associated with higher risk of new episodes of AKI and worse outcomes.[6,9]

DEFINITION OF ACUTE KIDNEY INJURY IN CIRRHOSIS

Traditionally, the diagnosis of renal failure in patients with cirrhosis was defined as an increase in serum creatinine (SCr) of greater than or equal to 50% from baseline to a final value of greater than 1.5 mg/dL (133 μmol/L).[10,11] Using this definition, however, at the time of diagnosis, most patients already had severely reduced glomerular filtration rate (GFR) (<30 mL/min), and the use of a fixed threshold did not capture the dynamic changes in SCr, limiting the differentiation between acute and chronic renal failure.[12] Consequently, the diagnosis of renal failure in patients with cirrhosis was modified according to Acute Kidney Injury Network criteria by the International Club of Ascites (ICA) in 2015.[13] According to the ICA-AKI criteria, AKI in cirrhosis is defined as an increase in SCr of greater than or equal to 0.3 mg/dL (≥26.5 μmol/L) within 48 hours or a percentage increase in SCr of greater than or equal to 50% from baseline, which is known, or presumed, to have occurred within the prior 7 days.[13] These criteria also classify AKI into different stages (AKI 1, AKI 2, and AKI 3) depending on the magnitude of change in SCr (**Table 1**) and provide definitions for the concepts of progression and regression of AKI and response to treatment. Several studies have validated the usefulness of AKI criteria in patients with cirrhosis and describe that AKI stages are useful for prognosis stratification because they correlate with mortality.[2,3,14,15]

Results from different studies have shown that the population of patients included in AKI stage 1 is heterogeneous and should be divided into 2 subgroups with different prognoses. These studies showed that patients with stage 1 and SCr at diagnosis less than 1.5 mg/dL, named AKI stage 1A, had significantly better prognosis than that of patients with stage 1 and SCr at diagnosis greater than or equal to 1.5 mg/

Table 1		
Diagnostic criteria and acute kidney injury stages		
Definition of acute kidney injury		
Increase in SCr ≥0.3 mg/dL (≥26.5 μmol/L) within 48 h; or, a percentage increase in SCr ≥50% from baseline, which is known, or presumed, to have occurred within the prior 7 d		
Acute kidney injury stages		
1A	Increase in SCr ≥0.3 mg/dL (26.5 μmol/L) from baseline to a value <1.5 mg/dL (133 μmol/L)	
1B	Increase in SCr ≥0.3 mg/dL (26.5 μmol/L) from baseline to a value ≥1.5 mg/dL (133 μmol/L)	
2	Increase in SCr >2-fold to 3-fold from baseline	
3	Increase in SCr >3-fold from baseline or SCr ≥4.0 mg/dL (353.6 μmol/L) with an acute increase ≥0.3 mg/dL (26.5 μmol/L) or initiation of RRT	

dL, named AKI stage 1B.[2,3,14] Patients with AKI stage 1A have significantly higher 90-day survival rates compared with that of patients with AKI stage 1B (82% vs 55%, respectively; $P = .001$). In addition, progression of AKI and development of acute-on-chronic liver failure (ACLF) are significantly more common in patients with AKI stage 1B compared with those with AKI stage 1A. In view of these results, it currently is recommended that patients with cirrhosis AKI stage 1 should be divided into 2 groups for better prognosis stratification.[16]

An important point derived from the new definition is the need of a baseline value of SCr. The ICA-AKI criteria arbitrarily defined baseline SCr for the diagnosis of AKI as the closest SCr value within 3 months before hospital admission.[13] In patients without a previous value available before hospitalization, the value at admission should be used. It should be taken into account that in this latter subgroup of patients, a diagnosis of AKI may be missed. Therefore, the management of that specific group of patients should be based not only on the AKI definition but also on clinical experience; if there is a precipitant event and SCr is greater than or equal to 1.5 mg/dL, it is reasonable to assume that these patients probably have an AKI episode and should be treated accordingly.

As discussed previously, AKI is defined by increase in SCr levels. It is well known, however, that SCr is an inaccurate marker of renal function in cirrhosis, because SCr could be underestimated due to sarcopenia found in patients with advanced cirrhosis.[17] Along the same lines, equations to estimate GFR are based on SCr and tend to overestimate true GFR.

In recent years, the use of plasma cystatin C has gained interest and could represent an alternative maker of renal function, not only for estimating GFR but also for predicting kidney dysfunction and mortality in patients with acute decompensation of cirrhosis.[9,18] Nevertheless, a reference method for cystatin C dosage is lacking, and genetic variability in cystatin C production or metabolism has been reported.[17] Thus, further investigation on cystatin C and new methods for an accurate assessment of renal dysfunction in patients with decompensated liver cirrhosis are needed.

DIFFERENTIAL DIAGNOSIS OF ACUTE KIDNEY INJURY: ROLE OF URINE BIOMARKERS

Hepatorenal syndrome (HRS)-AKI is a particular type of AKI that occurs only in patients with advanced cirrhosis. Patients with cirrhosis, however, may develop other causes of AKI, with hypovolemia-induced AKI and acute tubular necrosis (ATN) the most common, whereas others, such as nephrotoxicity, glomerulonephritis, and urinary tract obstruction, are less common.[1,10,19] Recently, different studies in hospitalized patients with cirrhosis have shown that the most frequent cause of AKI is hypovolemia (ranging between 48% and 75%), followed by ATN (12%–31%) and HRS-AKI (11%–29%).[5,9,20] Importantly, the etiology of AKI is associated with prognosis, with ATN and HRS the causes associated with the lowest 3-month survival.[3] Recent data showed that in patients with AKI stage 1A and 1B, the frequency of hypovolemia-induced AKI was higher than in patients with AKI stage 2 and 3, whereas the frequency of HRS and ATN was significantly higher in patients with AKI stage 2 and 3 compared with those with lower AKI stages.[14]

Hepatorenal Syndrome: Definition and New Diagnostic Criteria

HRS-AKI is a unique type of renal failure that occurs in patients with advanced cirrhosis characterized by severe impairment of kidney function due to marked vasoconstriction of renal arteries secondary to marked splanchnic vasodilation existing in patients with advanced cirrhosis. In addition, a systemic inflammatory response may be involved in the pathophysiology of the syndrome (discussed later).[11,21,22] Traditionally, HRS was classified into 2 clinical types: (1) type 1 HRS, a rapidly progressive form of acute renal failure with very poor short-term prognosis, defined when SCr value doubled from the baseline to a final value greater than or equal to 2.5 mg/dL in less than 2 weeks; and (2) type 2 HRS, a steadily progressive form of renal failure SCr values, usually ranging between 1.5 mg/dL and 2.5 mg/dL, that was associated with better short-term prognosis.[11,21] The new definition of AKI in cirrhosis led to changes in the diagnostic criteria of HRS. The new diagnostic criteria of HRS-AKI are shown in **Box 1**.[13] The only change with respect to the classical definition of HRS is the removal of the cutoff value of SCr that leads to early diagnosis and treatment of AKI-HRS. Therefore, the new definition includes not only patients with classic type 1 HRS (SCr >2.5 mg/dL) but also patients with SCr less than 2.5 mg/dL, fulfilling the new HRS-AKI criteria. The characteristics and outcomes of the latter patients are unknown and should be evaluated in future studies. The classic term type 2 HRS is not included in the current concept of HRS-AKI, because it is not an acute impairment but rather a chronic impairment of kidney function, and these patients do not fulfill AKI criteria. Therefore, type 2 HRS currently is considered a form of CKD (HRS-CKD) that is characteristic of cirrhosis.[13,16,23]

Differential Diagnosis of the Cause of Acute Kidney Injury

Differential diagnosis between the different causes of AKI is essential because they need different treatment approaches that should be initiated as soon as possible. To date, there is no specific laboratory test or marker for the diagnosis of HRS-AKI, and its diagnosis remains a diagnosis of exclusion of other causes of AKI. In many cases, a detailed clinical history (existence of infections, fluid losses, and gastrointestinal bleeding), physical examination (hemodynamics and volume status), blood tests and cultures, and evaluation of urine electrolytes are sufficient for establishing the cause. Nevertheless, in some cases, the differential diagnosis of the cause of AKI in daily clinical practice may be challenging, in particular, the differential diagnosis between AKI-HRS and ATN, because both usually occur in critically ill patients that frequently associate other complications that may act as confounders to establishing a correct clinical differential diagnosis.[16,22]

Box 1
Diagnostic criteria of hepatorenal syndrome according to International Club of Ascites - Acute Kidney Injury criteria

Cirrhosis with ascites

Diagnosis of AKI according to ICA-AKI criteria: acute increase in SCr $\geq$0.3 mg/dL ($\geq$26.5 μmol/L) within 48 hours; or, a percentage increase in SCr $\geq$50% from baseline, which is known, or presumed, to have occurred within the prior 7 days

No response after 2 consecutive days of diuretic withdrawal and plasma volume expansion with albumin (1 g per kg of body weight)

Absence of shock

No current or recent use of nephrotoxic drugs (NSAIDs, aminoglycosides, iodinated contrast media, etc.)

No macroscopic signs of structural kidney injury, defined as
• Absence of proteinuria (<500 mg/d)
• Absence of microhematuria (<50 red blood cells per high power field)
• Normal findings on renal ultrasonography

Urine biomarkers

In recent years, several urinary biomarkers have been studied for the differential diagnosis of AKI in patients with cirrhosis, especially to differentiate HRS-AKI from ATN.[24] In this context, classic urinary markers, such as urine sodium, fractional excretion of sodium (FeNa), and urine osmolality, generally are considered not useful in patients with cirrhosis because these can be influenced by diuretics. In addition, urinary sodium in advanced cirrhosis may be markedly low due to increased sodium retention.

In past decades, urinary biomarkers of tubular damage have been shown to be useful for the differential diagnosis of ATN, characterized by injury of tubular epithelial cells, from HRS, which is characterized by functional renal vasoconstriction with minimal renal abnormalities. Several urinary biomarkers have been studied in this setting, including urinary neutrophil gelatinase-associated lipocalin (NGAL), interleukin (IL)-18, albumin, kidney injury molecule-1 (KIM-1), and liver fatty acid–binding protein (L-FABP). Several studies consistently have shown that patients with hypovolemia-induced AKI have lower levels of NGAL, IL-18, albumin, and L-FABP compared with those of patients with HRS and ATN. On the contrary, patients with ATN have the highest levels of these biomarkers, and patients with HRS have intermediate levels but significantly lower levels than patients with ATN and significantly higher than levels of patients with hypovolemia-induced AKI.[5,25–28]

Among these biomarkers, urinary NGAL is the one that has shown most promising results. NGAL is a low-molecular-weight protein produced by tubular renal cells that also is expressed in neutrophils and cells of the liver/gastrointestinal tract.[29] Urinary NGAL levels rise significantly during AKI, prior to SCr elevation.[30] In 2012, 2 initial studies demonstrated the usefulness of urinary NGAL for the differential diagnosis of AKI in cirrhosis. Both studies showed that patients with ATN had the highest levels of NGAL compared with other causes of AKI (hypovolemia, HRS, and CKD).[26,31] Studies that have investigated several urinary biomarkers in addition to NGAL (ie, IL-18, KIM-1, L-FABP, and albumin, among others) have shown that these biomarkers are useful for the differential diagnosis of ATN from nontubular causes of AKI, but NGAL was the one performing the best.[27,28] Moreover, in a meta-analysis, including more than 1000 patients with cirrhosis, urine NGAL and IL-18 showed good accuracy to differentiate between ATN and other types of AKI (areas under the receiver operating characteristic [AUROCs] 0.89 and 0.88, respectively).[32]

Finally, a recent large prospective study, including 320 consecutive cases of AKI in hospitalized patients for decompensated cirrhosis, supports the use of urinary NGAL in clinical practice. This study showed that among different urinary biomarkers measured (NGAL, IL-18, albumin, FeNa, and β2-microglobulin), NGAL measured at day 3 of AKI after albumin administration had the greatest accuracy for the differential diagnosis between ATN and other types of AKI (AUROC 0.87 at a cutoff value of 220-µg/g creatinine).[5]

In addition, urinary biomarkers not only are useful for differential diagnosis of the cause of AKI but also can be useful to predict kidney and clinical outcomes of patients with cirrhosis. There are data derived from prospective studies and a meta-analyses showing that NGAL independently predicts short-term mortality in patients with cirrhosis and AKI.[5,32] Urine biomarkers also may detect AKI earlier than SCr and they also may predict the recovery of renal function after liver transplantation (LT). This should be confirmed, however, in future studies.[24,33,34]

In summary, there is large body of evidence showing that urine biomarkers are useful for the differential diagnosis and prognosis of patients with cirrhosis and AKI. Results suggest that NGAL can be used in clinical practice to help distinguish between ATN and HRS.[16]

PATHOPHYSIOLOGY OF HEPATORENAL SYNDROME

HRS represents the end stage of a circulatory dysfunction that occurs late in the natural history of decompensated cirrhosis.[22] Traditionally, HRS has been considered a type of renal failure of functional origin. The hallmark of HRS is the existence of marked renal vasoconstriction that leads to a reduction in renal blood flow that finally turns into a decrease in GFR with consequent functional AKI.[22] This functional nature of renal dysfunction in HRS with absence of renal parenchymal damages has been based on the decrease in renal blood flow assessed by Doppler ultrasound in patients with cirrhosis and ascites, the absence of significant histologic changes in renal postmortem studies after pharmacologic treatment, and the reversibility of renal dysfunction after LT.[22,35,36]

Impairment of systemic arterial circulation and activation of systemic and renal vasoconstrictor factors leading to HRS are the main physiologic responses to portal hypertension.[37,38] In addition to systemic circulatory dysfunction, impairment in cardiac function and systemic inflammation are factors that may play an important role in the development of HRS (**Fig. 1**).

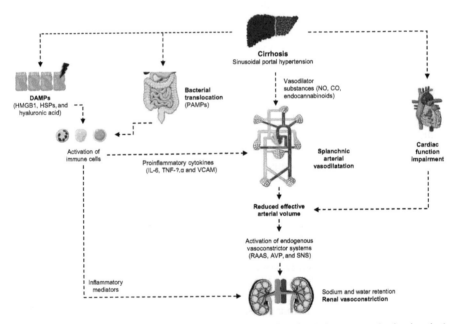

Fig. 1. Pathophysiology of HRS. Patients with advanced cirrhosis have a marked splanchnic arterial vasodilation triggered by portal hypertension. Splanchnic vasodilation leads to a decreased systemic vascular resistance with the development of effective arterial hypovolemia. The activation of vasoconstrictor systems leads to a marked renal vasoconstriction, low GFR, and development of HRS. In this advanced stage, there is a reduced cardiac output and decreased effective arterial blood volume. Systemic inflammation seems to play a role in the pathophysiology of complications of cirrhosis. PAMPs and DAMPs from bacterial translocation and injured liver, respectively, may lead to a marked inflammatory response. Inflammatory mediators lead to further systemic vasodilatation and also could cause direct kidney tissue damage. CO, carbon monoxide; HMGB1, high-mobility group box 1; HSPs, heat shock proteins; NO, nitric oxide. (*Adapted from* Ginès P, Solà E, Angeli P, Wong F, Nadim MK, Kamath PS. Hepatorenal syndrome. Nat Rev Dis Prim 2018;4:23. https://doi.org/10.1038/s41572-018-0022-7; with permission.)

Systemic Circulatory Dysfunction

Liver cirrhosis is characterized by the development of regenerative nodules that modify the normal architecture of the liver and cause an increase of intrahepatic vascular resistance and, consequently, portal pressure.[39] The increasing portal pressure is counteracted by the release of nitric oxide and other vasodilators substances (ie, carbon monoxide and endogenous cannabinoids) that induce splanchnic vasodilatation.[40] The accumulation of plasma volume in the splanchnic bed causes a decrease in the effective blood volume and mean arterial pressure (MAP) that initiates a compensatory response. This compensatory homeostatic response is mediated by the activation of the renin-angiotensin-aldosterone system (RAAS), the sympathetic nervous system (SNS), and arginine vasopressin (AVP).[41–43] The release of these vasoconstrictors systems is aimed at maintaining effective arterial blood volume and MAP within normal limits. The activation of systemic vasoconstrictor systems, however, leads to detrimental effects in the kidney, in particular sodium and water retention and, at advanced stages of the disease, renal vasoconstriction. In early stages of cirrhosis, the activation of vasoconstrictor systems is moderate, and local renal vasodilators can counteract the vasoconstrictor effect of RAAS, SNS, and AVP. The increasing amount of these vasoconstrictor hormones as the cirrhosis progress, however, finally leads to severe kidney vasoconstriction, leading to a decrease in GFR and the development of HRS.[38,44]

Reduced Cardiac Output

There are data suggesting that impaired cardiac function also plays an important role in the development of HRS.[45] As described previously, cirrhosis progression is associated with a decrease in effective arterial blood volume. In this context, cardiac output tends to increase to maintain systemic hemodynamic homeostasis.[46,47] In advanced cirrhosis, patients may develop systolic and diastolic cardiac dysfunction and conductance abnormalities that lead to a decrease in cardiac output. This cardiac dysfunction is known as cirrhotic cardiomyopathy.[48] Cirrhotic cardiomyopathy has been associated with a decrease in renal blood flow, decreased GFR, a higher probability of developing HRS among patients with advanced cirrhosis, and also lower 3-month and 12-month survival rates.[49,50]

Kidney Factors

Together with the increase of vasoconstrictor factors, an additional mechanism that may play a role in the development of HRS is a decrease in the production of renal vasodilators, in particular prostaglandins.[51] Prostaglandins are lipid mediators that have a vasodilator effect on the kidney circulation and may act by compensating the enhanced vasoconstrictor effects of the RAAS and the SNS. This mechanism is supported by the fact that treatment with nonsteroidal anti-inflammatory drugs (NSAIDs), which inhibit prostaglandin synthesis, may lead to the development of AKI, resembling HRS, in patients with cirrhosis and ascites.[52]

In addition, abnormalities in renal autoregulation can play a role. In healthy individuals, renal autoregulation maintains a constant renal blood flow independently of arterial pressure fluctuations. Patients with advanced cirrhosis, however, have a shift to the right of the renal autoregulation curve, meaning that for the same renal perfusion pressure, renal blood flow is lower than that of healthy subjects. This effect, which probably is related to the increased activity of the SNS, may increase the risk that patients with advanced cirrhosis have of developing AKI, in particular HRS.[53]

Systemic Inflammation

In recent years, there has been accumulating evidence showing that systemic inflammation may play an important role in the progression of cirrhosis and development of complications, including HRS.[54] Cirrhosis is associated with systemic inflammation that increases progressively with the severity of liver, circulatory, and renal dysfunction.[54,55]

Patients with decompensated cirrhosis develop bacterial translocation from the gut to mesenteric lymph nodes, which is associated with increased levels of proinflammatory cytokines.[56] It currently is accepted that systemic inflammation results from the activation of immune cells secondary to pathogen-associated molecular patterns (PAMPs) derived from bacterial translocation and/or damage-associated molecular patterns (DAMPs) released from the injured liver.[54,55]

Patients with decompensated cirrhosis show increased levels of white blood cells, plasma C-reactive protein, and circulating proinflammatory cytokines, such as IL-6, IL-8, and tumor necrosis factor (TNF)-α.[55,57–60] In addition, decompensated cirrhosis is associated with activated circulating neutrophils and monocytes.[55,61] Levels of inflammatory markers increase in parallel with disease severity and are markedly high in patients with ACLF, a syndrome that is characterized by the presence of multiple organ failures, including the kidney.[58–60,62] There are recent data showing that HRS-AKI is associated with marked systemic inflammation. Results from a recent study describe that HRS-AKI is associated with increased serum levels of proinflammatory cytokines, in particular IL-6, TNF-α, and vascular cell adhesion molecule 1 (VCAM-1), regardless of the presence of a bacterial infection. Levels of proinflammatory cytokines were markedly higher compared with patients with hypovolemia-related AKI and patients with decompensated cirrhosis without AKI. In addition, levels of VCAM were associated with increased short-term mortality.[63]

Bacterial infections, in particular spontaneous bacterial peritonitis (SBP), are leading triggers of HRS. There are data showing that patients with SBP who develop HRS-AKI have higher levels of IL-6 and TNF-α compared with those patients with SBP who do not develop HRS.[57]

MANAGEMENT OF HEPATORENAL SYNDROME–ACUTE KIDNEY INJURY
General Management of Acute Kidney Injury in Cirrhosis

The management of patients with cirrhosis and AKI depends on the cause. As described previously, early identification of the cause of AKI is the most important step in the management of AKI in cirrhosis. Management of AKI should be started as soon as possible, according to AKI stage, even in the absence of a definitive recognized etiology of AKI (**Fig. 2**).[16] Diuretic treatment should be discontinued and the potential precipitating factors of AKI should be identified and treated: screening and treatment of infections, volume expansion in case of fluid loss, and discontinuation of all nephrotoxic drugs (ie, NSAIDs).[13] Patients with fluid loss secondary to diarrhea or excessive diuresis due to diuretic treatment should be treated with crystalloids. Patients with acute gastrointestinal bleeding should be given packed red blood cells to maintain hemoglobin levels between 7 g/dL and 9 g/dL.[64,65] Patients with initial AKI stage 1B or greater and patients with initial AKI stage 1A that progresses to greater than or equal to AKI stage 1B despite initial management should receive volume expansion with intravenous albumin (1 g of albumin/kg of body weight; maximum dose of 100 g) for 2 consecutive days. At that step, if there is no response to albumin administration, a diagnosis of HRS-AKI should be considered. An algorithm for diagnosis and management of AKI in cirrhosis is shown in **Fig. 2**.

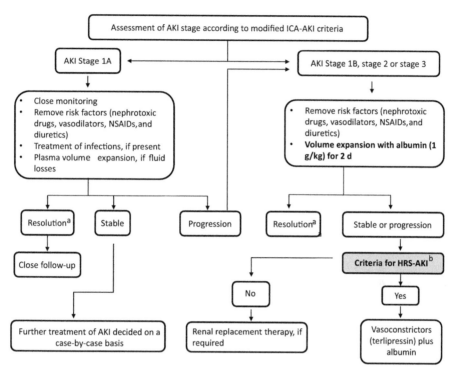

Fig. 2. Algorithm for the management of AKI in patients with cirrhosis. [a]Return of SCr levels to less than 0.3 mg/dL from baseline. [b]At this point, the use of new urine biomarkers, in particular NGAL, may help in the differential diagnosis of the type of AKI. (*Adapted from* Ginès P, Solà E, Angeli P, Wong F, Nadim MK, Kamath PS. Hepatorenal syndrome. Nat Rev Dis Prim 2018;4:23. https://doi.org/10.1038/s41572-018-0022-7; with permission. (Figure 4 in original).)

Management of Hepatorenal Syndrome–Acute Kidney Injury

The initial goal in the management of patient with HRS is to optimize the clinical status, with adequate management of fluid balance and close monitoring of blood pressure and other vital signs.[13,64] Patients need to be hospitalized and monitored closely. Intravenous fluids should be administered with caution to prevent pulmonary edema and development or worsening of hypervolemic hyponatremia. Patients with HRS-AKI are prone to developing other complications of cirrhosis, in particular bacterial infections; therefore, early identification and management of concurrent complications are essential. The use of a central venous catheter is recommended in patients who are going to receive pharmacologic therapy, because it involves the administration of volume expansion with albumin. The use of a bladder catheter is not recommended in all patients because it is associated with increased risk of urinary tract infections. Bladder catheterization is recommended only in patients with marked oliguria. Given that patients with advanced cirrhosis frequently are malnourished and require a sodium-restricted diet, a nutritionist should be a part of the team taking care of the patient.[16,66]

Specific treatment of HRS-AKI should be started as soon as possible. The only definitive treatment of HRS-AKI is LT. Therefore, all patients with HRS-AKI should be evaluated for LT. In candidates for LT, all efforts should be made to normalize renal function before transplantation. The treatment of choice for the management of AKI-HRS is vasoconstrictors and albumin.[16]

Pharmacologic therapy

Previous to the new definition of HRS-AKI, the type of HRS (type 1 vs type 2) was taken into account when considering treatment. All clinical trials evaluating the efficacy of vasoconstrictors and albumin available to date are based on those criteria. With the new definition of HRS-AKI, these criteria no longer are applied. As described previously, patients with type 1 HRS are included within the term HRS-AKI, whereas type 2 HRS is considered a type of CKD. Therefore, according to the new definition, there is no specific cutoff value of SCr for a diagnosis of HRS-AKI and to start pharmacologic treatment.[13,16] According to new definition and algorithm (see **Fig. 2**), vasoconstrictor therapy is recommended for those individuals with AKI stage 1B criteria or greater who meet HRS-AKI criteria.[16] These new criteria will lead to start pharmacologic treatment earlier. To date, there is no information on the efficacy and safety of treatment in this setting and these need to be evaluated in future trials.

Vasoconstrictors together with albumin currently is the most effective pharmacologic therapy for the management of AKI-HRS.[16] A combination of vasoconstrictors and albumin counteracts the intense vasodilation of the splanchnic circulation and improves effective arterial blood volume, leading to suppression of endogenous vasoconstrictor factors responsible for the development of HRS. Vasoconstrictors that have been evaluated for the management of HRS include terlipressin, noradrenaline, and the combination of midodrine and octreotide.[67–78]

Terlipressin. Terlipressin is the most widely studied drug for the management of HRS. It is a synthetic analog of vasopressin with a marked vasoconstrictor effect by acting on vasopressin V1 receptors, predominantly. Several studies, including randomized controlled trials and some meta-analyses, have shown that terlipressin in combination with albumin is significantly associated with improvement of kidney function in patients with type 1 HRS.[67–69,71–73] According to previous trials, overall reversal of type 1 HRS is achieved in approximately 40% to 60% of patients. In contrast to results from previous trials, a recent large, randomized, placebo-controlled, double-blind trial aimed at assessing the efficacy of terlipressin in the reversal of type 1 HRS conducted in North America (REVERSE Trial [NCT01143246]) did not show significant differences in the reversal of type 1 HRS between terlipressin plus albumin and placebo arms.[71] The study described some positive findings, however, in particular, a greater improvement of kidney function in patients treated with terlipressin, and survival was highly correlated with changes in SCr levels.

There are some reasons that could explain the negative results of this study in contrast to previous trials. First, the duration of treatment with terlipressin was relatively short in this study because up to one-third of patients received less than or equal to 3 days of treatment and only 6% completed the 14 days of therapy. In addition, renal replacement therapy (RRT) was used as a rescue therapy in a high proportion of patients in the early stages of treatment, considered one of the main reasons for treatment failure.[79]

Finally, recent results from a large North American randomized, placebo-controlled trial, including 300 patients with type 1 HRS, have been reported (CONFIRM Study [NCT02770716]). In this study patients were randomized 2:1 to receive terlipressin plus albumin versus placebo plus albumin. Results show that in patients treated with terlipressin plus albumin the reversal rate of type 1 HRS was significantly higher than in those patients treated with placebo plus albumin (36% vs 17%, respectively; $P<.001$).[80]

Classically, terlipressin has been administered by repeated intravenous boluses (starting dose of 0.5–1 mg every 4–6 h and increasing to a maximum of 2 mg every

4–6 h in cases of reduction of baseline SCr <25%). Recently, a randomized trial compared the efficacy and safety of terlipressin given by continuous intravenous infusion (dose 2 mg/d up to 12 mg/d) compared with intravenous boluses. Results of these trials showed that response rates between both groups were similar. Mean effective dose of terlipressin was significantly lower in the continuous infusion group, however, and, importantly, that was associated with a lower rate of adverse events.[69]

Treatment with terlipressin always should be associated with intravenous albumin. There is evidence showing that the combination terlipressin and albumin is more effective than terlipressin alone.[70] Although the dose of albumin has not been well established, a dose of 20 g/d to 40 g/d is recommended.[16]

The most common side effects associated with terlipressin are diarrhea and abdominal cramps. Severe adverse events, such as ischemic and cardiovascular events or arrhythmias, also may occur. The administration of albumin may be associated with circulatory overload and, therefore, should be administered with caution. Patients with established ischemic heart disease or peripheral vascular disease probably should not be treated with terlipressin.

Treatment with terlipressin plus albumin should be continued until complete response (SCr <1.5 mg/dL or close to the baseline value before diagnosis) or for a maximum of 14 days in patients with partial response or no response. Recurrence of HRS in responders has been reported in up to 20% of cases. Retreatment with terlipressin and albumin usually is effective; however, in some cases, continuous recurrent episodes occur. Patients who respond to treatment with terlipressin plus albumin show a better survival rate than nonresponders. In addition, data from 2 meta-analysis show that treatment of terlipressin and albumin is associated with improvement in short-term survival.[81–83]

Predictors of response to therapy. As described previously, treatment with terlipressin and albumin should be started as soon as possible after diagnosis of HRS-AKI. There are data showing that SCr at the time of starting treatment is an independent predictive factor of response to treatment.[84]

In addition, the improvement of kidney function in patients with HRS treated with vasoconstrictors closely correlates with the increase in MAP. Studies suggest that response to treatment with vasoconstrictors and albumin correlates with the increase in MAP.[84–86] There are data showing that patients who experience a significant increase in MAP during terlipressin treatment have higher probability of recovering kidney function compared with patients without increase in MAP.[87] Therefore, a goal-directed approach to the treatment of HRS based on targeting an increase in MAP during treatment may lead to better outcome. Nevertheless, prospective studies evaluating this approach are needed before incorporating it into clinical practice.

Finally, recent data show that besides SCr values and MAP, the presence and severity of ACLF also have an important impact on treatment response. Patients with ACLF grade 3 have significantly lower probability of response to treatment compared with patients with ACLF grade 1 or grade 2 (29% in ACLF grade 3, compared with 60% and 48% in ACLF grade 1 and ACLF grade 2, respectively; $P<.001$).[88]

Other vasoconstrictors. In countries where terlipressin is not available, the use of other vasoconstrictors represents an alternative for the management of HRS-AKI. Norepinephrine, midodrine, and octreotide have been assessed in this setting.

Noradrenaline is an α-adrenergic and β-adrenergic receptor agonist with vasoconstrictor effect activity on systemic and splanchnic circulation that can improve renal perfusion. It has been evaluated in several randomized controlled trials for the management of type 1 HRS compared with terlipressin.[74–76,89] In summary, noradrenaline seems as effective as terlipressin for the management of HRS; however, the quality of evidence available to date supporting the use of noradrenaline is low, according to a recent meta-analysis.[81] Therefore, noradrenaline should be considered a good alternative treatment if terlipressin is not available. Noradrenaline should be administered in intensive care units under continuous vital signs monitoring.

Midodrine, a selective α_1-adrenergic receptor agonist, in combination with octreotide, a somatostatin analog, also has been evaluated for the management of HRS. Nonrandomized studies showed an improvement in renal function and GFR together with suppression of vasoconstrictor systems in patients with HRS treated with the combination of midodrine plus octreotide.[85,90] A randomized controlled trial showed, however, that treatment with midodrine, octreotide, and albumin was associated with significantly lower response rate compared with treatment with terlipressin and albumin in patients with HRS (70.4 vs 28.6%, respectively).[91] Therefore, it should not be used as a first-line treatment of HRS.

Nonpharmacologic therapy

Liver transplantation. The most effective therapy for patients with HRS-AKI is LT because it represents the definitive treatment of portal hypertension and liver failure, which are responsible for the development of HRS. Patients with AKI-HRS have a very poor prognosis and, therefore, should be transferred to hospitals with LT programs for LT evaluation. Patients with AKI-HRS have high mortality on the waiting list and, therefore, they should be given higher priority.[92] Considering that sSCr is one of the variables included in the Model for End-stage Liver Disease (MELD) score, the use of MELD score as organ allocation system allows giving high priority to these patients. To avoid a reduction in MELD score in patients who respond to pharmacologic treatment with vasoconstrictors and albumin, which would lead to a delay in LT allocation, it has been suggested to maintain the MELD score calculated with the SCr value before treatment while these patients are on the waiting list (**Fig. 3**).[16,93]

The presence of type 1 HRS has a negative impact on survival after the LT.[94] There are data, however, showing that in patients with complete reversal of type 1 HRS after LT, renal function and survival are excellent at 1-year post-LT and comparable to patients undergoing LT without AKI.[94]

AKI-HRS is reversible after LT in most patients and, therefore, LT alone generally is recommended.[16,93] Nonetheless, renal dysfunction may persist in some patients after transplant. In this context, there is much debate on when simultaneous liver-kidney (SLK) transplantation should be recommended instead of LT alone. Recent recommendations for SLK in the United States are (1) patients with AKI with an estimated GFR of less than or equal to 5 mL/min/1.73 m^2 for 6 weeks or a period of dialysis greater than or equal to 6 weeks; (2) stage greater than or equal to 3B CKD (GFR <44 mL/min/1.73 m^2) for greater than 90 days; and (3) comorbidities and presence of metabolic diseases.[95] European guidelines suggest that SLK should be considered in patients with cirrhosis and CKD in the following conditions: (1) estimated GFR (using Modification of Diet in Renal Disease 6 equation) less than or equal to 40 mL/min or measured GFR using iothalamate clearance less than or equal to 30 mL/min; (2) proteinuria greater than or equal to 2 g/d; (3) kidney biopsy showing greater than 30% global glomerulosclerosis or greater than 30% interstitial fibrosis; and (4) inherited metabolic disease. SLK also should be indicated in patients with cirrhosis and sustained AKI irrespective of its type, including HRS-AKI

Hepatorenal Syndrome
Evaluation for liver transplantation

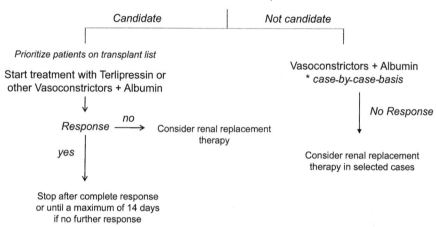

Fig. 3. Proposed algorithm for the management of AKI-HRS considering the evaluation and prioritization of patients for LT. (*Adapted from* Fagundes C, Ginès P. Hepatorenal syndrome: a severe, but treatable, cause of kidney failure in cirrhosis. Am J Kidney Dis. 2012 Jun;59(6):874-85. https://doi.org/10.1053/j.ajkd.2011.12.032. Epub 2012 Apr 4. PMID: 22480795; with permission. *Fagundes, Ginès. Am J Kidney Dis 2012.*[25])

without response to pharmacologic therapy, in the following conditions: (1) AKI on RRT for greater than or equal to 4 weeks and (2) estimated GFR less than or equal to 35 mL/min or measured GFR less than or equal to 25 mL/min greater than or equal to 4 week.[16,96]

Transjugular intrahepatic portosystemic shunt. Transjugular intrahepatic portosystemic shunt (TIPS) has been proposed as an alternative therapy for the management of HRS-AKI, because it reduces portal pressure, leading to an improvement of circulatory dysfunction, suppressing RAAS and SNS activity. The applicability of TIPS in patients with AKI-HRS, who have very advanced liver disease, is limited, however, because many patients have contraindications for the insertion of TIPS. There are data showing that TIPS decreases the activity of endogenous vasoconstrictor systems and, in consequence, improves kidney function in approximately 60% of patients with HRS.[97,98] These studies, however, excluded patients with Child-Pugh score greater than or equal to 12, with serum bilirubin greater than 5 mg/dL, and with previous hepatic encephalopathy. Therefore, considering that existing data are limited and the applicability of TIPS in these patients is very low, TIPS placement should not be recommended in the treatment of HRS-AKI.[16,99,100]

Renal replacement therapy and alternative dialysis methods. RRT should not be considered as the first-line therapy for patients with AKI-HRS. RRT should be considered in nonresponders to pharmacologic therapy. Indications for RRT are the same as in the general population, including severe and/or refractory electrolyte or acid-base imbalance, volume overload, and/or symptomatic azotemia. Published data on RRT in patients with cirrhosis is limited, however, with controversial effects on survival.[101,102]

Alternative dialysis methods, such as the molecular adsorbent recirculating system (MARS), which removes substances from plasma, such as bilirubin, bile acids, and cytokines, have been assessed. In a randomized controlled trial, including patients with type 1 HRS, treatment with MARS showed a significant reduction in SCr and mortality compared with patients treated with standard medical therapy.[103] Data about potential benefits of MARS in this setting still are limited, however, and this strategy should be considered an experimental therapy until further studies are available. Current guidelines do not recommend MARS for the management of AKI-HRS.[16]

PREVENTION

The administration of intravenous albumin together with antibiotics in patients with SBP is indicated to prevent the development of AKI-HRS.[16] Albumin counteracts the marked arterial splanchnic vasodilation triggered by the infection that further impairs the already existing systemic circulatory dysfunction. A randomized controlled trial showed that in patients with SBP receiving intravenous albumin (1.5 g/kg at diagnosis of infection and 1 g/kg at 48 h), the incidence of type 1 HRS was reduced to only 10% compared with 33% patients who received antibiotics alone. Moreover, in-hospital mortality was lower in the group treated with albumin (10% those who recieved albumin, against 29% in those who did not recieved albumin).[104] In infections other than SBP, albumin administration has not shown to prevent the development of AKI-HRS and, therefore, is not indicated. Finally, the administration of norfloxacin (400 mg/d) for prevention of SBP in patients with impaired liver function and low ascitic protein concentration also reduced the incidence of development of HRS-AKI.[105]

CLINICS CARE POINTS

- AKI is a common complication in patients with cirrhosis and has a poor prognosis.
- New diagnostic criteria takes into account slight increases of SCr and, therefore, allow early diagnosis of AKI.
- Treatment and prognosis differs between etiologies, so it is essential to early identify the etiology of AKI.
- Urine biomarkers could have a role in the differential diagnosis between ATN and HRS-AKI.
- HRS-AKI is one of the most common causes of AKI in patients with cirrhosis and has a very poor prognosis.
- In patients with HRS-AKI, vasoactive drugs, preferably Terlipressin, in combination with albumin, should be initiated as soon as possible.
- Liver transplantation should be considered in all patients developing HRS-AKI.
- The use of albumin in patients with SBP, or the prophylaxis with Norfloxacin in patients with advanced liver disease and low ascitic fluid protein concentration, prevent the development of HRS-AKI.

DISCLOSURES

Authors have nothing to disclose.

REFERENCES

1. Guadalupe G-T,RPC, Antonella V. Acute kidney injury in cirrhosis. Hepatology 2008;48:2064–77.

2. Piano S, Rosi S, Maresio G, et al. Evaluation of the acute kidney injury network criteria in hospitalized patients with cirrhosis and ascites. J Hepatol 2013;59: 482–9.
3. Fagundes C, Barreto R, Guevara M, et al. A modified acute kidney injury classification for diagnosis and risk stratification of impairment of kidney function in cirrhosis. J Hepatol 2013;59:474–81.
4. Tandon P, James MT, Abraldes JG, et al. Relevance of new definitions to incidence and prognosis of acute kidney injury in hospitalized patients with cirrhosis: a retrospective population-based cohort study. PLoS One 2016;11: e0160394.
5. Huelin P, Solà E, Elia C, et al. Neutrophil gelatinase-associated lipocalin for assessment of acute kidney injury in cirrhosis: a prospective study. Hepatology 2019;70:319–33.
6. Bassegoda O, Huelin P, Ariza X, et al. Development of chronic kidney disease after acute kidney injury in patients with cirrhosis is common and impairs clinical outcomes. J Hepatol 2020;72:1132–9.
7. Desai AP, Knapp SM, Orman ES, et al. Changing epidemiology and outcomes of acute kidney injury in hospitalized patients with cirrhosis – a US population-based study. J Hepatol 2020. https://doi.org/10.1016/j.jhep.2020.04.043.
8. Fede G, D'Amico G, Arvaniti V, et al. Renal failure and cirrhosis: a systematic review of mortality and prognosis. J Hepatol 2012;56:810–8.
9. Maiwall R, Pasupuleti SSR, Bihari C, et al. Incidence, risk factors, and outcomes of transition of acute kidney injury to chronic kidney disease in cirrhosis: a prospective cohort study. Hepatology 2020;71:1009–22.
10. Ginès P, Schrier RW. Renal failure in cirrhosis. N Engl J Med 2009;361:1279–90.
11. Arroyo V, Ginès P, Gerbes AL, et al. Definition and diagnostic criteria of refractory ascites and hepatorenal syndrome in cirrhosis. Hepatology 1996;23: 164–76.
12. Arroyo V, Terra C, Ginès P. Advances in the pathogenesis and treatment of type-1 and type-2 hepatorenal syndrome. J Hepatol 2007;46:935–46.
13. Angeli P, Ginès P, Wong F, et al. Diagnosis and management of acute kidney injury in patients with cirrhosis: revised consensus recommendations of the International Club of Ascites. J Hepatol 2015;62:968–74.
14. Huelin P, Piano S, Solà E, et al. Validation of a staging system for acute kidney injury in patients with cirrhosis and association with acute-on-chronic liver failure. Clin Gastroenterol Hepatol 2017;15:438–45.e5.
15. Belcher JM, Garcia-Tsao G, Sanyal AJ, et al. Association of AKI with mortality and complications in hospitalized patients with cirrhosis. Hepatology 2013;57: 753–62.
16. Angeli P, Bernardi M, Villanueva C, et al. EASL clinical practice guidelines for the management of patients with decompensated cirrhosis. J Hepatol 2018. https://doi.org/10.1016/j.jhep.2018.03.024.
17. Francoz C, Sola E. Assessment of renal function in cirrhosis: sarcopenia, gender and ethnicity matter. J Hepatol 2019;70:828–30.
18. Markwardt D, Holdt L, Steib C, et al. Plasma Cystatin C is a predictor of renal dysfunction, ACLF and mortality in patients with acutely decompensated liver cirrhosis. Hepatology 2017. https://doi.org/10.1002/hep.29290.
19. Moreau R, Lebrec D. Acute renal failure in patients with cirrhosis: perspectives in the age of MELD. Hepatology 2003;37:233–43.
20. Jaques DA, Spahr L, Berra G, et al. Biomarkers for acute kidney injury in decompensated cirrhosis: a prospective study. Nephrology (Carlton) 2019;24:170–80.

21. Salerno F, Gerbes A, Ginès P, et al. Diagnosis, prevention and treatment of hepatorenal syndrome in cirrhosis. Gut 2007;56:1310 LP–1318.

22. Ginès P, Solà E, Angeli P, et al. Hepatorenal syndrome. Nat Rev Dis Primers 2018;4:23.

23. Wong F, Nadim MK, Kellum JA, et al. Working party proposal for a revised classification system of renal dysfunction in patients with cirrhosis. Gut 2011;60: 702–9.

24. Allegretti AS, Solà E, Ginès P. Clinical application of kidney biomarkers in cirrhosis. Am J Kidney Dis 2020. https://doi.org/10.1053/j.ajkd.2020.03.016.

25. Fagundes C, Ginès P. Hepatorenal syndrome: a severe, but treatable, cause of kidney failure in cirrhosis. Am J Kidney Dis 2012;59:874–85.

26. Verna EC, Brown RS, Farrand E, et al. Urinary neutrophil gelatinase-associated lipocalin predicts mortality and identifies acute kidney injury in cirrhosis. Dig Dis Sci 2012;57:2362–70.

27. Ariza X, Solà E, Elia C, et al. Analysis of a urinary biomarker panel for clinical outcomes assessment in cirrhosis. PLoS One 2015;10:e0128145.

28. Belcher JM, Sanyal AJ, Peixoto AJ, et al. Kidney biomarkers and differential diagnosis of patients with cirrhosis and acute kidney injury. Hepatology 2013; 60:622–32.

29. Mishra J, Ma Q, Prada A, et al. Identification of neutrophil gelatinase-associated lipocalin as a novel early urinary biomarker for ischemic renal injury. J Am Soc Nephrol 2003;14:2534 LP–2543.

30. Koyner JL, Parikh CR. Clinical utility of biomarkers of AKI in cardiac surgery and critical illness. Clin J Am Soc Nephrol 2013;8:1034 LP–1042.

31. Fagundes C, Pépin M-N, Guevara M, et al. Urinary neutrophil gelatinase-associated lipocalin as biomarker in the differential diagnosis of impairment of kidney function in cirrhosis. J Hepatol 2012;57:267–73.

32. Puthumana J, Ariza X, Belcher JM, et al. Urine interleukin 18 and Lipocalin 2 are biomarkers of acute tubular necrosis in patients with cirrhosis: a systematic review and meta-analysis. Clin Gastroenterol Hepatol 2017;15:1003–13.e3.

33. Parikh CR, Coca SG, Thiessen-Philbrook H, et al. Postoperative biomarkers predict acute kidney injury and poor outcomes after adult cardiac surgery. J Am Soc Nephrol 2011;22:1748–57.

34. Levitsky J, Baker TB, Jie C, et al. Plasma protein biomarkers enhance the clinical prediction of kidney injury recovery in patients undergoing liver transplantation. Hepatology 2014;60:2017–26.

35. Mindikoglu AL, Pappas SC. New developments in hepatorenal syndrome. Clin Gastroenterol Hepatol 2018;16:162–77.e1.

36. Solé C, Solà E, Kamath PS, et al. Lack of evidence for a continuum between hepatorenal syndrome and acute tubular necrosis. J Hepatol 2020;72:581–2.

37. Møller S, Bendtsen F. The pathophysiology of arterial vasodilatation and hyperdynamic circulation in cirrhosis. Liver Int 2017;38:570–80. https://doi.org/10.1111/liv.13589.

38. Schrier RW, Arroyo V, Bernardi M, et al. Peripheral arterial vasodilation hypothesis: a proposal for the initiation of renal sodium and water retention in cirrhosis. Hepatology 2005;8:1151–7.

39. Tsochatzis EA, Bosch J, Burroughs AK. Liver cirrhosis. Lancet 2014;383: 1749–61.

40. Yasuko I, Groszmann RJ. The hyperdynamic circulation of chronic liver diseases: from the patient to the molecule. Hepatology 2006;43:S121–31.

41. Bernardi M, Domenicali M. The Renin-Angiotensin-Aldosterone System in Cirrhosis. In: Ginès P, Arroyo V, Rodés J, et al, editors. Ascites and Renal Dysfunction in Liver Disease; 2005.
42. Dudley FJ, Esler MD. The sympathetic nervous system in cirrhosis. Ascites Ren Dysfunct Liver Dis 2007. https://doi.org/10.1002/9780470987476.ch5.
43. Schrier RW. Water and sodium retention in edematous disorders: role of vasopressin and aldosterone. Am J Med 2006;119:S47–53.
44. Arroyo V, Terra C, Ginès P. New treatments of hepatorenal syndrome. Semin Liver Dis 2006;26:254–64.
45. Ginès P, Guevara M, Perez-Villa F. Management of hepatorenal syndrome: another piece of the puzzle. Hepatology 2004;40:16–8.
46. Angeli P, Merkel C. Pathogenesis and management of hepatorenal syndrome in patients with cirrhosis. J Hepatol 2008;48:S93–103.
47. Arroyo V, Fernandez J, Ginès P. Pathogenesis and treatment of hepatorenal syndrome. Semin Liver Dis 2008;28:81–95.
48. Møller S, Lee SS. Cirrhotic cardiomyopathy. J Hepatol 2018;69:958–60.
49. Krag A, Bendtsen F, Henriksen JH, et al. Low cardiac output predicts development of hepatorenal syndrome and survival in patients with cirrhosis and ascites. Gut 2010;59:105 LP–110.
50. Ruiz-del-Arbol L, Monescillo A, Arocena C, et al. Circulatory function and hepatorenal syndrome in cirrhosis. Hepatology 2005;42:439–47.
51. Arroyo V, Ginés P, Rimola A, et al. Renal function abnormalities, prostaglandins, and effects of nonsteroidal anti-inflammatory drugs in cirrhosis with ascites: an overview with emphasis on pathogenesis. Am J Med 1986;81:104–22.
52. Elia C, Graupera I, Barreto R, et al. Severe acute kidney injury associated with non-steroidal anti-inflammatory drugs in cirrhosis: a case-control study. J Hepatol 2015;63:593–600.
53. Stadlbauer VP, Wright GAK, Banaji M, et al. Relationship between activation of the sympathetic nervous system and renal blood flow autoregulation in cirrhosis. Gastroenterology 2008;134:111–9.e2.
54. Bernardi M, Moreau R, Angeli P, et al. Mechanisms of decompensation and organ failure in cirrhosis: from peripheral arterial vasodilation to systemic inflammation hypothesis. J Hepatol 2015;63:1272–84.
55. Albillos A, Lario M, Álvarez-Mon M. Cirrhosis-associated immune dysfunction: distinctive features and clinical relevance. J Hepatol 2014;61:1385–96.
56. Wiest R, Lawson M, Geuking M. Pathological bacterial translocation in liver cirrhosis. J Hepatol 2014;60:197–209.
57. Navasa M, Follo A, Filella X, et al. Tumor necrosis factor and interleukin-6 in spontaneous bacterial peritonitis in cirrhosis: relationship with the development of renal impairment and mortality. Hepatology 2003;27:1227–32.
58. Clària J, Stauber RE, Coenraad MJ, et al. Systemic inflammation in decompensated cirrhosis: characterization and role in acute-on-chronic liver failure. Hepatology 2016;64:1249–64.
59. Girón-González JA, Martínez-Sierra C, Rodriguez-Ramos C, et al. Implication of inflammation-related cytokines in the natural history of liver cirrhosis. Liver Int 2004;24:437–45.
60. Solé C, Solà E, Morales-Ruiz M, et al. Characterization of inflammatory response in acute-on-chronic liver failure and relationship with prognosis. Sci Rep 2016;6: 32341.

61. Waidmann O, Brunner F, Herrmann E, et al. Macrophage activation is a prognostic parameter for variceal bleeding and overall survival in patients with liver cirrhosis. J Hepatol 2013;58:956–61.

62. Moreau R, Jalan R, Gines P, et al. Acute-on-chronic liver failure is a distinct syndrome that develops in patients with acute decompensation of cirrhosis. Gastroenterology 2013;144:1426–37.e9.

63. Solé C, Solà E, Huelin P, et al. Characterization of inflammatory response in hepatorenal syndrome. relationship with kidney outcome and survival. Liver Int 2018;0. https://doi.org/10.1111/liv.14037.

64. Nadim MK, Durand F, Kellum JA, et al. Management of the critically ill patient with cirrhosis: a multidisciplinary perspective. J Hepatol 2016;64:717–35.

65. Villanueva C, Colomo A, Bosch A, et al. Transfusion strategies for acute upper gastrointestinal bleeding. N Engl J Med 2013;368:11–21.

66. Merli M, Berzigotti A, Zelber-Sagi S, et al. EASL clinical practice guidelines on nutrition in chronic liver disease. J Hepatol 2019;70:172–93.

67. Neri S, Pulvirenti D, Malaguarnera M, et al. Terlipressin and albumin in patients with cirrhosis and Type I hepatorenal syndrome. Dig Dis Sci 2008;53:830–5.

68. Sanyal AJ, Boyer T, Garcia–Tsao G, et al. A randomized, prospective, double-blind, placebo-controlled trial of terlipressin for type 1 hepatorenal syndrome. Gastroenterology 2008;134:1360–8.

69. Cavallin M, Piano S, Romano A, et al. Terlipressin given by continuous intravenous infusion versus intravenous boluses in the treatment of hepatorenal syndrome: a randomized controlled study. Hepatology 2015;63:983–92.

70. Ortega R, Ginès P, Uriz J, et al. Terlipressin therapy with and without albumin for patients with hepatorenal syndrome: results of a prospective, nonrandomized study. Hepatology 2003;36:941–8.

71. Boyer TD, Sanyal AJ, Wong F, et al. Terlipressin plus albumin is more effective than albumin alone in improving renal function in patients with cirrhosis and hepatorenal syndrome type 1. Gastroenterology 2016;150:1579–89.e2.

72. Martín–Llahí M, Pépin M, Guevara M, et al. Terlipressin and albumin vs albumin in patients with cirrhosis and hepatorenal syndrome: a randomized study. Gastroenterology 2008;134:1352–9.

73. Prashant S, Chawla A, Ramesh G, et al. Beneficial effects of terlipressin in hepatorenal syndrome: a prospective, randomized placebo-controlled clinical trial. J Gastroenterol Hepatol 2003;18:152–6.

74. Sharma P, Kumar A, Shrama BC, et al. An open label, pilot, randomized controlled trial of noradrenaline versus terlipressin in the treatment of Type 1 hepatorenal syndrome and predictors of response. Am J Gastroenterol 2008; 103:1689.

75. Singh V, Ghosh S, Singh B, et al. Noradrenaline vs. terlipressin in the treatment of hepatorenal syndrome: a randomized study. J Hepatol 2012;56:1293–8.

76. Alessandria C, Ottobrelli A, Debernardi-Venon W, et al. Noradrenalin vs terlipressin in patients with hepatorenal syndrome: a prospective, randomized, unblinded, pilot study. J Hepatol 2007;47:499–505.

77. Tavakkoli H, Yazdanpanah K, Mansourian M. Noradrenalin versus the combination of midodrine and octreotide in patients with hepatorenal syndrome: randomized clinical trial. Int J Prev Med 2012;3:764–9.

78. Uriz J, Ginès P, Cárdenas A, et al. Terlipressin plus albumin infusion: an effective and safe therapy of hepatorenal syndrome. J Hepatol 2000;33:43–8.

79. Ginès P. Management of hepatorenal syndrome in the era of acute-on-chronic liver failure: terlipressin and beyond. Gastroenterology 2016;150:1525–7.

80. Wong F, Curry MP, Reddy KR, et al. L05 - the confirm study: a north American randomized controlled trial (RCT) of terlipressin plus albumin for the treatment of hepatorenal syndrome type 1 (HRS-1). Late-breaking abstracts - presented at the 70th annual meeting of the American association f. Hepatology 2019; 70:1480A–1A.

81. Facciorusso A, Chandar AK, Murad MH, et al. Comparative efficacy of pharmacological strategies for management of type 1 hepatorenal syndrome: a systematic review and network meta-analysis. Lancet Gastroenterol Hepatol 2017;2: 94–102.

82. Israelsen M, Krag A, Allegretti AS, et al. Terlipressin versus other vasoactive drugs for hepatorenal syndrome. Cochrane Database Syst Rev 2017. https://doi.org/10.1002/14651858.CD011532.pub2.

83. Gluud LL, Christensen K, Christensen E, et al. Systematic review of randomized trials on vasoconstrictor drugs for hepatorenal syndrome. Hepatology 2010;51: 576–84.

84. Boyer TD, Sanyal AJ, Garcia-Tsao G, et al. Predictors of response to terlipressin plus albumin in hepatorenal syndrome (HRS) type 1: relationship of serum creatinine to hemodynamics. J Hepatol 2011;55:315–21.

85. Velez JCQ, Nietert PJ. Therapeutic response to vasoconstrictors in hepatorenal syndrome parallels increase in mean arterial pressure: a pooled analysis of clinical trials. Am J Kidney Dis 2011;58:928–38.

86. Velez JCQ, Kadian M, Taburyanskaya M, et al. Hepatorenal acute kidney injury and the importance of raising mean arterial pressure. Nephron 2015;131: 191–201.

87. Nazar A, Pereira GH, Guevara M, et al. Predictors of response to therapy with terlipressin and albumin in patients with cirrhosis and type 1 hepatorenal syndrome. Hepatology 2009;51:219–26.

88. Piano S, Schmidt HH, Ariza X, et al. Association between grade of acute on chronic liver failure and response to terlipressin and albumin in patients with hepatorenal syndrome. Clin Gastroenterol Hepatol 2018;16:1792–800.e3.

89. Indrabi RA, Javid G, Zargar SA, et al. Noradrenaline is equally effective as terlipressin in reversal of type 1 hepatorenal syndrome: a randomized prospective study. J Clin Exp Hepatol 2013;3:S97.

90. Florence W, Lavinia P, Kenneth S. Midodrine, octreotide, albumin, and TIPS in selected patients with cirrhosis and type 1 hepatorenal syndrome. Hepatology 2004;40:55–64.

91. Cavallin M, Kamath PS, Merli M, et al. Terlipressin plus albumin versus midodrine and octreotide plus albumin in the treatment of hepatorenal syndrome: a randomized trial. Hepatology 2015;62:567–74.

92. Cárdenas A, Ginès P. Management of patients with cirrhosis awaiting liver transplantation. Gut 2011;60:412 LP–421.

93. Angeli P, Gines P. Hepatorenal syndrome, MELD score and liver transplantation: an evolving issue with relevant implications for clinical practice. J Hepatol 2012; 57:1135–40.

94. Wong F, Leung W, Al Beshir M, et al. Outcomes of patients with cirrhosis and hepatorenal syndrome type 1 treated with liver transplantation. Liver Transpl 2014;21:300–7.

95. Formica RNJ. Simultaneous liver kidney transplantation. Curr Opin Nephrol Hypertens 2016;25(6):577–82.

96. Nadim MK, Sung RS, Davis CL, et al. Simultaneous liver–kidney transplantation summit: current state and future directions. Am J Transplant 2012;12:2901–8.

97. Guevara M, Ginès P, Bandi JC, et al. Transjugular intrahepatic portosystemic shunt in hepatorenal syndrome: effects on renal function and vasoactive systems. Hepatology 1998;28:416–22.
98. Brensing K, Textor J, Perz J, et al. Long term outcome after transjugular intrahepatic portosystemic stent-shunt in non-transplant cirrhotics with hepatorenal syndrome: a phase II study. Gut 2000;47(2):288–95.
99. Testino G, Ferro C, Sumberaz A, et al. Type-2 hepatorenal syndrome and refractory ascites: role of transjugular intrahepatic portosystemic stent-shunt in eighteen patients with advanced cirrhosis awaiting orthotopic liver transplantation. Hepatogastroenterology 2003;50:1753–5.
100. Guevara M, Ginès P, Bandi JC, et al. Transjugular intrahepatic portosystemic shunt in hepatorenal syndrome: effects on renal function and vasoactive systems. Hepatology 2003;28:416–22.
101. Sourianarayanane A, Raina R, Garg G, et al. Management and outcome in hepatorenal syndrome: need for renal replacement therapy in non-transplanted patients. Int Urol Nephrol 2014;46:793–800.
102. Staufer K, Roedl K, Kivaranovic D, et al. Renal replacement therapy in critically ill liver cirrhotic patients—outcome and clinical implications. Liver Int 2017;37:843–50.
103. Mitzner SR, Stange J, Klammt S, et al. Improvement of hepatorenal syndrome with extracorporeal albumin dialysis mars: results of a prospective, randomized, controlled clinical trial. Liver Transpl 2000;6:277–86.
104. Sort P, Navasa M, Arroyo V, et al. Effect of intravenous albumin on renal impairment and mortality in patients with cirrhosis and spontaneous bacterial peritonitis. N Engl J Med 1999;341:403–9.
105. Fernández J, Navasa M, Planas R, et al. Primary prophylaxis of spontaneous bacterial peritonitis delays hepatorenal syndrome and improves survival in cirrhosis. Gastroenterology 2007;133:818–24.

Invasive Procedures in Patients with Cirrhosis
A Clinical Approach Based on Current Evidence

Annabel Blasi, MD, PhD[a,b], Andres Cardenas, MD, MMSc, PhD[b,c,d,*]

KEYWORDS

- Cirrhosis • Coagulopathy • Thromboelastography • Platelet transfusion
- Plasma transfusion • Endoscopic band ligation • Invasive procedures
- Portal hypertension

KEY POINTS

- Patients with advanced liver disease have both pro- and antihemostatic pathways.
- All available laboratory tests of hemostasis have major limitations in patients with cirrhosis and lack data, especially as preprocedure risk measures.
- Platelet count values less than 50,000/μL may be associated with higher risk of bleeding, and platelet transfusion should be considered before high-risk procedures.
- Fresh frozen plasma should not be administered in patients with cirrhosis before an invasive procedure.

Patients with cirrhosis have several hemostatic disturbances. These are mainly caused by an altered synthetic capacity of the liver that leads to decreased concentrations of coagulation factors, inhibitors of coagulation, and fibrinolytic factors.[1] In addition, platelets are low because of decreased thrombopoietin (TPO) synthesis (mainly synthesized in the liver), platelet sequestration in the spleen, and increased platelet destruction. **Box 1** describes the multiple hemostatic derangements that occur in patients with cirrhosis. Hemostatic pathways in cirrhosis are for the most part rebalanced in an unstable manner, and this balance can tip in both directions, bleeding and thrombosis.[1,2] Hemostatic changes that lead to bleeding and clotting can occur at the same time; this explains why patients with thrombocytopenia can

Funding: A. Cárdenas is funded by the Instituto de Salud Carlos III and Plan Estatal de Investigación Ciéntifica y Técnica y de Innovación - Grant No PI19/00752 and has received funding for this work by Fundación Marta Balust."

[a] Anesthesia Department, Hospital Clinic of Barcelona, Villarroel 170, Barcelona 08036, Spain; [b] Institut d'Investigacions Biomèdiques August Pi-Sunyer (IDIBAPS) and Ciber de Enfermedades Hepáticas y Digestivas (CIBEREHD), Barcelona, Spain; [c] GI/Liver Unit, Institut Clínic de Malalties Digestives i Metabòliques, Hospital Clínic, Barcelona, Spain; [d] Department of Medicine, University of Barcelona, Spain
* Corresponding author. Institut de Malalties Digestives i Metaboliques, University of Barcelona, Hospital Clinic, Villarroel 170, Esc 3-2, Barcelona 08036, Spain.
E-mail address: acardena@clinic.cat

Box 1
Alterations in the hemostatic system of patients with cirrhosis

1. Defective hepatic synthetic capacity of coagulation factors, inhibitors of coagulation, and fibrinolytic factors
2. Low circulating platelets caused by a combination of decreased TPO synthesis, splenomegaly with sequestration, or accelerated platelet destruction
3. Elevated plasma levels of hemostatic proteins synthesized by endothelial cells
4. Increased consumption of hemostatic proteins
5. Acquired disorders in platelet function
6. Modification of hemostatic proteins (eg, fibrinogen) result in altered function

---

develop venous thrombosis. Patients with advanced liver disease have both pro- and antihemostatic pathways that are altered, but in balance, that is why it is so challenging to determine their real hemostatic status with currently available clinical tests. All available laboratory tests of hemostasis have major limitations in patients with cirrhosis and lack data, especially as preprocedure risk measures. Because of the multiple and intricate factors involved in hemostatic pathways, none of the commercially available blood tests are reliable for assessing the risk of bleeding this patient population.[3] In addition, the interpretation of many of these tests, mainly the platelet count and prothrombin time and international normalized ratio (INR), vary depending on different clinical situations (ie, infection, renal failure, volume status, and endothelial dysfunction). This article summarizes current concepts of coagulation in cirrhosis, available tests used to predict bleeding, procedures and risk of bleeding, and the rationale and expert-based recommendations of prophylactic measures for patients with cirrhosis who undergo invasive procedures.

COAGULATION TESTS IN CIRRHOSIS

Table 1 describes the current coagulation tests in cirrhosis. The platelet count has traditionally been considered a parameter that can help guide the risk of bleeding and provide assessment of transfusion of platelets before procedures. That said, it is not a robust test that provides accurate information about primary hemostasis. Low platelet counts in patients with cirrhosis are mainly caused by decreased thrombopoietin production and splenic sequestration. Thrombocytopenia, defined as a platelet count below 150,000, is common in patients with cirrhosis, but levels below 50,000 occur in less than 2% of patients with cirrhosis.[3] However, elevated levels of Von Willebrand factor (vWF) protein, involved in platelet adhesion and platelet aggregation, offset this low platelet count.[4] Moreover, there is increased platelet activity in circulating platelets of patients with cirrhosis.[5]

Another commonly used test is the prothrombin time and the INR, which measures procoagulant factors I, II, V, VII, and X, but does not evaluate the status of anticoagulant factors such as protein C, S, or antithrombin; thus, it cannot assess the global hemostatic status in these patients. The INR is a calculation of the prothrombin time that was created to monitor oral anticoagulation with warfarin. It is normalized against warfarin-treated patients based on the activity of an added and commercially available thromboplastin reagent. This causes significant variation between different laboratories depending on which thromboplastin is used.[6,7]

The factor VIII/protein C ratio, as a balance of pro/anticoagulants, has been used to assess secondary hemostasis in patients with cirrhosis; however, the clinical

Table 1 Coagulation tests in cirrhosis	
PT/INR	Designed for monitoring anticoagulation (warfarin) Does not help assess thrombin generation Does not help predict bleeding risk
Platelet count	Risk of spontaneous bleeding at very low levels (<15,000) Risk of bleeding after procedures <50,000
Fibrinogen levels	Not widely studied in cirrhosis, may help predict bleeding risk
Bleeding time	Does not predict the bleeding risk
Fibrinolysis	Not widely available
Global tests: thrombin generation Viscoelastic tests: thromboelastometry/ graphy	Ideal - clinical utility in cirrhosis is not well studied, mainly used in research Global viscoelastic tests (VETs) provide a more physiologic assessment of coagulation Thresholds have not been fully validated yet, do not predict bleeding risk

translation of this ratio is uncertain. Values in cirrhosis have a mean of 0.8, while in controls, it is of 0.66. Because the ratio correlates with the severity of liver disease, it allows differentiation between the presence of hepatic dysfunction from disseminated intravascular coagulation, which is associated with low levels of coagulation factors.[8]

Fibrinogen is a key step of the coagulation system, that can help predict the risk of bleeding. Target levels range from 100 to 200 mg/dL, but they are extrapolated from other settings.[9,10] Fibrinogen levels are typically low in patients with cirrhosis, because fibrinogen is synthesized by the liver. Additionally, the half-life of fibrinogen is shortened, and its function can be impaired in cirrhosis. Some patients with liver disease and prolonged thrombin times have a dysfibrinogenemia functionally characterized by an abnormality of fibrin monomer polymerization.[11,12] This deficiency is not reflected by the simple determination of fibrinogen plasma levels.

The whole blood tests, known as viscoelastic tests, include thromboelastography (TEG) and rotational thromboelastometry (ROTEM). These tests depend on changes of a blood clot in a specific rotational machine and better simulate in vivo activity of the hemostatic pathways.[13] In most patients with compensated cirrhosis, clot formation, clot thickness, and clot lysis are preserved.[14] However, anticoagulant pathways are not considered in either of these tests, and normal range values were defined on healthy controls, without a specific cut off for patients with liver disease. ROTEM and TEG have been shown to be useful to guide transfusion in patients with cirrhosis who are actively bleeding during liver transplant and undergoing invasive procedures, but their ability to predict bleeding remains unknown.[15,16] From a clinical standpoint, the main input of ROTEM/TEG in patients with liver disease is the negative predictive value. A normal value means that despite abnormal conventional indices, the etiology of bleeding is not the coagulopathy.[17] This information can avoid unnecessary administration of procoagulants.

There are several concomitant situations that significantly impact on hemostasis. They are not assessed by the laboratory tests but need to be acknowledged, because they can tip the balance.

1. Volume status, portal-collateral pressure, and flow are important considerations. Volume administration/restriction interferes with coagulation factors and platelet concentration. Most bleeding in cirrhosis is related to portal hypertension, which should be lowered as the first hemostatic measure.[18,19]

2. For rheological reasons, once the hematocrit level drops below 25%, the erythrocyte concentration is insufficient to adequately push platelets toward vessel walls, reducing the platelet - endothelium interaction.[20]

3. Infections can lead to an additional increase in vWF levels (abnormally high in patients with cirrhosis), which elevates the risk for clotting. vWF levels may proportionally increase with the lipopolysaccharide blood concentration.[21,22]

4. Renal failure reduces the adhesive and aggregative properties of platelets.[23] Acute kidney injury has been associated with an increased risk of bleeding after low-risk procedures such as paracentesis in patients with decompensated cirrhosis[24]

5. Occult bleeding from gastrointestinal origin is common in patients with cirrhosis and can lead to iron deficiency that may increase the risk of clotting. Hypercoagulability in children with iron deficiency can be detected by thromboelastometry.[25]

6. Although controversial, bleeding can be attributed to hyperfibrinolysis. Current laboratory measures do not assess fibrinolysis, and thromboelastometry may not be sensitive enough to detect it. Hyperfibrinolysis can cause spontaneous mucocutaneous and other unusual bleeding manifestations and is more common in patients with decompensated cirrhosis and in those with acute liver failure.[26]

THRESHOLDS AND BLEEDING RISK

INR was developed to monitor anticoagulation with warfarin. The administration of fresh frozen plasma before an invasive procedure can worsen portal hypertension and in addition does not change thrombin production.[27]

Platelets before an invasive procedure can be administered in certain patients. The idea behind platelet transfusion prior to an invasive procedure in cirrhosis stems from in vitro data that have shown that platelet levels over 50,000 μL promote thrombin generation.[28] The most accepted target for platelet prophylaxis is the cut off less than 50,000 μ/L platelets; however, there are no clinical studies that support this contention. Most experts and guidelines suggest that the thresholds vary depending on the risk of the procedure and concomitant clinical scenario (active bleeding, infection, renal failure).[24] This value has ranged between 30.000 and 75.000.[29–31]

The currently used target levels of fibrinogen are not well studied in cirrhosis. Nonetheless, in a series including 211 patients with cirrhosis admitted to the intensive care unit (ICU), fibrinogen and platelet count were identified as adequate routine coagulation parameters for prediction of new onset of major bleeding. Bleeding on admission, platelet count less than 30,000 u/L, fibrinogen level less than 60 mg/dL, and activated partial thromboplastin time values greater than 100 seconds were the strongest independent predictors for new onset of major bleeding in a multivariate regression analysis. Median plasma fibrinogen values within 24 hours prior to occurrence of bleeding were 110 (range 63–161) mg/dL.[9]

CLINICAL SCENARIOS

Bleeding after an invasive procedure in patients with cirrhosis may be the consequence of multiple factors including hemostatic dysfunction, portal hypertension, and type of procedure. Measures aimed at preventing and treating bleeding need to consider the etiology and the type of procedure. The most common procedures in patients with cirrhosis like paracentesis and endoscopy have a low risk of bleeding even with a high INR and thrombocytopenia (<50,000 μ/L). That said, bleeding risk assessment of any procedure is the first step to decide if prophylaxis is needed. This depends on the type of procedure, stage of cirrhosis (ie, Child class or model for end-stage liver disease [MELD] score), and other factors such as concomitant infection, renal failure, or endothelial dysfunction. There is no uniform classification for the risk of procedures, but procedure risk stratification should be based on specific procedure type when data are available. For instance, endoscopic band ligation in patients with cirrhosis is associated with delayed bleeding in less than 3% to 5% of patients after an ulcer falls off, and this usually occurs between 5 and 10 days after the procedure; thus the administration of platelets or other blood products does not protect the patient in that timeframe.[30,31] In a study of 150 patients with cirrhosis undergoing band ligation, platelet count and INR were not predictive of bleeding, but advanced cirrhosis (Child- C) was the most important predictor of bleeding.[32] The authors have adapted previously published guidelines,[30,31,33] dividing procedures into low, moderate, and high risk of bleeding (**Table 2**). The consequences of bleeding and the opportunity to quickly detect and control the bleeding should be considered in the assessment. This classification does not apply to pharmacologically anticoagulated patients and patients with renal failure who may be at increased risk for bleeding.

PROPHYLACTIC TRANSFUSION
Prophylaxis of Bleeding Before Invasive Procedures

There are no data to support a specific INR or platelet cutoff in which procedural bleeding risk is elevated. Therefore, because no solid data support transfusion thresholds, decisions need to be individualized.

Table 2
Procedural risk of bleeding in cirrhosis

Low-Moderate (<1.5–2%)	High (≥2%)
Polypectomy <1 cm	Mucosectomy/polypectomy ≥1 cm
Central line placement	Therapeutic bronchoscopy
Cardiac catheterization	Enteral or biliary dilatation, biliary sphincterotomy
Hepatic catheterization	Lumbar puncture/central nervous system procedures
Paracentesis	Balloon enteroscopy
Esophageal band ligation	Radiofrequency, transarterial chemoembolization of HCC
Endoscopy and colonoscopy	Percutaneous liver biopsy
Diagnostic endoscopic ultrasound	Therapeutic coronary angiography
Pacemaker/defibrillator placement	Endoscopic ultrasound- fine needle aspiration/FNB
Diagnostic bronchoscopy without biopsy	Percutaneous gastrostomy
Diagnostic thoracentesis	Percutaneous biopsy of extrahepatic organ
Transesophageal echocardiogram	All major surgery (cardiac, intra-abdominal, orthopedic) and dental extractions
Skin biopsy	Transjugular intrahepatic portosystemic shunt, transjugular liver biopsy
Other	Intraocular therapy

Data from Refs.[30,31,33]

Thrombocytopenia

As mentioned before, in vitro studies suggest that platelet levels greater than 50,000/µL are required for thrombin generation in cirrhosis, but these data did not consider hemostatic compensation by vWF and other endothelial-based components.[28] In addition, this cutoff has not been validated as a predictor of bleeding in cirrhosis. Platelet transfusions are commonly used in patients with less than 50,000/µL before invasive procedures, but their half-life is short, and transfusions carry a potential for infections and transfusion-related lung injury syndromes. Studies have shown that the platelet count before the procedure does not accurately predict procedural bleeding complications.[29] Current guidelines suggest that an individualized approach is needed for patients with thrombocytopenia before procedures because of the lack of data in regards for safety and efficacy of transfusions platelet counts in patients with cirrhosis.[33] Based on published data, the authors administer prophylactic platelet transfusions in patients with severe thrombocytopenia (<30,000 µ/L) in low-risk procedures and use a cutoff of 50,000 µ/L platelets in those undergoing a high-risk procedure.

Two medications, avatrombopag and lusutrombopag, were recently approved by the US Food and Drug Administration (FDA) and European Medication Agency (EMEA). Both increase platelet counts in patients with cirrhosis by acting as TPO receptor agonists that promote the bone marrow to produce platelets.[34,35] Experience with these agonists is limited outside clinical trials. The indication is for elevating the platelet count in patients with cirrhosis who are scheduled for an outpatient procedure. These drugs are given 5 days before the procedure in those individuals with a platelet count less than 50,000. Both are comparable and achieve platelet counts greater than 50,000/µL prior to the procedure, and the elevation in platelet counts lasts for up to 2 weeks, which may be desirable in patients who develop delayed bleeding after a procedure. Both drugs showed no statistical differences in thrombotic complications compared with placebo.[34,35] Despite increasing the platelet count, neither medication was evaluated for postprocedural bleeding events.

There are no data on platelet cut-offs prior to procedures, and general interventions to increase platelet counts to specifically prevent bleeding are not well studied and should be individualized.

Factor deficiencies

As discussed previously, the INR only assesses quantitative problems with procoagulant clotting factors and thus is not a reliable test of hemostatic balance and does not predict procedural bleeding risk. The INR should not be used to assess procedural bleeding risk in patients who are not taking warfarin. Fresh frozen plasma (FFP) transfusion prior to procedures is associated with risks and no proven benefits. Large volumes of fresh frozen plasma (15–20 mL x Kg) are required to reach an arbitrary INR target, with minimal effect on thrombin generation (because FFP contains both pro and anticoagulants).[36] This volume can worsen portal pressure, and FFP transfusions carry a risk of transfusion-related lung injury syndrome.[27,37]

Recombinant factor VIIa can normalize the INR in patients with cirrhosis. However, a randomized clinical trial showed no role in the setting of acute variceal bleeding, and because it may carry a risk of thrombosis, it is not recommended.[38] The authors do not administer vitamin K unless the patient has malnutrition or prolonged cholestasis, because vitamin K replacement has minimal effect on the INR in patients with cirrhosis.

INR is no longer considered relevant as a hemostatic parameter, and as such there is no place for FFP administration before an invasive procedure.[30-33] The authors consider is use deleterious and advice against is use as a prophylactic measure prior to invasive procedures in patients with cirrhosis.

Low fibrinogen

As mentioned before, low fibrinogen levels (<100 mg/dL) can be associated with spontaneous and procedure-related bleeding in critically ill patients with cirrhosis.[9] That said, it is believed that the low levels are mostly caused by critical illness and not liver dysfunction per se.[33] Hyperfibrinolysis is also uncommon in patients with cirrhosis, but there are no commercially available tests to evaluate hyperfibrinolysis in clinical practice.

There are scarce data on the use of fibrinogen-rich products in cirrhosis. These include cryoprecipitates and fibrinogen concentrate. Both increase fibrinogen levels in patients with cirrhosis, but there are no data to indicate that they prevent bleeding. Fibrinogen concentrate contains 1 g per vial, and the doses are based on baseline fibrinogen level (usually <100 mg/dL) and range from 2 to 4 g with a half-life of 2 to 3 days. The data on fibrinogen replacement are derived from experience in active bleeding during major surgery and liver transplantation but not in prophylactic bleeding for bleeding in patients with cirrhosis. That said, the authors and other experts do consider fibrinogen replacement in patients with cirrhosis and low levels of fibrinogen (<100 mg/dL) who will undergo a high risk procedure.

Prophylaxis and Active Bleeding

It should be considered that in most cases active bleeding in cirrhosis patients is related to portal hypertension. The authors use transfusion thresholds similar to those for high-risk procedures and during an acute bleed, the authors aim for a platelet count greater than 50,000 and fibrinogen levels above 100 mg/dL. Hemoglobin of 7 to 8 g/dL is the recommended target transfusion for red blood cells. Fluid administration and hemodynamic monitoring should be considered as a part of hemostatic treatment. It is now well documented that a restrictive fluid management strategy during bleeding is likely beneficial..[39] If fluids are needed (ie, hypotension/shock), the authors favor the use of crystalloids. Vasoactive drugs (somastostatin, terlipressin) are recommended to maintain mean arterial pressure greater than 65 mm Hg.

CURRENT RECOMMENDATIONS BASED ON AVAILABLE EVIDENCE

Most available data on testing for bleeding risk in cirrhosis are not validated. The standard tests used for the evaluation of hemostasis are the platelet count and fibrinogen. The INR level is not recommended as a test that predicts bleeding risk. Global tests of clot formation, such as ROTEM and TEG, are promising but need to be validated, and they need to evaluate the risk of bleeding, not only thresholds for transfusion. The authors do not routinely correct thrombocytopenia and coagulopathy before common low-risk procedures such as diagnostic paracentesis and routine upper endoscopy. The transfusion of platelets or fibrinogen carries a risk of transfusion-related acute lung injury and/or transfusion reactions. The authors advise against using FFP as it does not improve hemostasis and can cause circulatory overload. The authors do consider transfusion of platelets and/or fibrinogen for management of active bleeding and/or low- to high-risk procedures. They aim for a hemoglobin level greater than 7 g/L, platelet count greater than 30,000 to 50,000 μ/L, and fibrinogen greater than 100 mg/dL. Thrombopoietin agonists are promising and an adequate replacement of platelet transfusion in scheduled procedures. **Table 3** summarizes the authors' current practice, which is only based on their interpretation of the current data, expertise, and consensus among different specialties.

Table 3
Prophylaxis transfusion in cirrhosis

Low-Risk Procedure	High-Risk Procedure	Active Bleeding

• INR – not relevant
• Platelets ≤30.000
• Slant
  ◦ Platelets or TPO agonist
	• INR – not relevant
	• Fibrinogen <100 mg/dL
	• Platelets ≤50.000
	• Slant
	  ◦ Fibrinogen 50 mg/kg
	  ◦ Platelets or TPO agonist
		• INR – not relevant
		• Fibrinogen <100 mg/dL
		• Platelets ≤50.000
		• Slant
		  ◦ Fibrinogen 50 mg/kg
		  ◦ Platelets or TPO agonist

CLINICS CARE POINTS

- INR and prothrombin time do not measure bleeding risk in cirrhosis. Fresh frozen plasma should not be administered.
- Platelet count values less than 50,000/μL may be associated with higher risk of bleeding, and platelet transfusion should be considered before high-risk procedures, but this practice lacks supportive data.
- Viscoelastic tests are not standardized/do not appear to fully predict bleeding or thrombosis.
- Thrombopoietin agonists in patients with thrombocytopenia (<50,000 μ/L) may have a role in pre-planned procedural prophylaxis.

DISCLOSURE

A. Cárdenas is a consultant for Mallinckrodt Pharmaceuticals, Boston Scientific Corp, Shionogi Inc., Sobi Pharmaceuticals and has participated on Advisory Boards for Mallinckrodt Pharmaceuticals and has received grant support from Mallinckrodt and Boston Scientific Corp.

REFERENCES

1. Lisman T, Porte RJ. Rebalanced hemostasis in patients with liver disease: Evidence and clinical consequences. Blood 2010;116(6):878–85.
2. Fisher C, Patel VC, Stoy SH, et al. Balanced haemostasis with both hypo- and hyper-coagulable features in critically ill patients with acute-on-chronic-liver failure. J Crit Care 2018;43:54–60.
3. Blasi A. Coagulopathy in liver disease: lack of an assessment tool. World J Gastroenterol 2015;21(35):10062–71.
4. Lisman T, Bongers TN, Adelmeijer J, et al. Elevated levels of von Willebrand factor in cirrhosis support platelet adhesion despite reduced functional capacity. Hepatology 2006;44(1):53–61.
5. Davì G, Ferro D, Basili S, et al. Increased thromboxane metabolites excretion in liver cirrhosis. Thromb Haemost 1998;79(4):747–51.
6. Trotter JF, Brimhall B, Arjal R, et al. Specific laboratory methodologies achieve higher model for endstage liver disease (MELD) scores for patients listed for liver transplantation. Liver Transplant 2004;10(8):995–1000.
7. Magnusson M, Sten-Linder M, Bergquist A, et al. The international normalized ratio according to Owren in liver disease: interlaboratory assessment and determination of international sensitivity index. Thromb Res 2013;132(3):346–51.

8. Tripodi A, Primignani M, Chantarangkul V, et al. An imbalance of pro- vs anti-coagulation factors in plasma from patients with cirrhosis. Gastroenterology 2009;137(6):2105–11.

9. Drolz A, Horvatits T, Roedl K, et al. Coagulation parameters and major bleeding in critically ill patients with cirrhosis. Hepatology 2016;64(2):556–68.

10. Bolliger D, Szlam F, Molinaro RJ, et al. Finding the optimal concentration range for fibrinogen replacement after severe haemodilution: an in vitro model. Br J Anaesth 2009;102(6):793–9.

11. Palascak JE, Martinez J. Dysfibrinogenemia associated with liver disease. J Clin Invest 1977;60(1):89–95.

12. Miesbach W, Schenk J, Alesci S, et al. Comparison of the fibrinogen Clauss assay and the fibrinogen PT derived method in patients with dysfibrinogenemia. Thromb Res 2010;126(6):e428–33.

13. Abeysundara L, Mallett SV, Clevenger B. Point-of-care testing in liver disease and liver surgery. Semin Thromb Hemost 2017;43(4):407–15.

14. Kleinegris MC, Bos MHA, Roest M, et al. Cirrhosis patients have a coagulopathy that is associated with decreased clot formation capacity. J Thromb Haemost 2014;12(10):1647–57.

15. De Pietri L, Bianchini M, Montalti R, et al. Thrombelastography-guided blood product use before invasive procedures in cirrhosis with severe coagulopathy: a randomized, controlled trial. Hepatology 2016;63(2):566–73.

16. De Pietri L, Bianchini M, Rompianesi G, et al. Thromboelastographic reference ranges for a cirrhotic patient population undergoing liver transplantation. World J Transplant 2016;6(3):583.

17. Thai C, Oben C, Wagner G. Coagulation, hemostasis, and transfusion during liver transplantation. Best Pract Res Clin Anaesthesiol 2020;34(1):79–87.

18. Massicotte L, Carrier FM, Denault AY, et al. Development of a predictive model for blood transfusions and bleeding during liver transplantation: an observational cohort study. J Cardiothorac Vasc Anesth 2018;32(4):1722–30.

19. Weeder PD, Porte RJ, Lisman T. Hemostasis in liver disease: Implications of new concepts for perioperative management. Transfus Med Rev 2014;28(3):107–13.

20. Fernandez F, Goudable C, Sie P, et al. Low haematocrit and prolonged bleeding time in uraemic patients: effect of red cell transfusions. Br J Haematol 1985;59(1):139–48.

21. Mandorfer M, Schwabl P, Paternostro R, et al. Von Willebrand factor indicates bacterial translocation, inflammation, and procoagulant imbalance and predicts complications independently of portal hypertension severity. Aliment Pharmacol Ther 2018;47(7):980–8.

22. Kalambokis GN, Oikonomou A, Christou L, et al. von Willebrand factor and pro-coagulant imbalance predict outcome in patients with cirrhosis and thrombocytopenia. J Hepatol 2016;65(5):921–8.

23. Lutz J, Menke J, Sollinger D, et al. Haemostasis in chronic kidney disease. Nephrol Dial Transplant 2014;29:29–40.

24. Patel IJ, Rahim S, Davidson JC, et al. Society of Interventional Radiology consensus guidelines for the periprocedural management of thrombotic and bleeding risk in patients undergoing percutaneous image-guided interventions—part II: recommendations: endorsed by the Canadian Association for Interventional Radiology and the Cardiovascular and Interventional Radiological Society of Europe. J Vasc Interv Radiol 2019;30(8):1168–84.e1.

25. Özdemir ZC, Düzenli Kar Y, Gündüz E, et al. Evaluation of hypercoagulability with rotational thromboelastometry in children with iron deficiency anemia. Hematology 2018;23(9):664–8.
26. Hu KQ, Yu AS, Tiyyagura L, et al. Hyperfibrinolytic activity in hospitalized cirrhotic patients in a referral liver unit. Am J Gastroenterol 2001;96(5):1581–6.
27. Zimmon DS, Kessler RE. The portal pressure-blood volume relationship in cirrhosis. Gut 1974;15:99–101.
28. Tripodi A, Primignani M, Chantarangkul V, et al. Thrombin generation in patients with cirrhosis: the role of platelets. Hepatology 2006;44(2):440–5.
29. Giannini EG, Greco A, Marenco S, et al. Incidence of bleeding following invasive procedures in patients with thrombocytopenia and advanced liver disease. Clin Gastroenterol Hepatol 2010;8(10):899–902.
30. O'Leary J, Greenberg CS, Patton HM, et al. AGA clinical practice update: coagulation in cirrhosis. Gastroenterology 2019;157(1):34–43.e1.
31. Intagliata NM, Argo CK, Stine JG, et al. Concepts and controversies in haemostasis and thrombosis associated with liver disease: proceedings of the 7th international coagulation in liver disease conference. Thromb Haemost 2018;118(8): 1491–506.
32. Vieira da Rocha EC, D'Amico EA, Caldwell SH, et al. A prospective study of conventional and expanded coagulation indices in predicting ulcer bleeding after variceal band ligation. Clin Gastroenterol Hepatol 2009;7:988–93.
33. Northup PG, Garcia-Pagan JC, Garcia-Tsao G, et al. Vascular liver disorders, portal vein thrombosis, and procedural bleeding in patients with liver disease: 2020 practice guidance by the American Association for the Study of Liver Diseases. Hepatology 2020. https://doi.org/10.1002/hep.31646.
34. Peck-Radosavljevic M, Simon K, Iacobellis A, et al. Lusutrombopag for the treatment of thrombocytopenia in patients with chronic liver disease undergoing invasive procedures (L-PLUS 2). Hepatology 2019;70:1336–48.
35. Terrault N, Chen YC, Izumi N, et al. Avatrombopag before procedures reduces need for platelet transfusion in patients with chronic liver disease and thrombocytopenia. Gastroenterology 2018;155:705–18.
36. Rassi AB, d'Amico EA, Tripodi A, et al. Fresh frozen plasma transfusion in patients with cirrhosis and coagulopathy: effect on conventional coagulation tests and thrombomodulin-modified thrombin generation. J Hepatol 2020;72:85–94.
37. Kleinman S, Caulfield T, Chan P, et al. Toward an understanding of transfusion-related acute lung injury: statement of a consensus panel. Transfusion 2004;44: 1774–89.
38. Bosch J, Thabut D, Albillos A, et al. Recombinant factor VIIa for variceal bleeding in patients with advanced cirrhosis: a randomized, controlled trial. Hepatology 2008;47:1604–14.
39. Massicotte L, Lenis S, Thibeault L, et al. Reduction of blood product transfusions during liver transplantation. Can J Anaesth 2005;52(5):545–6.

Current Concepts of Cirrhotic Cardiomyopathy

Manhal J. Izzy, MD[a],*, Lisa B. VanWagner, MD, MSc[b,c]

KEYWORDS

- Cirrhotic cardiomyopathy • Diastolic dysfunction • Heart failure
- Liver transplantation • Heart disease • Cardiovascular events • Echocardiogram
- Transjugular intrahepatic portosystemic shunt

KEY POINTS

- The criteria for diagnosis of cirrhotic cardiomyopathy were recently revised in 2020 to reflect the improved performance of echocardiography for diagnosis of abnormal cardiac structure and function.
- Cirrhotic cardiomyopathy may increase the risk for major cardiac events after transjugular intrahepatic portosystemic shunt placement and after liver transplant.
- Echocardiographic follow-up of patients with cirrhotic cardiomyopathy is warranted.

 Video content accompanies this article at http://www.liver.theclinics.com.

INTRODUCTION

Cirrhosis accounts for 1.16 million deaths worldwide annually, making it the 11th most common cause of death globally.[1] Cirrhosis deaths are expected to increase over the next decade because of the ongoing epidemics of obesity and alcohol-related liver disease.[1] The primary physiologic complication in patients with cirrhosis is elevated pressure in the portal venous system (ie, portal hypertension). This elevated pressure can manifest as ascites, hepatic hydrothorax, hepatorenal syndrome, or portal hypertensive gastropathy and gastroesophageal varices with bleeding. These complications are markers of hepatic decompensation and are associated with 50% mortality at 1 year, especially in Child C patients.[2]

[a] Department of Medicine, Division of Gastroenterology, Hepatology, and Nutrition, Vanderbilt University Medical Center, 1660 The Vanderbilt Clinic, Nashville, TN 37232, USA;
[b] Department of Medicine, Division of Gastroenterology and Hepatology, Northwestern University Feinberg School of Medicine, 676 North St Clair, Suite 1400, Chicago, IL 60611, USA;
[c] Department of Preventive Medicine, Division of Epidemiology, Northwestern University Feinberg School of Medicine, 676 North St Clair, Suite 1400, Chicago, IL 60611, USA
* Corresponding author.
E-mail address: manhal.izzy@vumc.org

Clin Liver Dis 25 (2021) 471–481
https://doi.org/10.1016/j.cld.2021.01.012
1089-3261/21/© 2021 Elsevier Inc. All rights reserved.

The cardiovascular effects of portal hypertension result in hyperdynamic circulation characterized by low systemic vascular resistance and high-cardiac output. Cirrhotic cardiomyopathy (CCM) is characterized by intrinsic subclinical alterations in myocardial structure and function in the absence of overt structural abnormalities owing to other causes (eg, ischemia).[3] CCM is usually latent, but it can become unmasked under stress, such as an acute change in hemodynamic loading conditions, leading to clinical heart failure.[4] CCM is related to both portal hypertension and cirrhosis, irrespective of the underlying cause of end-stage liver disease (ESLD), although some diseases (eg, alcohol, nonalcoholic steatohepatitis, iron overload) may have further impact on cardiac function.[5]

In the following review, the authors discuss the epidemiology, pathophysiology, diagnostic criteria, and clinical implications of CCM. They focus particularly on aspects of clinical care for screening, surveillance, and management of CCM in the context of liver transplantation and transjugular intrahepatic portosystemic (TIPS) placement. Finally, the authors address the major unmet needs and research priorities surrounding CCM.

EPIDEMIOLOGY

There is limited information on the epidemiology of CCM, as its diagnosis is difficult because of near normal cardiac function at rest. Typically, the syndrome is not recognized until clinical decompensation occurs, at which time patients often present with features of high-output heart failure or diastolic heart failure.[6] With regard to heart failure, there are 4 stages for its development; stage A: the presence of risk factors (eg, hypertension, diabetes mellitus); stage B: the presence of structural changes (eg, remodeling) without clinical features; stage C: clinical presentation; and stage D: refractory clinical presentation[7] (**Table 1**). Although accurate identification and staging of heart failure owing to CCM are challenging, echocardiography, which is used

Table 1			
Cirrhotic cardiomyopathy in the spectrum of heart failure			
	ACCF/AHA HF Stage[7]	**CCM Correlate**	**Therapeutic Target**
Early stage	Stage A	Patients with cirrhosis or metabolic syndrome and its components without structural heart disease	Risk factor modification (eg, control blood pressure, weight loss as needed)
	Stage B	LV remodeling and/or systolic or diastolic dysfunction on imaging *without* HF symptoms	Treat structural heart disease to prevent progression to symptomatic HF (stage C)
Late stage	Stage C	LV remodeling and/or systolic or diastolic dysfunction + prior or current HF symptoms	GDMT to prevent progression to stage D HF
	Stage D	Refractory HF requiring specialized interventions	GDMT to reduce mortality

Abbreviations: ACCF, American College of Cardiology Foundation; AHA, American Heart Association; GDMT, guideline-directed medical therapy; HF, heart failure; LV, left ventricle.

Data from Izzy M, VanWagner LB, Lin G, et al. Redefining Cirrhotic Cardiomyopathy for the Modern Era [published correction appears in Hepatology. 2020 Sep;72(3):1161]. Hepatology. 2020;71(1):334-345. https://doi.org/10.1002/hep.30875.

clinically to identify cardiac correlates of early-stage heart failure (stage A or B), is operator dependent, and accuracy and reproducibility can be limited by the acoustic window. In late-stage heart failure (stage C or D), clinical heart failure symptoms may be masked or confounded by those of advanced cirrhosis (eg, low functional capacity, shortness of breath, and fluid overload). Therefore, accurate staging of heart failure owing to CCM may require sophisticated investigation beyond standard echocardiography to identify changes in myocardial tissue structure, function, and flow before the onset of cardiac decompensation (see *Diagnosis*).

Because of the latent nature of the disease, the actual prevalence, incidence, and natural history of CCM are largely unknown. Attempts have been made to extrapolate the prevalence of CCM by looking at the prevalence of QT interval prolongation in patients with cirrhosis, which previously was touted as the most common manifestation of CCM.[3,6] The prevalence of QT interval prolongation increases with severity of portal hypertension from 25% in Child A cirrhosis to up to 60% in Child C cirrhosis.[5] However, QT can be prolonged because of a variety of causes (eg, thyroid disease, obesity, medications[8]), which limits its use as an accurate surrogate for CCM. In patients undergoing liver transplantation, up to 50% of waitlist candidates show signs of cardiac dysfunction, and 7% to 24% of early deaths after liver transplantation result from overt heart failure.[5,9–11] Similarly, the leading cause of death after TIPS in patients with cirrhosis is cardiac decompensation, and 20% of patients can have a heart failure hospitalization within 1 year of TIPS.[12]

CLINICS CARE POINTS

- The true prevalence, incidence, and natural history of CCM is unknown.
- Detection of CCM requires a high index of clinical suspicion.

PATHOPHYSIOLOGY

The long recognized characteristic cardiovascular finding in ESLD is hyperdynamic circulation in view of low systemic vascular resistance and high-cardiac-output state (**Fig. 1**).[13] With portal hypertension and cirrhosis, a constellation of changes in vasoactive mediator levels occurs, the result of which is a vasodilatory state; there is also an increased vascular response to vasodilators and a decrease in responsiveness to vasoconstrictors. These changes occur in the systemic circulation and splanchnic circulation but not in the hepatic microcirculation.[14] The vasodilation and associated hypotension lead to activation of vasoconstrictor systems, including the renin-angiotensin system and the sympathetic nervous system, resulting in renal vasoconstriction and sodium and fluid retention. These changes in turn expand circulating volume, further exacerbating the hyperdynamic circulation. With this, structural and functional changes occur in the heart, including left ventricular remodeling.[15] Diastolic dysfunction (DD) develops, as does systolic dysfunction; blunted responses to stress are seen, as is chronotropic incompetence.[5,16] At a structural level, changes consistent with diffuse myocardial fibrosis have been described.[17]

Although patients with cirrhosis often exhibit total body volume overload, increased arterial compliance leads to a functional hypovolemia, and therefore, a decrease in cardiac preload. In CCM, the heart fails to increase cardiac output in response to the decrease in effective circulating volume, which may in part be attributed to high peripheral arterial vasodilation. This cardiac insufficiency may also be masked by

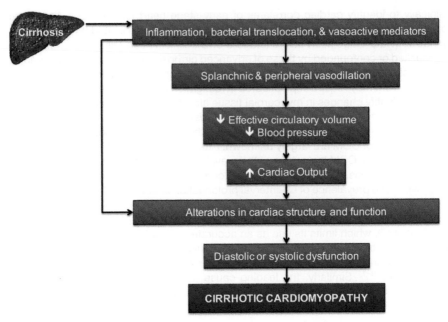

Fig. 1. The role of cirrhosis physiology in the development of CCM.

splanchnic arterial vasodilation, which further unloads the ventricle by increasing splanchnic blood flow. Other contributors to the blunted cardiac response in CCM include autonomic dysfunction and impaired volume and baroreceptor reflexes. In animal models, the cardiac alterations that characterize CCM have been attributed to a variety of molecular causes, including biophysical changes in the cardiomyocyte membrane through altered K^+ channels, altered L-type Ca^{2+} channels, and altered Na^+/Ca^{2+} exchanger, attenuation of the stimulatory β-adrenergic system, and overactivity of negative inotropic systems mediated via increases in cyclic GMP.[18]

CLINICS CARE POINT

- CCM develops over time in response to chronic exposure to hyperdynamic circulation.

DIAGNOSIS
2005 Criteria

The first attempt to devise diagnostic criteria for CCM was in 2005 during the World Congress of Gastroenterology. The proposed criteria at that time described the systolic component of CCM (ie, systolic dysfunction) as having reduced left-ventricular ejection fraction (LVEF) less than 55% or having suboptimal contractile response to pharmacologically or physiologically induced stress. The 2005 criteria described the diastolic component of CCM (ie, diastolic dysfunction) as low early to late diastolic transmitral flow velocity (E/A) less than 1, isovolumetric relaxation time greater than 200 milliseconds, or deceleration time greater than 80 milliseconds (**Fig. 2**).[4] Although that attempt to characterize CCM was an important first step in the right direction, applying 2005 criteria to clinical practice can be challenging for multiple reasons.

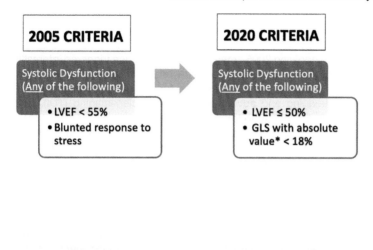

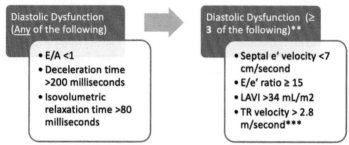

Fig. 2. The Revised Criteria for Cirrhotic Cardiomyopathy. LVEF, left ventricular ejection fraction; GLS, global longitudinal strain; E/A, early to late diastolic transmitral flow velocity; e, early diastolic mitral annular tissue velocity; LAVI, left atrial volume index, TR, tricuspid regurgitation. *GLS is a negative value reflecting myocardial fiber shortening during systole. To avoid confusion, using the absolute value is recommended to describe changes in GLS. **Presence of only 2 abnormalities suggests diastolic dysfunction of indeterminate grade. Further evaluation is needed using E/A ratio change during Valsalva, pulmonary vein velocity, GLS, left atrial strain, and isovolumetric relaxation time. *** This criterion is only applicable in the absence of primary pulmonary hypertension or portopulmonary hypertension.

The remarkable vasodilatory state for patients with ESLD significantly decreases afterload, which can result in an exaggerated, hard-to-interpret LVEF. Therefore, LVEF may not be reliably used as a sole surrogate for detection of systolic dysfunction in these patients. Applying depressed contractile response to stress to daily practice is limited by lack of unanimous definition or characterization of what depressed contractile response to stress entails. Furthermore, the frequent use of nonselective beta-blockers, which lower cardiac output by reducing heart rate, for variceal bleeding prophylaxis in patients with ESLD is another limitation for applying the 2005 CCM criterion. The aforementioned DD criteria have shortcomings as well. They tend to exhibit U-shaped phenomenon where measurements on both ends of the spectrum (ie, in normal DD and in advanced DD) can look alike.[19] In addition, volume overload and its effect on preload impede the utility of the E/A ratio, because it is relatively preload dependent.[3] It is noteworthy that the 2005 criteria included a set of cardiac surrogates to support the diagnosis of CCM, such as prolonged QT interval, which has been the most studied supportive criterion of CCM. However, as mentioned above, QT can be prolonged because of a variety of causes, which limits its diagnostic potential for CCM.

2020 Criteria

The challenges in applying 2005 criteria to clinical practice triggered interest in revising them, and the evolution in echocardiography technology paved the path for the revision. This evolution was most remarkable for clinical implementation of speckle tracking strain imaging and advancing tissue Doppler imaging (TDI). In 2015, the American Society of Echocardiography (ASE) and European Association of Cardiovascular Imaging (EACVI) recommended considering myocardial strain, specifically global longitudinal strain (GLS), assessment in addition to ejection fraction in the evaluation of left-ventricular contractile function.[20] GLS reflects the myocardial fiber strain defined by proportional shortening in fiber length during systole in relation to diastole, and hence, it is a negative value (Video 1). In 2016, ASE and EACVI revised the DD evaluation criteria, some of which are only obtainable via TDI, which has become a routinely applied technology in clinical practice.[19] In early 2020, the Cirrhotic Cardiomyopathy Consortium (CCMC), an international multidisciplinary consortium, published the revised CCM criteria.[3] The systolic component of CCM was characterized as reduced LVEF (≤50%) or decline in GLS (absolute value <18). The diastolic component was defined by having at least 3 of the following: early diastolic transmitral flow to early diastolic mitral annular tissue velocity (E/e') ≥15, left atrial volume index (LAVI) greater than 34 mL/m², septal e' less than 7 cm/s, or tricuspid regurgitation maximum velocity greater than 2.8 m/s in the absence of pulmonary hypertension. When DD is diagnosed, the severity can be determined using E/A ratio (0.8–2 = grade II and >2 = grade III). Patients with only 2 out of the 4 criteria need further echocardiographic evaluation to define DD grade. This additional evaluation entails assessing E/A ratio change during Valsalva, pulmonary vein velocity, GLS, left atrial strain, and isovolumetric relaxation time. Although 2020 criteria did not include supportive criteria like those of 2005, the CCMC suggested studying the diagnostic utility of a group of variables (eg, abnormal chronotropic or inotropic response, myocardial mass change, and serum biomarkers) that may have future potential in the management of CCM.[3]

CLINICS CARE POINTS

- GLS needs to be incorporated in systolic function assessment, in addition to LVEF in patients with ESLD.
- E/e', septal e', LAVI, and tricuspid regurgitant velocity should be evaluated to determine diastolic function in patients with ESLD.

PRETRANSPLANT IMPLICATIONS

The data are scarce regarding impact of CCM in its new definition on pretransplant outcomes or outcomes in patients with ESLD. However, the individual components of the new CCM criteria have been studied in relation to these outcomes. Lee and colleagues[21] described in 44 patients with decompensated cirrhosis who were prospectively followed for a median of 22 months that E/e' greater than 10 was associated with reduced survival (28 vs 37 months). Another prospective study evaluated cardiac decompensation within 1 year after TIPS in 100 patients and showed that elevated E/e' (11 in cardiac decompensation group vs 7 in others) or LAVI (40 vs 29 mL/m²) pre-TIPS was associated with higher risk of cardiac decompensation post-TIPS.[12] Jansen and colleagues[22] retrospectively reviewed the 2-year clinical course of 114 patients who underwent TIPS and found that decreased left ventricular contractility detected as depressed GLS absolute value less than 16.6% was associated with development of acute on chronic liver failure and impaired survival. These studies demonstrate the prognostic value for the new CCM individual criteria. It is important to note that because these studies predate the new CCM criteria, evaluation of CCM as a whole entity was not possible, and only some of the CCM criteria (eg, LAVI, E/e', and GLS) were evaluated. It is possible that some of the patients with elevated LAVI or E/e' in these studies had normal values for the other 3 variables of DD, which, in the presence of normal systolic function, rules out CCM. Therefore, future studies are needed to evaluate the prevalence of the recently redefined CCM and its impact on the clinical course of patients with decompensated cirrhosis, including those undergoing TIPS placement.

Data about utility of other cardiac imaging modalities relating to CCM in pretransplant care are even more limited. Wiese and colleagues[17] showed in 52 patients with cirrhosis that increased myocardial extracellular volume on cardiac MRI, reflecting myocardial fibrosis possibly owing to CCM, is associated with increased risk of death or receiving liver transplant during 2 years of observation. Interestingly, the study showed that increased myocardial extracellular volume corresponds with higher Child-Pugh scores in the cohort, which suggests that CCM can worsen as liver disease progresses.

POSTTRANSPLANT IMPLICATIONS

There have been emerging data about the impact of CCM, DD, or their individual echocardiographic surrogates on posttransplant outcomes. A recently presented retrospective study at the American Transplant Congress (May 2020) showed in 141 patients who were followed for a median of 4.5 years posttransplant that meeting 2020 criteria for CCM increases the risk of major cardiovascular outcomes (coronary artery disease, congestive heart failure, arrhythmia, and stroke) by more than 2-fold.[23] There was a trend toward association between CCM and heart failure occurring more than 90 days posttransplant. It is notable that CCM affected one-third of the study cohort in whom DD was the predominant feature for CCM.[23] Other studies have evaluated the individual criteria of CCM in relation to posttransplant outcomes. Dowsley and colleagues[24] showed that increased LAVI (>40) and increased E/e' (>10) are associated with posttransplant early heart failure (within 2.6 months). The study also showed that abnormal LAVI predicts poor survival at 1- and 5-year posttransplant. Although CCM was initially thought to reverse after transplant,[25] subsequent studies, using contemporary echocardiographic criteria, did not validate this finding.[9,24]

CLINICS CARE POINTS

- E/e' greater than 10 can be associated with poor outcomes post-TIPS and posttransplant.
- Reduced GLS may negatively impact TIPS outcomes.

PROPOSED MANAGEMENT

CCM typically indicates subclinical structural and functional cardiac changes in patients with ESLD, which places these patients in stage B on the path toward heart failure, which can become evident as the burden on the heart increases after TIPS placement or after liver transplant. TIPS placement results in increased preload, which in the setting of CCM may lead to overt heart failure (ie, cardiac decompensation). Therefore, if TIPS is performed in a patient with CCM, it may be beneficial to obtain a surveillance echocardiography within the first few months to ensure that there is no subclinical worsening in cardiac function that may warrant initiation of anti-remodeling therapy.

This risk for heart failure can be further augmented after liver transplant when increasing number of patients develop metabolic syndrome or at least some of its components.[26] At that point, effective management of hypertension, diabetes mellitus, dyslipidemia, and obesity will be critical in mitigating the risk of developing heart failure as well as other major cardiovascular outcomes. To this end, a recent study showed that arterial hypertension was adequately managed in less than one-third of liver transplant recipients and that adequate control was associated with improved survival and decreased incidence of cardiovascular events.[27]

Echocardiographic surveillance of transplant candidates with CCM was recently recommended by the CCMC.[3] The recommended surveillance interval for comprehensive echocardiography is every 6 months among liver transplant candidates on the waitlist. Among liver transplant recipients, surveillance is recommended every 6 months for 2 years following liver transplantation. This surveillance can potentially detect asymptomatic further decline in cardiac function, which can affect candidacy to remain on the waitlist. Conversely, in patients with ESLD without transplant potential, surveillance is unlikely to be of benefit given the poor expected survival and high rate of liver-related decompensation relative to cardiac events.[28,29] In the

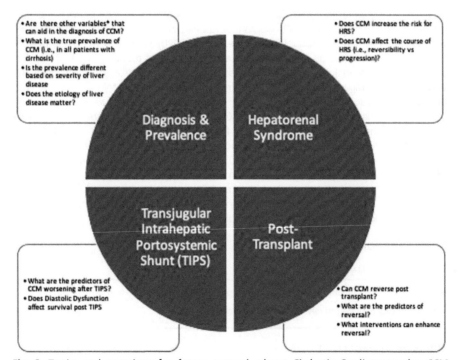

Fig. 3. Topics and questions for future research about Cirrhotic Cardiomyopathy. CCM, cirrhotic cardiomyopathy; HRS, hepatorenal syndrome; TIPS, transjugular intrahepatic portosystemic shunt. *Examples: abnormal chronotropic or inotropic response, electrocardiographic changes, electromechanical uncoupling, myocardial mass change, changes on cardiac magnetic resonance imaging, and serum biomarkers.

posttransplant setting, surveillance can detect subclinical significant decline in systolic for example can trigger therapeutic interventions (eg, angiotensin-converting enzymes inhibitors, beta-blockade) that may improve survival.

CLINICS CARE POINTS

- If TIPS is performed in a patient with CCM, post-TIPS echocardiography may be of benefit.
- Once CCM is diagnosed in a liver transplant candidate, echocardiographic surveillance should be considered every 6 months while on the waitlist and continue until 24 months posttransplant.

FUTURE DIRECTIONS

Although the knowledge of CCM has been advancing over the past few years, multiple unanswered questions remain with multiple opportunities for future investigations (**Fig. 3**). The true prevalence of CCM in all comers with decompensated cirrhosis remains unknown, as studies have focused predominantly on liver transplant candidates. CCM has been historically associated with hepatorenal syndrome[30]; however, this association needs to be reevaluated according to the new criteria. The evolution of CCM after liver transplant and factors predicting reversal versus persistence of CCM need to be explored to potentially identify patients who can benefit from early intervention.

SUMMARY

There are new criteria for CCM which assessment needs to be incorporated in the standard echocardiographic examinations performed in patients with ESLD. CCM and its components appear to negatively impact outcomes in patients while awaiting liver transplant, after TIPS, or after liver transplant. Therefore, close follow-up is warranted in these patients. Prospective studies are critically needed to further evaluate pretransplant and posttransplant outcomes in CCM patients.

DISCLOSURE

M.J. Izzy has nothing to disclose. L.B. Vanwagner receives investigator-initiated grant support and is on the speaker's bureau for W.L. Gore & Associates, is on the speaker's bureau for Salix Pharmaceuticals, and consults for Gilead Sciences outside of the submitted work.

SUPPLEMENTARY DATA

Supplementary data related to this article can be found online at https://doi.org/10.1016/j.cld.2021.01.012.

REFERENCES

1. Mokdad AA, Lopez AD, Shahraz S, et al. Liver cirrhosis mortality in 187 countries between 1980 and 2010: a systematic analysis. BMC Med 2014;12(1):145.
2. Runyon BA, Aasld. Introduction to the revised American Association for the Study of Liver Diseases Practice Guideline management of adult patients with ascites due to cirrhosis 2012. Hepatology 2013;57(4):1651–3.

3. Izzy M, VanWagner LB, Lin G, et al. Redefining cirrhotic cardiomyopathy for the modern era. Hepatology 2020;71(1):334–45.

4. Izzy M, Oh J, Watt KD. Cirrhotic cardiomyopathy after transplantation: neither the transient nor innocent bystander. Hepatology 2018;68(5):2008–15.

5. Zardi EM, Zardi DM, Chin D, et al. Cirrhotic cardiomyopathy in the pre- and post-liver transplantation phase. J Cardiol 2016;67(2):125–30.

6. Zardi EM, Abbate A, Zardi DM, et al. Cirrhotic cardiomyopathy. J Am Coll Cardiol 2010;56(7):539–49.

7. Yancy CW, Jessup M, Bozkurt B, et al. 2013 ACCF/AHA guideline for the management of heart failure: a report of the American College of Cardiology Foundation/American Heart Association Task Force on practice guidelines. J Am Coll Cardiol 2013;62(16):e147–239.

8. van Noord C, Eijgelsheim M, Stricker BH. Drug- and non-drug-associated QT interval prolongation. Br J Clin Pharmacol 2010;70(1):16–23.

9. Sonny A, Ibrahim A, Schuster A, et al. Impact and persistence of cirrhotic cardiomyopathy after liver transplantation. Clin Transplant 2016;30(9):986–93.

10. VanWagner LB, Lapin B, Levitsky J, et al. High early cardiovascular mortality after liver transplantation. Liver Transpl 2014;20(11):1306–16.

11. VanWagner LB, Serper M, Kang R, et al. Factors associated with major adverse cardiovascular events after liver transplantation among a national sample. Am J Transpl 2016;16(9):2684–94.

12. Billey C, Billet S, Robic MA, et al. A prospective study identifying predictive factors of cardiac decompensation after transjugular intrahepatic portosystemic shunt: the Toulouse algorithm. Hepatology 2019;70(6):1928–41.

13. Kowalski HJ, Abelmann WH. The cardiac output at rest in Laennec's cirrhosis. J Clin Invest 1953;32(10):1025–33.

14. Moller S, Henriksen JH. Cardiovascular complications of cirrhosis. Gut 2008; 57(2):268–78.

15. Lossnitzer D, Steen H, Zahn A, et al. Myocardial late gadolinium enhancement cardiovascular magnetic resonance in patients with cirrhosis. J Cardiovasc Magn Reson 2010;12:47.

16. Reddy YNV, Melenovsky V, Redfield MM, et al. High-output heart failure: a 15-year experience. J Am Coll Cardiol 2016;68(5):473–82.

17. Wiese S, Hove J, Mo S, et al. Myocardial extracellular volume quantified by magnetic resonance is increased in cirrhosis and related to poor outcome. Liver Int 2018;38(9):1614–23.

18. Gaskari SA, Honar H, Lee SS. Therapy insight: cirrhotic cardiomyopathy. Nat Clin Pract Gastroenterol Hepatol 2006;3(6):329–37.

19. Nagueh SF, Smiseth OA, Appleton CP, et al. Recommendations for the evaluation of left ventricular diastolic function by echocardiography: an update from the American Society of Echocardiography and the European Association of Cardiovascular Imaging. Eur Heart J Cardiovasc Imaging 2016;17(12):1321–60.

20. Lang RM, Badano LP, Mor-Avi V, et al. Recommendations for cardiac chamber quantification by echocardiography in adults: an update from the American Society of Echocardiography and the European Association of Cardiovascular Imaging. J Am Soc Echocardiogr 2015;28(1):1–39 e14.

21. Lee SK, Song MJ, Kim SH, et al. Cardiac diastolic dysfunction predicts poor prognosis in patients with decompensated liver cirrhosis. Clin Mol Hepatol 2018;24(4):409–16.

22. Jansen C, Schröder A, Schueler R, et al. Left ventricular longitudinal contractility predicts acute-on-chronic liver failure development and mortality after transjugular intrahepatic portosystemic shunt. Hepatol Commun 2019;3(3):340–7.
23. Izzy MJSA, Sun X, Angirekula M, et al. Refined criteria for cirrhotic cardiomyopathy predict post liver transplant cardiac events [abstract]. Am J Transpl 2020; 20(suppl 3).
24. Dowsley TF, Bayne DB, Langnas AN, et al. Diastolic dysfunction in patients with end-stage liver disease is associated with development of heart failure early after liver transplantation. Transplantation 2012;94(6):646–51.
25. Torregrosa M, Aguade S, Dos L, et al. Cardiac alterations in cirrhosis: reversibility after liver transplantation. J Hepatol 2005;42(1):68–74.
26. Laish I, Braun M, Mor E, et al. Metabolic syndrome in liver transplant recipients: prevalence, risk factors, and association with cardiovascular events. Liver Transpl 2011;17(1):15–22.
27. VanWagner LB, Holl JL, Montag S, et al. Blood pressure control according to clinical practice guidelines is associated with decreased mortality and cardiovascular events among liver transplant recipients. Am J Transpl 2020;20(3):797–807.
28. Patel S, Siddiqui MB, Chandrakumaran A, et al. Progression to cirrhosis leads to improvement in atherogenic milieu. Dig Dis Sci 2020;66(1):263–72.
29. Shroff H, Rinella ME. Thanks to CLD for small favors: reduced CVD risk in patients awaiting liver transplantation. Dig Dis Sci 2020;66(1):7–9.
30. Angeli P, Garcia-Tsao G, Nadim MK, et al. News in pathophysiology, definition and classification of hepatorenal syndrome: a step beyond the International Club of Ascites (ICA) consensus document. J Hepatol 2019;71(4):811–22.

Moving?

Make sure your subscription moves with you!

To notify us of your new address, find your **Clinics Account Number** (located on your mailing label above your name), and contact customer service at:

Email: journalscustomerservice-usa@elsevier.com

800-654-2452 (subscribers in the U.S. & Canada)
314-447-8871 (subscribers outside of the U.S. & Canada)

Fax number: 314-447-8029

Elsevier Health Sciences Division
Subscription Customer Service
3251 Riverport Lane
Maryland Heights, MO 63043

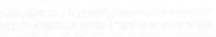

Printed and bound by CPI Group (UK) Ltd, Croydon, CR0 4YY

14/10/2024

01773929-0001